# The Ultimate Consumer's Guide to Diets and Nutrition

# The
# Ultimate
# Consumer's Guide
# to Diets
# and Nutrition

———

## James Marti

Executive Director,
Holistic Medicine Research Foundation

A MARINER ORIGINAL
HOUGHTON MIFFLIN COMPANY
Boston · New York   1997

For information about permission to reproduce
selections from this book, write to
Permissions, Houghton Mifflin Company,
215 Park Avenue South, New York,
New York 10003.

*Library of Congress Cataloging-in-Publication Data*
Marti, James.
   The ultimate consumer's guide to diets and
nutrition / James Marti.
     p.    cm.
   "A Mariner book."
   Includes bibliographical references and index.
   ISBN 0-395-72860-6
   1. Reducing diets — Handbooks, manuals, etc.
I. Title.
RM222.2.M365    1997
613.2'5 — dc21    96-53266    CIP

Printed in the United States of America

Book design by Joyce Weston

QUM 10 9 8 7 6 5 4 3 2 1

The table on pages 26 and 27, "Recommended Dietary Allowances,"
is reprinted with permission from *Recommended Dietary Allowances,*
10th Edition. Copyright © 1989 by the National Academy of Sciences.
Courtesy of the National Academy Press, Washington, D.C.

The author is grateful for permission to reproduce the table on pages 171
and 172, "Recommended Daily Allowances of Nutrients for Normal Children."
This table is reprinted from Shils, Maurice, et al., *Modern Nutrition in
Health and Disease,* 7th Edition, copyright © Lea & Febiger, 1994.

The members of the Medical Advisory Board of this book have dedicated their careers to helping thousands of patients, often without financial reward or recognition. Their lifelong commitment to holistic healing is exemplary of the best in American medicine, and this book is dedicated to them.

# Contents

Preface    ix
Introduction    1

PART ONE

1. Healthful Nutrition    9
2. Analyzing Your Current Nutritional Status    28
3. Assessing Your Current Physical Status    38
4. Defining Your Diet Goals    49

PART TWO

5. Medically Supervised Diet Programs: Very-Low-Calorie-
   Diet Programs    73
6. Commercial Weight-Loss Diet Programs    97
7. Weight-Loss Support Groups    113
8. Over-the-Counter Botanical Diet Programs    121
9. Popular Book Diet Programs    129

PART THREE

10. Diets for Women    153
11. Diets for Children    164
12. Diets for the Elderly    185

13. Vegetarian Diet Programs   204
14. High-Performance Sports Diets   222


PART FOUR

15. Diets for Osteoporosis   249
16. Diets for Arthritis   264
17. Diets for Coronary Artery Disease   280
18. Diets for Type I and Type II Diabetes   298
19. Food Allergy Elimination Diets   316
20. Diets for Hypertension (High Blood Pressure)   336
21. Diets for Hypoglycemia   355
22. Diets for Irritable Bowel Syndrome   373
23. Multiple Sclerosis Diets   391
24. Cancer and Chemotherapy Diets   408

References and Resources   434
Index   459

# Preface

As a teacher and researcher, I have been privileged to witness the miraculous effects of diet and nutrition in healing. The first dramatic instance occurred in 1970 when I was a professor of nonviolence studies at Syracuse University. My course was based on the nonviolence philosophy of Mahatma Gandhi, who believed that the one way to decrease violence was to stop eating meat. Gandhi argued that meat increased bodily hormones such as estrogen and testosterone, which, he said, had been linked with violence. As a result, I and many students in my course experimented with a vegetarian diet. Surprisingly, many of us found that we lost weight, increased our vigor, slept less, and experienced fewer stomach discomforts.

In those days, vegetarians were treated as second-class diners on campus, nibbling our carrots, tofu, and nutburgers, while all around us the carnivores indulged in a banquet of cow meat and gravy. But our vegetarian diet gradually won over adherents and changed epicurean attitudes. Our follow-up studies revealed that the vegetarian dieters not only had lower estrogen and testosterone levels, but lower systolic and diastolic blood pressure levels as well. Equally as important, when we resumed eating meat, our blood pressure returned to pretest levels after several weeks.

This astonished me. I wondered if a meatless diet wouldn't also lower my cholesterol levels. Keep in mind this was 1972, and we didn't know then what we do now about cholesterol. Indeed, I found that by consuming half a pound of beef a day, my cholesterol levels rose 19 percent — and I had deliberately chosen the leanest cuts of meat.

After resuming a meatless diet, I regained my low cholesterol levels in two weeks.

Today we have proof that a vegetarian diet lowers the risk of certain cancers, gallstones, diabetes, and osteoporosis. The San Francisco Medical

Research Foundation (SFMRF) has documented that vegetarian women excrete two to three times as much estrogen as meat-eaters, and their lower estrogen levels protect them from osteoporosis. In 1988, when I served as SFMRF's executive director, we circulated the first studies to reveal that women who are fifty to eighty years of age who are vegetarians lose an average of only 18 percent bone mineral mass, while women of this age who consume meat lose 35 percent bone mineral mass. Vegetarian women are also less likely to develop gallstones and diabetes, because meat appears to interfere with insulin metabolism.

We also know that dietary protocols can treat certain cancers. In 1990 my mother was diagnosed with cancer, and, like many people, she asked if she should undergo chemotherapy. Unlike many holistic practitioners, I urged her to undergo chemotherapy, but only on the condition that she follow a radical high-fiber, anticarcinogenic diet, which I believe strengthens the immune system. For several months, I dutifully sent her care packages that included seven-day menu plans, recipes, and exotic healing foods and supplements like spirulina, vitamin C crystals, Green Magma, and liquid chlorophyll. My mother's cancer went into remission three months later.

Today it's not difficult to convince the average citizen that the foods one eats contain extremely important chemical nutrients that have the ability to heal. Fortunately, some of these foods are quite delicious. Perhaps you'll think it strange, but wild yams happen to be one of my favorite edibles. The noble yam can be puréed into a soup or baked as a pumpkin-like bread — and it has remarkable healing properties. Wild yams contain a compound called diosgenin, which is essentially a progesterone molecule with a small molecule addition. The natural progesterone in wild yams has many of the same benefits as synthetic progesterone (progestin) but none of its deleterious side effects. Progesterone, by countering estrogen in the body, can help heal premenstrual syndrome, uterine fibroids, urinary tract infections, ovarian cysts, endometriosis, and fibrocystic breasts, all of which are aggravated by estrogen.

In 1987, SFMRF first began advising women patients to eat wild yams or use progesterone-based skin creams. When the women who did so later measured their lumbar spine densities, they found they'd increased their bone mass. In some cases, the effects were striking. One patient had had a pathological arm fracture at age seventy-two, and as a result of adding wild yams to her diet, at age eighty-four she had increased her bone density by 40 percent. She had no fractures, and she also felt better. Other women found their fibrocystic breast symptoms decreased. And some women who consumed wild yams or took supplements began to lose weight and found a renewed interest in sex. In the Trobriand Islands off New Guinea, the yam is a dietary staple. It's also a totem signifying good health.

I continue to personally experiment with foods because the adventure of stalking nature for miracle nutrients that heal me intrigues me no end. The chewy pumpkin seeds that I snack on contain saw palmetto and zinc, which serve as counteragents to prostate problems. My morning black walnut (*Juglans nigra*) tea contains the highest natural source of serotonin, which elevates my mood and increases my concentration. I also drink a blended beverage of spirulina and aloe vera juice in the morning because it contains all the essential amino acids and may prevent some cancers. In addition, I take L-glutamine capsules because Dr. Jean Fryer, a Stanford neuropsychologist, told me many years ago that it helped her brain injury patients recover their memory — and my memory can use all the help it can get!

I hope you'll enjoy reading this *Guide* as much as I enjoyed writing it, and that you will discover the healing powers of foods. Hundreds of diet organizations, research institutions, and diet formulators responded to our queries for information, and I only wish I could thank them all. I am especially grateful to the authors of the diet programs reviewed in this book, who patiently answered my questions and corrected our summaries of their diets.

I owe an immense debt of gratitude to Dr. George L. Blackburn, Professor of Surgery at Harvard Medical School and Chief of the Nutrition/Metabolism Laboratory of the Cancer Research Institute, who critiqued the chapter drafts and added suggestions. He, along with the other members of *The Ultimate Consumer's Guide to Diets and Nutrition* Medical Advisory Board, improved the content of the book immeasurably.

However you use this book, I urge you to consult your physician before beginning any diet. Each person is unique, and diets, like prescriptions, affect each of us differently. The trick is to design a diet that matches your own biochemical makeup. I wish you luck in your path of personal discovery.

James Marti
Holistic Medicine Research Foundation
San Francisco, California

# Introduction

The contemporary dieter is confronted with a bewildering array of options from which to choose, some medically sound, others of dubious value, most with some sort of commercial slant. The consumer's dilemma is the same as that confronting the prospective purchaser of a new automobile: deciding among multiple brands based upon such considerations as ease of use, personal appeal, track record, availability, distinguishing features, and cost. And while both can involve a substantial investment of time and money over the long term, unlike the choice of a car, a diet almost always entails making lifestyle changes. For example, adopting new eating habits or severely limiting calories is bound to impact a dieter's personal and professional life to some degree. Equally important, diets and the foods that they contain or do not contain invariably affect a person's overall health and well-being.

Foods are essential nutrients as well as essential pleasures, and anyone's decision to adopt a particular diet should be based on sound medical information. With this in mind, *The Consumer's Guide to Diets and Nutrition* was written to provide discriminating consumers with a concise survey of legitimate weight loss and medical diets. It is designed to help people choose the most appropriate diet for their needs after they have analyzed their nutritional and physical fitness status and taken into account any preexisting medical conditions (such as diabetes or high blood pressure) that might affect dietary choices. For once people know where they are, nutritionally speaking, they are in a much better position to define where they want to go and how best to get there.

## BASIS OF COMPARISON

In 1994, the Holistic Medicine Research Foundation solicited from its Medical Advisory Board a list of more than two hundred popular diets. Diet plans and programs were then comparatively analyzed in terms of the following categories:

1. Goals. What is the diet intended to help dieters do?
2. Eligibility. For whom is the diet appropriate, given its basic nutritional approach? Is the diet safe and effective, for example, for pregnant women, children, or the elderly?
3. Basic nutritional approach. What nutritional premises underlie the diet in terms of accomplishing its goals?
4. Credentials. What are the credentials of the developer(s) of the diet and the staff (in group programs) that implements it?
5. Required and recommended food groups or foods. What foods are required or recommended in order for the diet to be effective?
6. Eliminated or restricted foods. What foods are eliminated or restricted on the diet?
7. Daily meal plans, sample menus, and recipes. Does the diet outline daily meal plans, sample menus, or recipes? If so, are they consistent with the diet's basic nutritional approach?
8. Vitamin and mineral supplements. Does the diet provide the recommended dietary allowances (RDAs) for essential vitamins, minerals, and trace elements? If not, does it counsel dieters to take vitamin and mineral supplements?
9. Smoking and alcohol. What recommendations does the diet make to restrict or eliminate smoking and drinking, both of which affect the absorption of nutrients?
10. Physical activity. What recommendations does the diet make in terms of exercise?
11. Behavioral modification. Does the diet require people to change their eating or lifestyle habits in any way? If so, how are these changes reinforced?

It should be noted that not all diet programs specifically mention required or recommended food groups or foods. In addition, diet formulators are often somewhat imprecise in their terminology. Some, for example, refer to "protein" or "carbohydrate" as recommended foods. But they are, more accurately, nutrients. Nevertheless, to be fair to the diet formulator, we have used their terms and categories throughout our book. Also, not all diets specifically eliminate or restrict certain foods. Some include daily meal plans, sample menus, or recipes in their diets.

We only discuss a diet's prohibition against smoking if the formulator specifically states that it impacts the success of their nutritional program. The same is true for alcohol, physical activity, and behavioral modification. If diet formulators formally include these in their nutritional program, we list their recommendations in the *Guide*.

## GETTING STARTED

*The Consumer's Guide* consists of four parts. Part One, Chapters 1 through 4, discusses the fundamentals of nutrition and provides readers with helpful guidelines to assess their own nutritional status and physical fitness levels, and to identify their dietary goals.

More than 65 million Americans diet each year, and the vast majority of them do so to lose weight. Part Two, Chapters 5 through 9, compares medically supervised weight loss diet plans, commercial programs, nonprofit enrollment programs, over-the-counter (OTC) botanical products, and weight-loss books recommended for review by our medical board. Each type differs in the intensity of treatment provided, cost, the nature of the invention(s), and degree of involvement of health care providers.

Part Three, Chapters 10 through 14, reviews diets specifically designed for women, children, the elderly, vegetarians, and athletes — groups with their own special nutritional needs. Finally, Part Four, Chapters 15 through 24, analyzes diet plans developed to treat specific medical conditions: arthritis, osteoporosis, coronary artery disease (CAD), diabetes, food allergies, hypertension, hypoglycemia, irritable bowel syndrome (IBS), multiple sclerosis (MS), and cancer.

Before buying an automobile, careful consumers familiarize themselves with the basic principles underlying how it performs under a variety of conditions. They learn what kind of fuel the car needs and how much, the number of miles it can run per gallon, and any other relevant information to help this important commodity operate at peak performance. Likewise, before adopting any particular diet, people would do well to acquaint themselves with the basics of nutrition. Once armed with an understanding of the essentials of nutrition, prospective dieters are better able to assess their own nutritional status.

In addition to consulting with their physician, this book recommends that anyone considering adopting a particular diet perform their own initial assessment of their nutritional status. This is important because, regardless of the diet strategy either a physician or nutritionist may recommend, the dieter is always responsible for implementing it on a day-to-day basis. The better people are able to monitor the effects of the diet, the more successful they will be in realizing beneficial results. For this reason, a food diary is provided in Chapter 2 to help prospective dieters analyze their current nutritional status.

In human nutrition, there is a delicate interaction between the quantity and quality of the nutrient fuels taken into the body and the efficiency by which each body metabolizes that fuel. Both are equally important; each influences the other. The more physically fit people are, for example, the better they are able to utilize the essential nutrients they consume in a particular diet. Chapter 3 thus provides a physical status worksheet which readers can use to assess their diet readiness.

Once prospective dieters have analyzed their current nutritional status and physical fitness status, they are ready to define their dietary goals. Chapter 4 suggests a variety of medically safe diet goals and "target diets" which readers might wish to pursue given their nutritional and physical fitness status. Once they have defined their diet objectives, they can then turn to subsequent chapters which describe a variety of weight-loss and medical specialty diets.

Tens of millions of Americans are dieting at any one time either to lose weight, improve their appearance, or improve their health. Over the past several decades, dieters have become better informed about their nutritional options and more discriminating about which diets are medically and nutritionally sound and which are not. *The Consumer's Guide* provides comprehensive information about a variety of weight-loss and medical specialty diets that helps readers formulate an individualized diet plan based on their personal nutritional goals and lifestyle. The *Guide* does not recommend a diet. Its purpose is rather to help you assess a variety of clinical, nonclinical, commercial, and noncommercial diet programs currently available. The book should not be used as a substitute for seeking the advice of a physician, nutritionist, or dietitian. In some cases, the safest, most effective, and least expensive diet program may be one designed and monitored by a primary care physician or health professional.

The information in this book, however, will help you communicate with your health specialist. Good health is almost always a team effort between patients and their doctors. With the help of the *Guide*, the discriminating reader can become a more active participant in designing and implementing an optimum diet.

# Part One

# 1

## Healthful Nutrition

One way to illustrate the critical link between nutrition and health is to think of the human body as being composed of millions of tiny engines. Some of these work in unison, some function independently, and virtually all of them are on call twenty-four hours a day. Each of the engines, in order to run smoothly, requires specific fuels. When the wrong blend of fuel is given, the engine will not perform to its maximum capacity. If the fuel is of poor grade, the engine will sputter and hesitate, creating a loss of power. And if the engine is given no fuel at all, it will eventually stop running.

Because the body cannot produce most of the chemical constituents it needs to sustain life and function properly, the majority of fuel the human body uses comes directly from the nutrients contained in foods. The combination and amounts of foods that a person consumes on a daily basis constitute his or her nutrition.

How specific foods nourish the body depends largely on each person's biological makeup. Nevertheless, scientists have estimated the average minimum levels of essential nutrients which different groups of people require for long-term health. This chapter briefly surveys these essential nutrients and the food sources that supply them. Some people, including pregnant women, the elderly, and persons with medical disorders, may be deficient in one or more essential nutrients, and after consulting with their physician or health practitioner, may find it advisable to take vitamin or mineral supplements.

## NUTRIENTS

There are six categories of nutrients present in foods. In order of predominance, they are water, fats, carbohydrates, proteins, vitamins, and minerals. The body is composed of similar materials in approximately the same order of predominance. Thus, the body of a person who weighs 130 pounds contains approximately 75 pounds of water, 25 pounds of fat, and approximately 30 pounds of protein, carbohydrates, vitamins, and minerals. The body requires varying amounts of all six types of nutrients to maintain body heat, move (exertion), and build and restore bones and tissues.

### Calories

Fuel supplied by nutrients is measured in calories. When a person consumes more calories than their body burns up during basic body functions or exercise, the excess is stored primarily as fat. Therefore, in general, good nutrition involves consuming sufficient amounts of nutrients the body needs without adding excess fat. To obtain all the essential nutrients without consuming excess calories, a person must learn to select foods wisely. Foods that provide more nutrients than calories are said to have a high nutrient density; these foods are often referred to as "nutrient-dense." For example, three ounces of sardines and three ounces of steak provide the same amount of iron, but three ounces of sardines contain only 175 calories and three ounces of steak contain 330 calories. With respect to iron, the sardines are considered more nutrient-dense than steak.

### Water

Water, which constitutes 55 to 60 percent of an adult's body weight, is essential to life because every cell in the body contains water. Water is needed to digest food and transport nutrients, build and repair tissues, eliminate wastes and regulate body temperature.

Water, however, does not supply all the chemicals the body requires to grow, maintain its chemical structure and rejuvenate itself. The other necessary substances are proteins, carbohydrates, and lipids (fats), which must be metabolized (broken down) into smaller chemical constituents before they can be utilized, as well as vitamins and minerals, which are absorbed directly into the body. How much of these substances people require depends upon their age, sex, heredity (their unique genetic structure), the amount of exercise they get, and the amount of toxins that exist in their bodies.

## Proteins

The word "protein" in Greek means "of first importance," and indeed protein — which, next to water, makes up the greatest portion of human body weight — is involved in virtually every chemical process in the human body. Protein substances make up the muscles, ligaments, tendons, organs, glands, nails, hair, body fluids (except for bile and urine), enzymes, hormones, and genes.

Protein is not a single simple substance but a complex chain of amino acids that form many different chemical configurations and combine with other substances. Twenty-two amino acids have been identified in the proteins of the human body, twenty of which are required by the human body to function. Eighty percent of these are produced by the liver, and the remaining 20 percent — termed "essential amino acids" — must be obtained from the diet, primarily from animal and plant foods. If these eight essential amino acids that the body cannot produce internally are not present, some normal body processes can be impaired.

Adults need approximately 50 to 60 grams of protein daily to supply the essential amino acids, and most Americans eat enough meat, fish, eggs, and dairy products to fulfill this requirement. While both meat and plant foods contain proteins, meat is a better source because it contains all eight essential amino acids. Most vegetables lack in at least one essential amino acid; as a result, vegetarians usually must consume both grains and legumes to meet their amino acid requirements.

## Carbohydrates

Carbohydrates are the body's chief source of energy. They are also used in the synthesis of some cell components such as DNA (acids found in the chromosomes of the nucleus of all cells). An immense variety of foods, most of them derived from plants, supply carbohydrates.

Nutritionists distinguish two types of carbohydrates: simple carbohydrates and complex carbohydrates. Simple carbohydrates are called sugars, including fructose, glucose (also called dextrose), maltose, lactose, and sugar alcohols such as sorbitol and xylitol. Sugars are sometimes identified by their sources, such as maple syrup, honey, molasses, and corn syrup.

Foods containing sugars which people consume every day do not always taste sweet. Processed foods, for example, such as soups, spaghetti sauces, fruit drinks, cereals, yogurts, and frozen dinners often contain sugars.

Complex carbohydrates, which are primarily starches, are large chains of glucose molecules. Starch is the storage form of carbohydrates in plants, comparable to the glycogen in humans and animals. The primary sources of complex carbohydrates are grains, bread, rice, pasta, and vegetables such as potatoes and beans.

Both simple and complex carbohydrates produce glucose or glycogen, which, among other things, are essential for normal brain functioning. Simple carbohydrates, however, are high in calories and low in essential nutrients. Complex carbohydrate foods usually contain more vitamins and minerals as well as water and dietary fiber. Some, like legumes, contain protein as well.

## Fats

Most people are aware that excessive amounts of fat in one's diet have been linked with heart disease, cancer, and other medical disorders. Since fat contains about twice as many calories by weight as carbohydrates and protein, high-fat foods can contribute to obesity.

Nevertheless, balanced amounts of fat are absolutely essential for the normal functioning of the human body. Fats supply essential fatty acids which the body cannot make and thus must derive from foods. Linoleic acid is the most important of these because it is required for the proper growth and development of infants. Essential fatty acids also form the basic components of several hormone-like compounds, including prostaglandins, which help control blood pressure, blood clotting, inflammation, and other bodily functions.

The fats that most people eat in ordinary foods come in three principal forms: cholesterol, saturated fats (found primarily in animal products), and unsaturated fats — either polyunsaturated fats (as found in sunflower and safflower oil) or monounsaturated fats (as found in olive and canola oil). In general, saturated fats raise cholesterol levels in the blood, while unsaturated fats appear to reduce cholesterol, including LDL ("bad") cholesterol, without adverse side effects.

Saturated fats are found in animal foods (beef, pork, lamb, veal, egg yolks, whole milk, cream, cheese, ice cream, butter, and lard), chocolate, coconuts, and the fats normally used in processed foods such as coconut, palm, and palm-kernel oils. Many studies have shown a relationship between dietary fat consumption and cancer of the breast, colon, and prostate gland, which is one reason nutritionists recommend eating no more than 10 percent of calories in the diet as saturated fat.

## CHOLESTEROL

Cholesterol helps produce hormones, contributes to development of the brain, and aids the functioning of the nervous system. Cholesterol is not soluble in water and, because it cannot mix with blood, is carried through the bloodstream in protein "packets" called lipoproteins. The two most common kinds of lipoproteins are low-density lipoproteins (LDL) and high-density lipoproteins (HDL). While everyone needs a certain amount of HDL cholesterol, it is not necessary to consume high levels of cholesterol in foods because the liver manufactures all that the body needs.

Most of the cholesterol typically circulating in the bloodstream is carried by LDL — often called "bad" cholesterol because the portion not used by the body in its normal functions tends to collect on the lining of blood vessels and can cause atherosclerosis (buildup of fatty deposits, or plaque, in the arteries). Atherosclerosis reduces the supply of blood carrying oxygen and other vital nutrients to the heart and other organs, and can cause heart disorders, brain disorders, and strokes.

HDL cholesterol is usually called "good" cholesterol because it is more easily eliminated by the body. It also appears to help prevent the formation of fatty plaques in the arteries, and thus may protect against atherosclerosis.

Cholesterol is highly concentrated in egg yolks and organ meats such as liver, and is also found in milk, dairy products, poultry, and seafood. Only animal products contain cholesterol, although prepared foods including crackers or bakery goods may have high-cholesterol ingredients such as lard, eggs, or butter. And while it is not clear whether cholesterol alone, especially bad cholesterol, is harmful, medical experts concur that a diet high in LDL and saturated fats should be avoided.

## FIBER

Fiber is not a single substance but a large group of widely different compounds. Fiber is the part of plants that cannot be digested by enzymes in the human intestinal tract. Nutritionists usually distinguish two types of fiber: those that are soluble in water and those that are insoluble in water.

Most plant foods contain both types in varying amounts, although certain foods are particularly rich on one or the other. The most important component of fiber is cellulose, which, although it cannot be digested, can assist the digestive process. In addition, fibers such as cellulose and bran add bulk to the feces, thereby helping to prevent constipation and related disorders such as hemorrhoids.

Nutritionists recommend that people consume 20 to 30 grams of fiber daily. Good sources include vegetables, whole grains (such as bran and uncooked oats), fruits, and legumes.

## VITAMINS

Vitamins are essential for such important body functions as digestion, tissue formation and repair, and normal nerve functioning. They also aid in regulating metabolism and assist in many of the biochemical processes that release energy from digested foods. Vitamins are considered "micronutrients" because the body needs them in relatively small amounts compared with other nutrients such as carbohydrates.

To obtain sufficient vitamins, most nutritionists recommend that a daily diet include multiple servings of cereal or bread; dairy products (milk, cheese, ice cream, cottage cheese); meat, fish, or eggs; and vegetables and fruits.

### Vitamin A

Vitamin A promotes good vision, particularly vision in dim light, by generating pigments necessary for the proper functioning of the retina. In addition, vitamin A is required for adequate immune system response, builds the body's resistance to respiratory infections, and helps form and maintain healthy skin, hair, and mucous membranes.

Vitamin A is available in several forms. Retinols are a derivative of vitamin A found in foods that come from animals (meat, milk, and eggs), as well as fish liver oils, cheese, and butter. Beta-carotene, a previtamin that is converted by the body into vitamin A, is found in vegetables and fruits such as beets, broccoli, cantaloupe, carrots, apricots, alfalfa, asparagus, Swiss chard, dandelion greens, garlic, kale, papayas, parsley, peaches, red peppers, sweet potatoes, spinach, spirulina, pumpkin and yellow squash, turnip greens, and watercress.

## Vitamin B1 (Thiamin)

Vitamin B1 (thiamin) plays an essential role in regulating the body's metabolism, helping cells convert carbohydrates into energy. It is necessary for normal brain and nerve functioning, helps keep mucous membranes healthy, and replaces deficiencies caused by alcoholism (cirrhosis). It also appears to help regulate the thyroid, prevent infections, improve breast-feeding, and reduce prolonged diarrhea.

Natural sources of vitamin B1 include whole-grain products, dried beans (kidney, garbanzo, navy, and soy), sunflower seeds, brewer's yeast, bran, brown rice, wheat germ, and salmon.

## Vitamin B2 (Riboflavin)

Like vitamin B1, vitamin B2 (riboflavin) helps release energy from carbohydrates. It is essential for growth and the production of red blood cells, and it acts as a component in two coenzymes (flavin mononucleotide and flavin adrenin dinucleotide), both of which are needed for normal tissue growth. It also maintains healthy mucous membranes lining the respiratory, digestive, circulatory, and excretory tracts when used in conjunction with vitamin A. In addition, vitamin B2 appears to decrease a craving for sugar and thus may help prevent diabetes.

Natural sources of vitamin B2 include milk and dairy products, lean meats, nuts (especially almonds), green leafy vegetables, liver, kidney, and chicken. Cereals fortified with this vitamin are also excellent sources.

## Vitamin B3 (Niacin)

Two chemicals contain vitamin B3 properties: nicotinic acid (niacin) and niacinamide (nicotinamide adrenin dinucleotide). Both are necessary for releasing energy from foods, for the utilization of fats, and for tissue respiration. In addition, niacin helps control blood fat levels and is important for the proper functioning of skin and nerves. It also promotes growth, maintains normal functioning of the gastrointestinal tract, and is necessary for metabolism of sugar. Niacinamide is generally used in treatment because, unlike niacin, it does not cause burning, flushing, or itching of the skin.

Natural sources of vitamin B3 include nuts, sunflower seeds, dairy products, chicken, beef, liver, lean meats such as turkey or veal, brewer's yeast, wheat products, yeast, green vegetables and beans, halibut, salmon, swordfish, tuna, peanuts, and pork. Strict vegetarians who eat no animal foods must rely on nuts and legumes for niacin.

## Vitamin B5 (Pantothenic Acid)

Like vitamin B3, vitamin B5 (pantothenic acid) is essential for normal growth and development. It aids in the release of energy from foods, plays a critical role in the production of adrenal hormones, and helps synthesize numerous body materials.

Vitamin B5 is found in lentils, liver, lobster, peanuts, peas, blue cheese, brewer's yeast, corn, eggs, soybeans, sunflower seeds, wheat germ, whole-grain products, and meats of all kinds. It is also a primary component of mother's milk.

## Vitamin B6 (Pyridoxine)

Vitamin B6 is important in many chemical reactions of proteins and protein components. Along with vitamin B3 (niacinamide), vitamin B6 (pyridoxine) helps the body utilize fats by absorbing proteins and assists in the formation of red blood cells. Vitamin B6 is also essential in maintaining normal functioning of the brain, maintaining a chemical balance among body fluids, regulating excretion of water, synthesizing RNA and DNA (nucleic acids), which contain the genetic instructions for the reproduction of all cells, and aiding energy production and resistance to stress.

Vitamin B6 is found in milk and milk products, whole-grain breads and cereals, walnuts, peas, blackstrap molasses, brown rice, cabbage, cantaloupe, avocados, bananas, bran, brewer's yeast, carrots, hazelnuts, lentils, rice, salmon, shrimp, soybeans, sunflower seeds, tuna, and wheat germ.

## Vitamin B9 (Folic Acid)

Vitamin B9 (folic acid) has several essential functions. It controls cell growth and repair and it acts as a coenzyme for normal DNA synthesis. It also interacts with vitamin B12 to produce red blood cells. In addition, it maintains nervous system integrity and intestinal tract functions. In pregnant mothers, vitamin B9 helps regulate embryonic and fetal development of nerve cells.

Natural sources include dark green leafy vegetables, citrus fruits and juices, beans and other legumes, wheat bran and other whole grains, pork, poultry, and calves' liver.

Folic acid deficiency, the most common vitamin deficiency in the world, is prevalent in pregnant women. Vitamin B9 is vital to cell reproduction within the fetus, and without a constant source of vitamin B9, birth defects will result. The FDA now recommends that foods, preferably enriched flour, be fortified with folic acid to prevent neural tube defect, a common birth defect that occurs when the spinal column fails to close completely during the first six weeks of pregnancy.

## Vitamin B12 (Cobalamin)

Vitamin B12 (cobalamin) aids in red blood cell formation and helps maintain the central nervous system. It assists in the production of nucleic acid; nucleic acid helps preserve nerve tissue and prevent anemia. It is also required for protein synthesis and metabolism of carbohydrates and fats. In addition, it is important for the production of DNA and RNA.

Vitamin B12 is made from bacteria and is only present in foods that contain the bacteria or foods from animals that have ingested bacteria. Thus, most B12 foods come from animal products, and strict vegetarians may need to take B12 supplements. Excellent sources include beef and beef liver, clams, flounder, herring, liverwurst, mackerel, sardines, blue and swiss cheese, eggs, and milk.

## Vitamin C

Vitamin C (also known as ascorbic acid) plays many roles in the body. It helps promote healthy gums and teeth, aids in iron absorption, maintains normal connective tissue (collagen), and is essential for the healing of wounds. In addition, it is important in preserving the structural integrity of capillary walls, fighting bacterial infections, and protecting the circulatory system from fat deposits. It may also relieve emotional and environmental stress. Aggressive use of vitamin C has been used to treat cancer and other diseases in which the optimizing of immune function is a critical therapeutic goal.

Natural food sources of vitamin C include citrus fruits, tomatoes, potatoes, and green leafy vegetables such as broccoli, Brussels sprouts, collards, turnip and mustard greens, spinach, Swiss chard, watercress, parsley, and cabbage. It is also found in asparagus, avocados, cantaloupe, currants, mangoes, onions, oranges, papayas, green peppers, pineapple, raisins, rose hips, and strawberries. Relative to other nutrients, it is one of the safest substances known.

## Vitamin D

Vitamin D is essential for the normal formation and maintenance of bones and teeth, and for the absorption of calcium and phosphorus in the gastrointestinal tract. Vitamin D is also called cholecalciferol and is available from both natural and synthetic sources.

Small amounts of vitamin D are present in natural foods, especially milk and dairy products. Other sources of vitamin D include halibut, salmon, sardines and herring, organ meats, sweet potatoes, fish-liver oils, and egg yolks. Vitamin D is also obtained through exposure to sunlight.

## Vitamin E

Vitamin E, also called tocopherol, is an antioxidant that protects tissues and organs against the damage of oxidation. It is essential for the formation of red blood cells and the utilization of vitamins A, C, and K. Vitamin E also promotes normal blood clotting and healing, reduces scarring from some wounds, reduces blood pressure, improves athletic performance, relieves leg cramps, and may help prevent cataracts.

Nutrient sources of vitamin E include vegetable oils (soybean, cottonseed, sunflower, corn); vegetable oil products such as margarine; spinach, asparagus, and other green leafy vegetables; wheat germ; liver, sunflower seeds, walnuts, hazelnuts, almonds, butter, eggs, cashews, and soy lecithin. Salad oils, margarine, and shortening provide about 64 percent of vitamin E in the average U.S. diet; fruits and vegetables about 11 percent; and grains and grain products about 7 percent.

## Vitamin K (Phylloquinone)

Vitamin K is needed for blood clotting and plays an important role in bone formation. Concentrated amounts are found in dark green leafy vegetables, bran, alfalfa, vegetable oils, and tomatoes. Other foods that contain vitamin K include wheat, oatmeal, oats, rye, liver, egg yolks, cauliflower, cabbage, Brussels sprouts, and blackstrap molasses.

## Vitamin Deficiencies and Toxicities (Excesses)

A balanced diet usually provides all the necessary vitamins (and minerals) without the need for supplements. However, certain people are deficient in one or several vitamins and may need to take vitamin supplements. Pregnant and nursing women, newborns and growing children, and elderly and ill persons have special needs for vitamins, and may find their daily intake either below the RDAs or not sufficient to prevent deficiency symptoms. These people might consider taking vitamin supplements.

However, vitamin supplements alone will not take the place of a good diet. Nor will vitamin supplements provide direct sources of energy because, as enzyme components, vitamins can act only in the presence of nutrients contained in food. Thus, people taking vitamin supplements should ensure that they consume only the recommended amounts (RDAs) of vitamins (see Table 1), because excessive intakes can be toxic. The following list gives common symptoms and disorders that have been linked with vitamin deficiencies and toxicities (excess intakes).

### Symptoms Associated with Vitamin Deficiencies and Toxicities

**Vitamin A.** *Deficiency:* night blindness; triangular gray spots on eyes; softening of the cornea; skin dryness; infections; diarrhea; bone pain; dental decay; anemia; nerve damage. *Excess:* Loss of appetite; skin problems; swelling of ankles and feet; bone abnormalities; slowed clotting time; stopping of menstruation; headache; nausea; loss of hair; enlarged liver; jaundice.

**Vitamin B1** (thiamin). *Deficiency:* mental confusion; weakness; peripheral paralysis; enlarged heart; cardiac failure; calf muscle pain; edema; wasting.

**Vitamin B2** (riboflavin). *Deficiency:* eye and skin problems; reddening of eyes; hypersensitivity to light; dermatitis around lips and nostrils and cracking at corners of the mouth.

**Vitamin B3** (niacin). *Deficiency:* dermatitis; mental confusion; irritability; diarrhea; pellagra.

**Vitamin B5** (pantothenic acid). *Deficiency:* vomiting; malaise; abdominal cramps; insomnia.

**Vitamin B6** (pyridoxine). *Deficiency:* dermatitis; irritation of sweat glands; difficulty sleeping; abnormal brainwave patterns; convulsions.

**Vitamin B9** (folic acid). *Deficiency:* diarrhea and other gastrointestinal disorders; anemia.

**Vitamin B12** (cobalamin). *Deficiency:* pernicious anemia; nervous system malfunctions; heightened sensitivity of skin; loss of sensation in fingers and toes.

**Vitamin C.** *Deficiency:* scurvy (degeneration of teeth, bones, and gums); impaired wound healing; heart degeneration; pain in joints; anemia; depression. *Excess:* nausea, diarrhea, cramps.

**Vitamin D.** *Deficiency:* rickets (bone deformities); bone deterioration in adults. *Excess:* loss of appetite; thirst; nausea; weight loss; kidney damage; irritability; stones in soft tissue.

**Vitamin E.** *Deficiency:* anemia; possible nerve cell destruction; edema in infants. *Excess:* impaired blood clotting; gastrointestinal disorders.

**Vitamin K** (phylloquinone). *Deficiency:* severe bleeding.

## MINERALS AND TRACE ELEMENTS

Minerals and trace elements are essential parts of enzymes that participate in many biochemical and physiological processes, including the transportation of oxygen to the cells. If the human body requires more than 100 milligrams daily, the substance is labeled a mineral. If the body requires less than 100 milligrams each day, the substance is labeled a trace element. Of the trace elements — which include chromium, cobalt, copper, fluoride, germanium, iodine, lithium, manganese, molybdenum, selenium, and silicon — the two most important for the optimal functioning of the body are iron and zinc.

Unlike most vitamins, minerals are inorganic substances that are usually not destroyed by cooking, food processing, or exposure to air or acid. However, they sometimes combine with other substances in food to form insoluble salts that cannot be absorbed by the human digestive tract. The body utilizes at least eighty-four different minerals and trace elements, and when any one of these is deficient or an absorption interference occurs, malfunctions may result in the part of the body that depends on that mineral.

Most minerals and trace elements are widely found in foods, especially fresh fruits and vegetables, and severe deficiencies are unusual. However, iron deficiency occurs frequently in infants, children, and pregnant women, while zinc and copper deficiencies are common among the elderly.

## Calcium

Calcium, the major constituent of the structural framework of bones, is the body's most abundant mineral. For both men and women, 98 percent of the body's calcium is found in the bones, 1 percent in the teeth, and the remaining 1 percent in soft body tissues, where it performs a variety of essential functions.

In addition to supporting the growth and continued strength of bones and teeth, calcium helps regulate the heartbeat and other muscle contractions and maintain cell membranes. It is also essential to proper blood clotting, and assists in regulating the transport of ions in and out of cells, making muscular contractions and relaxation possible. Along with other nutrients, calcium has been used with moderate success to reduce the risk of angina and heart disease, and is also prescribed by naturopaths for mild allergies.

The richest food sources of calcium are milk and dairy products, including yogurt and hard cheeses. Canned sardines and salmon, caviar, almonds and Brazil nuts, molasses, shrimp, soybeans, tofu, and leafy green vegetables (particularly collard and dandelion greens and spinach) are also good sources, although oxalic acid in spinach renders much of the vegetable's calcium insoluble and nonabsorbable.

## Chloride

Chloride, which enters the body primarily through table salt, is a necessary constituent of stomach acid (hydrochloric acid). In addition, it interacts with sodium, potassium, and carbon dioxide to maintain an acid-base balance in body cells and fluids. It is vital for normal health.

Most people consume more than adequate amounts of chloride in salt substitutes (potassium chloride), sea salt, and table salt (sodium chloride). Only those on a severe salt-restricted diet need to be concerned about the amount of chloride they consume, and should consider using a salt substitute.

## Magnesium

Magnesium is important for many metabolic processes. It plays an essential role in the release of energy from glycogen (stored muscle fuel), the manufacture of proteins, the regulation of body temperature, and the proper functioning of nerves and muscles. In addition, it aids bone growth and helps maintain normal heart rhythms. Low intakes of magnesium have been linked not only to irregular heart rhythms but also to high blood pressure. Magnesium also strengthens tooth enamel, keeps metabolism steady, and works as a laxative in large doses.

Good sources of magnesium include whole-grain breads and cereals, nuts (particularly almonds and cashews), fish, molasses, soybeans, sunflower seeds, wheat germ, bananas, apricots, and leafy green vegetables.

## Phosphorus

Phosphorus is essential for energy production, the building and maintenance (in combination with calcium) of healthy bones and teeth, and the formation of cell membranes and genetic material. It is found in every cell of the body as a component of nucleic acids. In addition, it helps in the metabolism of carbohydrates and in the transport of fats throughout the body.

Phosphorus is present in almost all foods. Foods especially rich in phosphorus include meat, fish, poultry, milk, nuts, legumes, and whole-grain cereals and breads. Most people consume more than enough phosphorus from the large amount of meat they eat and from phosphorus salts used in processed foods. Prolonged use of antacids can lead to a harmful loss of phosphorus, and frequent consumption of carbonated drinks (which contain phosphorus) can distort the crucial ratio of calcium to phosphorus. If a diet contains too much phosphorus, calcium is not utilized efficiently.

## Potassium

Potassium is important for the proper functioning of muscles, including the heart. It is a crucial regulator of the amount of water in cells, which determines their ability to function properly. Potassium also helps transmit nerve impulses, is a buffer for body fluids, and catalyzes the release of energy from carbohydrates, proteins, and fats. As noted in Chapter 21, it may also help prevent hypertension (high blood pressure).

Natural sources of potassium include milk, bananas, avocados, dried fruits, citrus fruits, lentils, molasses, nuts, parsnips, potatoes, raisins, canned sardines, fresh spinach, and whole-grain cereals. A recommended daily allowance for potassium has not been established.

## Sodium

Sodium is an electrolyte present in all cells of the body. Its most important function is to regulate the balance of water inside and outside the cells. Sodium also plays a crucial role in maintaining blood pressure, aiding muscle contraction and nerve transmission, and regulating the body's acid-base balance.

Natural sources of sodium include bacon and ham, milk, beef, margarine and butter, bread, clams, green beans, canned sardines, and tomatoes. Most people consume sodium as sodium chloride in ordinary table salt. A recommended daily allowance for sodium has not been established.

## Sulfur

Sulfur is important in the body because it binds protein molecules, and therefore is a crucial constituent of proteins in hair, fingernails, toenails, and skin. It also functions as an antioxidant and aids the secretion of bile in the liver.

Sulfur is found in fish, eggs, cabbage, dried beans, milk, wheat germ, soybeans, turnips, onions, lean beef, kale, garlic, clams, and Brussels sprouts. A recommended daily allowance has not been established, and deficiencies in humans are unknown because sulfur is widespread in protein foods.

## Iron

Iron is essential to the formation of hemoglobin (which carries oxygen to the blood) and myoglobin (which carries oxygen in the muscle). It is also a key component of several enzymes and proteins.

Heme iron, which is found only in animal foods such as beef, liver, fish, and poultry, is better absorbed by humans than non-heme vegetable sources such as peas, beans, nuts, dried fruits, and leafy green vegetables. Consuming foods that contain iron along with foods rich in vitamin C (such as citrus fruits, tomatoes, or green peppers) can enhance iron absorption. Conversely, several foods and beverages contain substances that inhibit iron absorption, including tea, coffee, wheat bran, and egg yolks. Overuse of antacids and calcium supplements also decreases iron absorption.

## Zinc

Zinc is a component of nearly one hundred human enzymes involved in major metabolic processes, most of which work with red blood cells to move carbon dioxide from the tissues to the lungs. Zinc forms a component of many enzymes needed for cell division, growth, and repair (wound healing), as well as the proper functioning of the immune system. In addition, zinc functions as an important antioxidant, maintains normal levels of vitamin A in the blood, and helps synthesize DNA and RNA.

Natural sources include lean beef, egg yolks, fish, lamb, milk, oysters, pork, sesame and sunflower seeds, soybeans, turkey, wheat bran and germ, and whole-grain products.

## Iodine

Iodine is necessary for normal cell metabolism, and helps the thyroid gland synthesize and secrete the thyroid hormones thyroxine and levothyroxine. A deficiency of iodine can cause a goiter, an enlargement of the thyroid gland.

Most people consume adequate amounts of iodine in iodized table salt. Other excellent sources include dairy products, vegetables grown in iodine-rich soils, seafoods, and seaweed.

## Selenium

Selenium is a component of several enzymes which act as antioxidants and help fight cell damage caused by oxygen-deprived compounds. It is essential for the proper functioning of the heart muscle and in the maintenance of the immune system. As a result, it may protect against certain cancers.

Excellent sources include red meat, grains, fish, shellfish, eggs, garlic, chicken, and liver. It is also found in many vegetables, especially those grown in selenium-rich soils.

## RECOMMENDED DIETARY ALLOWANCES (RDAS) FOR VITAMINS AND MINERALS

Many people find it difficult to understand and identify the foods they should eat. To help the public understand basic nutrition and prepare healthy meals, the federal government periodically publishes a list of recommended dietary allowances, or daily intakes of the six nutrients, based on studies which many national agencies have conducted and reviewed. It also sets guidelines for average caloric needs to maintain certain weights according to an individual's height and age. The latest RDAs appear in Table 1. RDAs are generally set about 30 percent higher than the average amount the body requires, which, on a statistical basis, usually accommodates most healthy individuals. RDAs are designed for people who are in good health, are not suffering from clinical disease, and are not under an unusual amount of stress. The RDA also lists nutrient requirements for children and for pregnant and lactating women. By eating a balanced diet of natural foods each day, most people are able to acquire the essential nutrients in amounts recommended by the RDAs.

# Table 1. Recommended Dietary Allowances

| Category | Age (years) or Condition | Weight (kg) | Weight (lb) | Height (cm) | Height (in) | Protein (g) | Vitamin A (μg re)[c] | Vitamin D (μg)[d] | Vitamin E (mg α-te)[e] | Vitamin K (μg) |
|---|---|---|---|---|---|---|---|---|---|---|
| | | | | | | | | Fat-Soluble Vitamins | | |
| Infants | 0.0–0.5 | 6 | 13 | 60 | 24 | 13 | 375 | 7.5 | 3 | 5 |
| | 0.5–1.0 | 9 | 20 | 71 | 28 | 14 | 375 | 10 | 4 | 10 |
| Children | 1–3 | 13 | 29 | 90 | 35 | 16 | 400 | 10 | 6 | 15 |
| | 4–6 | 20 | 44 | 112 | 44 | 24 | 500 | 10 | 7 | 20 |
| | 7–10 | 28 | 62 | 132 | 52 | 28 | 700 | 10 | 7 | 30 |
| Males | 11–14 | 45 | 99 | 157 | 62 | 45 | 1,000 | 10 | 10 | 45 |
| | 15–18 | 66 | 145 | 176 | 69 | 59 | 1,000 | 10 | 10 | 65 |
| | 19–24 | 72 | 160 | 177 | 70 | 58 | 1,000 | 10 | 10 | 70 |
| | 25–50 | 79 | 174 | 176 | 70 | 63 | 1,000 | 5 | 10 | 80 |
| | 51+ | 77 | 170 | 173 | 68 | 63 | 1,000 | 5 | 10 | 80 |
| Females | 11–14 | 46 | 101 | 157 | 62 | 46 | 800 | 10 | 8 | 45 |
| | 15–18 | 55 | 120 | 163 | 64 | 44 | 800 | 10 | 8 | 55 |
| | 19–24 | 58 | 128 | 164 | 65 | 46 | 800 | 10 | 8 | 60 |
| | 25–50 | 63 | 138 | 163 | 64 | 50 | 800 | 5 | 8 | 65 |
| | 51+ | 65 | 143 | 160 | 63 | 50 | 800 | 5 | 8 | 65 |
| Pregnant | | | | | | 60 | 800 | 10 | 10 | 65 |
| Lactating | 1st 6 months | | | | | 65 | 1,300 | 10 | 12 | 65 |
| | 2nd 6 months | | | | | 62 | 1,200 | 10 | 11 | 65 |

[a]The allowances, expressed as average daily intakes over time, are intended to provide for individual variations among most normal persons as they live in the United States under usual environmental stresses. Diets should be based on a variety of common foods in order to provide other nutrients for which human requirements have been less well defined. See text for detailed discussion of allowances and of nutrients not tabulated.
[b]Weights and heights of reference adults are actual medians for the U.S. population of the designated age, as reported by NHANES II. The median weights and heights of those under 19 years of age were taken from Hamill et al. (1979) (see pages 16–17). The use of these figures does not imply that the height-to-weight ratios are ideal.

# Table 1. Recommended Dietary Allowances (continued)

| | Water-Soluble Vitamins | | | | | | | Minerals | | | | | | |
|---|---|---|---|---|---|---|---|---|---|---|---|---|---|---|
| Vitamin C (mg) | Thiamin (mg) | Riboflavin (mg) | Niacin (mg NE) | Vitamin B6 (mg) | Folate (μg) | Vitamin B12 (μg) | Calcium (mg) | Phosphorus (mg) | Magnesium (mg) | Iron (mg) | Zinc (mg) | Iodine (μg) | Selenium (μg) |
| 30 | 0.3 | 0.4 | 5 | 0.3 | 25 | 0.3 | 400 | 300 | 40 | 6 | 5 | 40 | 10 |
| 35 | 0.4 | 0.5 | 6 | 0.6 | 35 | 0.5 | 600 | 500 | 60 | 10 | 5 | 50 | 15 |
| 40 | 0.7 | 0.8 | 9 | 1.0 | 50 | 0.7 | 800 | 800 | 80 | 10 | 10 | 70 | 20 |
| 45 | 0.9 | 1.1 | 12 | 1.1 | 75 | 1.0 | 800 | 800 | 120 | 10 | 10 | 90 | 20 |
| 45 | 1.0 | 1.2 | 13 | 1.4 | 100 | 1.4 | 800 | 800 | 170 | 10 | 10 | 120 | 30 |
| 50 | 1.3 | 1.5 | 17 | 1.7 | 150 | 2.0 | 1,200 | 1,200 | 270 | 12 | 15 | 150 | 40 |
| 60 | 1.5 | 1.8 | 20 | 2.0 | 200 | 2.0 | 1,200 | 1,200 | 400 | 12 | 15 | 150 | 50 |
| 60 | 1.5 | 1.7 | 19 | 2.0 | 200 | 2.0 | 1,200 | 1,200 | 350 | 10 | 15 | 150 | 70 |
| 60 | 1.5 | 1.7 | 19 | 2.0 | 200 | 2.0 | 800 | 800 | 350 | 10 | 15 | 150 | 70 |
| 60 | 1.2 | 1.4 | 15 | 2.0 | 200 | 2.0 | 800 | 800 | 350 | 10 | 15 | 150 | 70 |
| 50 | 1.1 | 1.3 | 15 | 1.4 | 150 | 2.0 | 1,200 | 1,200 | 280 | 15 | 12 | 150 | 45 |
| 60 | 1.1 | 1.3 | 15 | 1.5 | 180 | 2.0 | 1,200 | 1,200 | 300 | 15 | 12 | 150 | 50 |
| 60 | 1.1 | 1.3 | 15 | 1.6 | 180 | 2.0 | 1,200 | 1,200 | 280 | 15 | 12 | 150 | 55 |
| 60 | 1.1 | 1.3 | 15 | 1.6 | 180 | 2.0 | 800 | 800 | 280 | 15 | 12 | 150 | 55 |
| 60 | 1.0 | 1.2 | 13 | 1.6 | 180 | 2.0 | 800 | 800 | 280 | 10 | 12 | 150 | 55 |
| 70 | 1.5 | 1.6 | 17 | 2.2 | 400 | 2.2 | 1,200 | 1,200 | 300 | 30 | 15 | 175 | 65 |
| 95 | 1.6 | 1.8 | 20 | 2.1 | 280 | 2.6 | 1,200 | 1,200 | 355 | 15 | 19 | 200 | 75 |
| 90 | 1.6 | 1.7 | 20 | 2.1 | 260 | 2.6 | 1,200 | 1,200 | 340 | 15 | 16 | 200 | 75 |

[c] Retinol equivalents. 1 retinol equivalent = 1 μg retinol or 6 μg β-carotene. See text for calculation of vitamin A activity of diets as retinol equivalents.

[d] As cholecalciferol. 10 μg cholecalciferol = 400 IU of vitamin D.

[e] α-Tocopherol equivalents. 1 mg d-α tocopherol = 1 α-TE. See text for variation in allowances and calculation of vitamin E activity of the diet as α-tocopherol equivalents.

[f] 1 NE (niacin equivalent) is equal to 1 mg of niacin or 60 mg of dietary tryptophan.

# 2

## Analyzing Your Current Nutritional Status

"There is only one good, knowledge," Socrates once said, "and one evil, ignorance." His observation is certainly true about nutrition, because the nutrients we consume — or do not consume — each day determine our health, our risk of developing chronic diseases, and even our life span.

While these claims may seem extreme, they are, in fact, the conclusions of the largest research effort ever conducted on how nutrition directly affects health. For four years, U.S. nutrition experts in the federal government, aided by hundreds of colleagues in universities, professional schools, industries, communities, and state and local government agencies, examined the results of more than 2,500 scientific studies in order to determine the links between diet and disease. Their conclusions were released in 1988 in the first *Surgeon General's Report on Nutrition and Health:* "What we eat may affect our risk for several of the leading causes of death for Americans, notably coronary heart disease, stroke, atherosclerosis, diabetes, and some types of cancer. These disorders together now account for more than two-thirds of all deaths in the United States."

The report's main conclusion is that overconsumption of certain dietary components is now a major concern for Americans. While many food factors are involved, chief among them is the disproportionate consumption of foods high in fats, often at the expense of foods high in complex carbohydrates and fiber that may be more conducive to health.

This chapter details the key recommendations contained in the *Surgeon General's Report* and summarizes dietary guidelines subsequently issued by four respected U.S. agencies. It also shows people how to administer their own nutritional assessment so as to be able to intelligently monitor their current diet and their daily food and nutrient intake. The central

## RECOMMENDATIONS OF THE
## *SURGEON GENERAL'S REPORT*

### Issues for Most People:

- **Fats and cholesterol:** Reduce consumption of fat (especially saturated fat) and cholesterol. Choose foods relatively low in these substances, such as vegetables, fruits, whole-grain foods, fish, poultry, lean meats, and lowfat dairy products. Use food preparation methods that add little or no fat.

- **Energy and weight control:** Achieve and maintain a desirable body weight. To do so, choose a dietary pattern in which energy (caloric) intake is consistent with energy expenditure. To reduce energy intake, limit consumption of foods relatively high in calories, fats and sugars, and minimize alcohol consumption. Increase energy expenditure through regular and sustained physical activity.

- **Complex carbohydrates and fiber:** Increase consumption of whole-grain foods and cereal products, vegetables (including dried beans and peas), and fruits.

- **Sodium:** Reduce intake of sodium by choosing foods relatively low in sodium and limiting the amount of salt added in food preparation and at the table.

- **Alcohol:** To reduce the risk for chronic disease, take alcohol only in moderation (no more than two drinks a day), if at all. Avoid drinking any alcohol before or while driving, operating machinery, taking medications, or engaging in any other activity requiring judgment. Avoid drinking alcohol while pregnant.

### Issues for Some People:

- **Fluoride:** Community water systems should contain fluoride at optimal levels for prevention of tooth decay. If such water is not available, use other appropriate sources of fluoride.

- **Sugars:** Those who are particularly vulnerable to dental cavities, especially children, should limit their consumption and frequency of use of food high in sugars.

- **Calcium:** Adolescent girls and adult women should increase consumption of foods high in calcium, including lowfat dairy products.

- **Iron:** Children, adolescents, and women of childbearing age should be sure to consume foods that are good sources of iron, such as lean meats, fish, certain beans, iron-enriched cereals, and whole-grain products.

## GUIDELINES FOR NUTRITION*

- **General Recommendations:** Eat a diet rich in whole "natural" and un-processed foods such as fruits, vegetables, grains, beans, seeds, and nuts. These foods contain valuable nutrients as well as dietary fiber.
- **Proteins:** Eat moderate quantities of protein, especially animal protein. Fish and many shellfish are excellent sources of lowfat protein.
- **Fats:** Maintain total fat intake at or below 30 percent of total caloric intake and saturated fats at less than 10 percent. Eat leaner cuts of meat, trim off excess fat, remove skin from poultry, and consume smaller portions.
- **Carbohydrates:** Carbohydrates should comprise between 60 and 70 percent of total caloric intake. Only 10 percent of carbohydrates should be refined or concentrated sugars such as honey, fruit juices, dried fruit, sugar, or white flour. Foods high in calories, such as whole-grain cereals and bread, are more healthful than foods or drinks containing sugar.
- **Dairy Products:** Eat dairy products for calcium, but avoid excessive amounts of whole milk, whole-milk cheeses, yogurt, ice cream, and other milk products that are high in saturated fats.

*Source: Marti J., and A. Hine, *Alternative Health and Medicine Encyclopedia* (Detroit, MI: Gale Research Inc., 1995).

component of this assessment is a food diary that encourages people to assume an active role in achieving their dietary goals.

## THE "GOOD DIET"

After the publication of the *Surgeon General's Report on Nutrition and Health,* several U.S. agencies — the American Council on Science and Health, the National Academy of Sciences, the U.S. Department of Agriculture, and the U.S. Department of Health and Human Services — issued their own dietary guidelines, as summarized below.

## PROFESSIONALLY ADMINISTERED NUTRITIONAL ASSESSMENTS

Physicians, nutritionists, and dietitians use several techniques, including physical examinations, to assess a person's nutritional status. Compiling a medical and diet history helps detect nutritional imbalances, deficiencies, usual eating habits and food preferences, and intake of medications, nutritional supplements, and alcohol. Biochemical or clinical laboratory tests (including blood and urine samples) can also directly measure nutrients and detect deficiencies, while other laboratory tests, such as the Schilling test of vitamin B12, detect how well a person absorbs certain essential nutrients. Immune function tests measure the type and amount of white blood cells present, which provides an indicator of both the body's nutritional status and resistance to disease.

## SELF-ADMINISTERED NUTRITIONAL ASSESSMENT

In addition to consulting with their physician, people can also conduct a self-administered nutritional assessment to intelligently monitor their current diet and their daily food and nutrient intake. One of the most effective is a food diary, which helps determine factors associated with food consumption such as time of day, place eaten, level of hunger, and mood. Among the advantages of this alternative (another alternative is a food frequency checklist) are that it encourages one to assume an active role in achieving dietary goals and to become conscious of the lifestyle and home factors that affect food choices and consumption patterns.

### How to Keep a Food Diary

To keep the diary, people record everything they eat for at least three days — the minimum period in which reliable information can be gathered on nutritional intake and food consumption patterns. Completing the diary for seven days is better, and using it for a thirty-day period is even more helpful. Nutritionists recommend that people keep the diary with them wherever they go so they can write down the required information immediately after eating throughout the day.

A sample one-day food diary appears below. It can be xeroxed and the additional pages stapled or bound together to make a diary for longer periods of time.

To make entries: 1) Record the date and type and amount of each food you consume in a twenty-four-hour period. 2) Using a calorie-counting guide, nutritional handbook, or computer diet software program, calculate the number of calories and nutrient composition for each food eaten. 3) Record the time when, and locale where, you ate, and whether the food was a meal or a snack. 4) Note how hungry you were, and what, if any, mood was associated with eating.

*Foods and Amounts.* In the "food consumed" column, record the type of *every* food and beverage you consumed during the course of the day and its product name. For example, if you ate cereal, toast, and coffee for breakfast, record in column 1:

**Food**
Grape-Nuts cereal
Whole-wheat toast
Coffee with cream

In the "amount" column, enter the amount of each food or beverage you consumed. Thus, in the second column you would enter:

| **Food** | **Amount** |
| --- | --- |
| Grape-Nuts cereal | 1 serving |
| Whole-wheat toast | 2 slices |
| Coffee with cream | 1 cup with 2 tablespoons cream |

*Calories.* While not all of the diets reviewed in this book "count" calories, it is a good idea, particularly at the beginning of any diet, to know how many calories you consume each day. By way of comparison, carbohydrates and proteins supply approximately four calories per gram, while fats supply approximately nine calories per gram.

In May 1994 the Food and Drug Administration began requiring companies that produce packaged foods to provide substantial information about fat content, calories, and other nutritional values in large type on a "nutrition facts" panel on their labels, and to show how items fit into a daily diet of 2,000 calories. The new rules, which took ten years to develop, also make it more difficult for companies to make claims for their products (such as "lowfat" or "high fiber") because they now have to substantiate them. This newly required information will help dieters filling out a food diary calculate the amounts of various nutrients — listed as grams or milligrams, as well as a percentage of recommended daily intake — they are consuming.

It should be noted that the purpose of counting calories is not to make people feel guilty or deprived. Rather, it provides an accurate assessment of the essential nutrients, vitamins, and minerals that they are or are not eating each day. Over time dieters will become more aware of their food consumption patterns. People suffering from obesity, or any of the medical disorders discussed in Chapters 15 through 24, must be particularly accurate in recording their daily calorie levels. Studies show that obese subjects often underreport their caloric intake and overestimate their levels of physical activity, which works against their weight-loss success.

*Protein.* Identifying the protein content of foods is important in order to determine if you are receiving adequate daily amounts of essential amino acids. Most Americans now consume twice the amount of protein they actually need, two-thirds of which comes from meat. As noted, national dietary guidelines now recommend that people consume moderate quantities of protein, especially animal protein, and suggest that fish, while low in saturated fat, is an excellent source of protein.

*Fats and Saturated Fats.* Recording total daily fat and saturated fat intake is especially important for people on weight-loss diets. Normally, when people consume excessive amounts of fat (more than 30 percent of daily calories), they experience weight gain. However, there are exceptions, and paying close attention to this column in the food diary will help people determine how well their bodies metabolize fat. Some dieters may find that even if they restrict fats to 20 percent of calories, they still gain weight. For example, studies by Swinburn and Ravussin have shown that not all obese individuals have elevated fat intakes. In general, however, over a long period of time (17 to 20 weeks), a high-fat diet will substantially increase weight.

It should also be noted that saturated fats tend to increase blood cholesterol levels, as most foods high in saturated fat are often high in cholesterol as well. However, dietary fat should not be eliminated altogether. Not only is this nutrient essential for energy, but it plays a crucial role in the consumption of fat-soluble vitamins.

*Cholesterol.* Cholesterol is directly linked with many diseases, particularly coronary artery disease (see Chapter 17). According to the *Surgeon General's Report*, a 1 percent reduction in total blood cholesterol is accompanied by a 1.5 percent reduction in heart disease risk. National dietary guidelines currently recommend that Americans consume no more than 300 milligrams of cholesterol per day. People who suspect that they may be at risk of heart disease should further restrict their cholesterol intake to less than 200 milligrams daily.

*Carbohydrates.* The two principal types of carbohydrates are complex carbohydrates and simple sugars (found predominantly in fruit). Complex carbohydrates are present in such foods as grains (wheat, rice, corn, oats, and barley), legumes (peas and beans), vegetables, and some animal tissues. National dietary guidelines currently recommend that 60 to 70 percent of total daily caloric intake should consist of complex carbohydrates.

*Fiber.* Fiber foods are important because they provide cellulose, which helps in digesting food and preventing several disorders of the gastrointestinal tract. Nutritionists recommend that people consume 20 to 30 grams of fiber daily.

*Sugar.* Sugar is not considered to be harmful when consumed in the proper amounts. However, sugar flavors many manufactured food products, and Americans tend to consume it to excess. To quantify, the average American is estimated to take in almost a third of a pound of refined sugar each day in synthetic foods. Refined sugars, which are rich in calories and do not provide essential nutrients, also deplete other essential nutrients in the bloodstream and prevent nonsugar foods from being easily metabolized.

*Alcohol.* It is very important to monitor your daily intake of alcohol. Heavy drinkers tend to overconsume sugar-rich foods and underconsume nutrient-dense, nonsugar foods. Since alcohol contains the energy equivalent of seven calories per gram, a few beers or mixed drinks several evenings a week can also substantially increase weight and body fat. In addition, alcohol irritates and damages the digestive tract, interferes with the body's use of many nutrients, and depletes tissue stores of protein, B vitamins, and essential minerals.

*Meal or Snack.* Recording the number of meals and snacks consumed each day will help identify food patterns that may be counterproductive. For example, eating one large meal a day, which supplies the majority of caloric intake, increases the difficulty of losing weight. Instead nutritionists recommend eating smaller amounts of food more frequently. Many of the diets reviewed in this book stress the importance of eating three balanced meals and consuming small, nutritious snacks throughout the day. This pattern tends to stabilize blood sugar and blood fat levels. Eating a balanced breakfast is crucial to weight loss. Studies indicate that dieters who eat breakfast compared to those who do not have more healthful dietary patterns overall.

*Hunger Level.* Everyone becomes hungry during the day when the body signals that it needs nutrients to provide energy for its many physiological processes. Keep in mind that hunger is different than appetite. Appetite is defined as the brain's psychological perception that it needs food (often as a response to external cues), while hunger is the body's physiological demand for sustenance. Healthy people respond only to hunger.

To record your hunger level in the food diary, use a scale of 0 to 10 — 0 being empty, 5 being comfortable, and 10 being completely full. Note at what level of hunger you were when you ate a particular food. You may find that your brain sometimes tricks your appetite to convince you that you need food when, in fact, you may already be satiated.

Many overweight individuals find that their eating behavior is triggered by external stimuli that are unrelated to feelings of hunger or satiety. For example, some people eat at predetermined times each day, regardless of whether or not they are hungry. Mealtimes are often an important form of socializing, and family gatherings or taking a break from work can trigger appetite.

In addition, some people are "recreational" eaters, meaning that their principal forms of recreation — playing cards, for example — include eating food. Again, these people do not necessarily eat because they are hungry, but because it is part of the social ritual surrounding that form of recreation.

*Time of Day.* It is also essential to record the time of day you consume each food and beverage because foods are metabolized differently depending on when they are ingested. Foods consumed at breakfast, for example, are more quickly metabolized — that is, the calories are burned — because most people perform some physical activity (even if it is just going to work) immediately following breakfast. A large meal eaten just before going to bed, on the other hand, is not metabolized as quickly because sleeping involves very little physical exertion.

*Place.* Locale can also influence when and how much people eat. Studies have shown, for example, that certain rooms in a house are often subconsciously linked with eating. People who spend a lot of time in the kitchen tend to eat more — and often overeat. Many people eat more when they are close to a refrigerator, while others are more susceptible to overeating when they shop for food. Eating at the home of friends, at family gatherings, at parties and at restaurants also encourages people to indulge beyond their natural appetites, especially in foods rich in fats and sugars, including alcohol.

In addition, watching television tends to encourage people to eat, even after they have consumed a large meal and presumably are no longer hungry. Murray and Pizzorno state in the *Encyclopedia of Natural Medicine* that next to prior obesity, television watching is the strongest predictor of subsequent obesity. In fact, there is a dose effect; the more TV that is watched, the greater the degree of obesity.

In addition, one national study cited by Dr. David Nieman in *Fitness and Your Health* found that teenagers who watched more than five hours of television per day were twice as likely to be obese as teens who watched less than one hour a day. The researchers suggested that TV watching reduced the opportunity for exercise, and also prompted more snacking because of the food advertisements. In a study of adults, the 2-to-1 obesity ratio held when comparing those who watched television more than three hours and those who watched less than one hour per day.

*Mood.* Many people with weight problems are unaware of the emotional cues that can trigger overeating. Psychologists have observed, for example, that stress, anxiety, and feeling lonely, bored, or angry can prompt food cravings. Unfortunately, giving in to these cravings ultimately tends to make a person feel worse, because it can lead to weight gain and guilt, and may even contribute to wavering self-esteem.

Several studies by Goldman and Mitchel found that a .84 correlation exists between stress and overeating. That is, of 100 people who ate excessively, 84 did so in response to a stressful event in their lives. They also found that if these people discussed their stress-related problems with friends, family members, or a support group, they subsequently ate less because seeking support allowed them to process their personal problems so they did not attempt to cope by overeating.

Some people derive a kind of emotional comfort from ingesting food. This may be because, starting as infants when nursing, most people learn to associate eating with receiving love, affection, and comfort. This strong association may persist throughout life, as reinforced by the fact that our culture's major events revolve around food, while socializing and celebrating are synonymous with eating. As a result, overindulgence can become a generalized behavioral pattern for dealing with psychological distress.

In the "mood" column, write down the mood that best summarizes your emotional status each time you consumed food or beverages.

The food diary outlined in this chapter will help dieters and nondieters monitor their daily food intake. Two types of assessments are essential to the success of any diet: nutritional status (how much food one consumes) and physical fitness status (how fast and efficiently one's body metabolizes foods). The next chapter discusses physical fitness and provides a physical status worksheet.

# 3

Assessing Your Current
Physical Status

Although many people think that the key to losing weight or maintaining an ideal body weight rests on caloric intake (or the amount of calories coming into the body), an equally important determinant is caloric expenditure (or the number of calories going out). Put in simple terms, if energy intake (calories in food) is greater than energy expenditure (calories used in basic functions such as digestion, exercise, and physical labor), body fat will be gained. If the intake is less than the expenditure, body fat will be lost.

However, weight measurement alone cannot always accurately determine a person's body fat composition. This chapter uses a number of other reliable determinants, all of which can be listed on the easy-to-fill-out worksheet provided, to help readers assess their current physical status.

## BODY WEIGHT

According to Dr. David Nieman in *Fitness and Your Health*, the best method of measuring body weight is to use a balance beam scale with movable weights, while wearing minimal clothing and no shoes. If you do not have access to one, use an ordinary floor scale. He advises calculating your body weight immediately upon rising in the morning before you have eaten breakfast. When repeating body weight measurements, make sure to weigh yourself under exactly the same conditions and at the same time of day because the weight of an average adult can vary by as much as 4 to 5 pounds within any one day. Consistent measurements at regular intervals will help you assess how any diet you choose impacts your body weight.

## PHYSICAL STATUS WORKSHEET

Date _____

Age _____

Height _____

Weight _____

Frame size (circle one): small, medium, large

Waist-to-hip ratio (WHR) _____

Body mass index (BMI) _____

Ideal body weight _____

Pounds overweight _____

Basal metabolic rate (BMR) _____

Physical energy expenditure (PEE) _____

Digestive metabolism _____

Total daily caloric requirements _____

## BODY HEIGHT

Nieman suggests that when measuring your height, stand erect without shoes and with your back as straight as possible, heels together, with your heels, buttocks, shoulders, and head touching a wall. Evenly distribute your weight on both feet, hang your arms freely at your sides, and look straight ahead. Just before being measured, inhale deeply and hold your breath. Have someone calculate the highest point on your head. The ideal instrument for this purpose is a vertical ruler with a horizontal headboard called a stadiometer, which is available in both fixed and portable versions. An alternative is to affix a measuring ruler to the wall and use a right-angle measuring block (such as a clipboard) to measure straight back from the crown of the head.

## FRAME SIZE

Frame size is most commonly determined by measuring the width of the elbow. Other measures have been proposed, Nieman explains, including the diameter of the chest and wrist circumference, but national norms are not yet available for these measurements.

When measuring your elbow width, stand erect, extend your arm, and bend the forearm upward at a 90-degree angle. Keep your fingers straight up, palm facing your body. The widest bony width of the elbow should be

**Table 2**

| Height (in inches, no shoes) | Elbow Breadth (in inches) |
|---|---|
| Men | |
| 61–62 | 2 1/2–2 7/8 |
| 63–66 | 2 5/8–2 7/8 |
| 67–70 | 2 3/4–3 |
| 71–74 | 2 3/4–3 1/8 |
| 75 | 2 7/8–3 1/4 |
| Women | |
| 57–58 | 2 1/4–2 1/2 |
| 59–62 | 2 1/4–2 1/2 |
| 63–66 | 2 3/8–2 5/8 |
| 67–70 | 2 3/8–2 5/8 |
| 71 | 2 1/2–2 3/4 |

measured, ideally with a sliding caliper, with pressure firm enough to compress soft tissue over the bone.

The following standards (from Metropolitan Life Insurance Company) represent elbow measurements for medium-framed men and women of various heights. Measurements smaller than those listed indicate that you have a small frame; larger measurements indicate a large frame.

## BODY COMPOSITION

Whether your weight is "healthy" depends on your body composition — how much of your weight is fat, where the fat is located, and whether you have weight-related medical problems (such as high blood pressure) or a family history of such problems.

Although no precise ways to determine healthy weight have yet been developed, the U.S. Department of Agriculture established a table of suggested weights for adults in 1990, which is considered by many experts as the best one currently available. The higher weights in the ranges shown below generally apply to men, who tend to have more muscle and bone; the lower weights more often apply to women, who have less muscle and bone.

## WAIST-TO-HIP RATIO (WHR)

According to the USDA, "Body shape as well as weight is important to health. Excess fat in the abdomen is believed to be of greater health risk

### Table 3. Suggested Weights for Adults[1]

| Height[2] | Weight in Pounds[3] | |
| --- | --- | --- |
| | 19 to 34 years | 35 years and over |
| 5'0" | 97–128 | 108–138 |
| 5'1" | 101–132 | 111–143 |
| 5'2" | 104–137 | 115–148 |
| 5'3" | 107–141 | 119–152 |
| 5'4" | 111–146 | 122–157 |
| 5'5" | 114–150 | 126–162 |
| 5'6" | 118–155 | 130–167 |
| 5'7" | 121–160 | 134–172 |
| 5'8" | 125–164 | 138–178 |
| 5'9" | 129–169 | 142–183 |
| 5'10" | 132–174 | 146–188 |
| 5'11" | 136–179 | 151–194 |
| 6'0" | 140–184 | 155–199 |
| 6'1" | 144–189 | 159–205 |
| 6'2" | 148–195 | 164–210 |
| 6'3" | 152–200 | 168–216 |
| 6'4" | 156–205 | 173–222 |
| 6'5" | 160–211 | 177–228 |
| 6'6" | 164–216 | 182–234 |

1. Source: "Nutrition and Your Health: Dietary Guidelines for Americans." In *Home and Garden Bulletin* 232 (Washington, D.C.: U.S. Department of Agriculture, November 1990).
2. Without shoes.
3. Without clothes.

than that in the hips and thighs." Many of the health problems of obesity, including hypertension, high serum cholesterol levels, cardiovascular disease, and diabetes have been associated with excess fat in the abdominal area.

Nieman suggests that a reliable method of determining whether you have too much fat in the abdominal area is to calculate your waist-to-hip ratio. To do this:

1. Measure around your waist near your navel while you stand relaxed, without pulling in your stomach.
2. Measure around your hips, over the buttocks, where they are largest.
3. Divide the waist measurement by the hips measurement to determine your waist-to-hip ratio (WHR).

According to Nieman, a man's risk of disease increases steeply when his WHR rises above 0.9. A woman's risk increases when her WHR rises above 0.8.

## BODY MASS INDEX

Body mass index (BMI) is another reliable indicator of whether a person is underweight, at an ideal weight, or overweight, and is more precise than weight tables. A variety of procedures both simple and complex are used to measure body fat, including the tape measure test, skinfold calipers, bio-electrical impedance, and hydrostatic, or underwater, weighing.

An easy way to calculate approximate BMI is by recording your height and weight and marking them on Table 4, Nomogram for body mass index (BMI), which appears on page 43. Then use a straight edge such as a ruler to connect the two points, circle the spot where this straight line crosses the center line (BMI), and enter the number on your physical status worksheet.

Physiologist Dr. David Parker has developed a useful table, which appears on page 44 as Table 5, for determining the maximum amount of body fat a healthy adult should have. Parker notes that athletes, or anyone who exercises aerobically three or four times a week, should be 2 or 3 percent less than the ideal in the table.

Dr. George L. Blackburn of Harvard Medical School, one of the nation's leading nutrition experts, notes in a September 1993 issue of the *Annals of Internal Medicine* that "healthy weights are generally associated with a body mass index (BMI) of 19 to 25 in those 19 to 34 years of age, and 21 to 27 in those 35 years of age and older. Beyond these ranges, health risks increase as BMI increases."

## DETERMINING IDEAL BODY WEIGHT

Once body fat has been calculated, you can determine your ideal weight. To illustrate the formula, the example of a 50-year-old man who weighs 175 pounds is used.

1. Using a scale, the man determines that his present weight is 175 pounds.
2. Using one of the available tests, such as the Nomogram for body mass index, he identifies his body fat percentage as 25 percent.

## Table 4. Nomogram for Body Mass Index

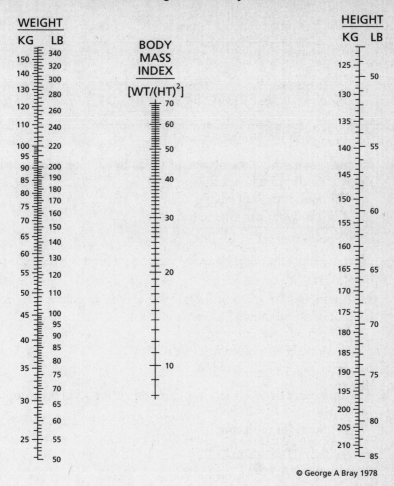

© George A Bray 1978

**Table 5. Ideal Body Fat Percentage\***

| Age | Males | Females |
|---|---|---|
| 16–19 | 15% | 19% |
| 20–29 | 16 | 20 |
| 30–39 | 17 | 21 |
| 40–49 | 18 | 22 |
| 50–59 | 19 | 23 |
| 60 and over | 20 | 24 |

\*Source: David C. Niemen, *Fitness and Your Health* (Palo Alto, CA: Bull Publishing, 1993).

3. By multiplying his present weight (175) by .25, he calculates how many pounds of fat he is carrying.

   175 pounds present weight
   × .25 body fat percentage (actual)
   
   44 pounds of fat

4. Next, he finds the ideal body fat percentage for a 50-year-old male is 19 percent.

5. He multiplies his present weight by .19 to calculate how many pounds of fat he should be carrying.

   175 pounds present weight
   × .19 body fat percentage (ideal)
   
   33 pounds of fat

6. The difference between actual and ideal pounds of fat is the amount he is "overfat."

   44 pounds of fat (actual)
   − 33 pounds of fat (ideal)
   
   11 pounds overfat

7. Subtracting the pounds of excess fat (11) from his present weight, he determines his ideal weight.

   175 pounds present weight
   − 11 pounds overfat
   
   164 pounds ideal weight

## MEASURING CALORIC NEED

Caloric intake has a great deal to do with attaining an ideal body weight. This is because body weight is not only a result of how much you eat, but how effectively your body metabolizes nutrients which are burned as calories while resting, exercising, and digesting foods.

The three measurements used to assess the total caloric requirements of the body are basal metabolic rate, physical energy expenditure, and digestive metabolism.

## Basal Metabolic Rate

Basal metabolism, or the basal metabolic rate (BMR), reflects the number of calories needed when the body is at rest. Even in this state, the lungs, heart, brain, and other vital organs are at work and require energy in the form of calories to maintain normal body functions such as respiration and circulation. Other terms used for this expenditure of energy include resting metabolic rate (RMR) and resting energy expenditure (REE).

The BMR varies as much as 30 percent among people of the same age, sex, and body weight. Much of this variance, according to Nieman, is due to body composition differences, with people having the highest amount of muscle and bone and the lowest amount of fat having the higher BMR. As people get older, their BMR drops, primarily because they lose muscle and bone mass from not exercising as much. Also, obese people have daily BMRs approximately 500 calories higher than nonobese people, because they have more muscle and bone to carry the extra weight.

According to the Food and Nutrition Board, the average adult male requires between 1,440 and 1,728 calories daily to meet the needs of his basal metabolism. For an average female, the range is 1,296 to 1,584 calories a day.

### Table 6. Conversion of Pounds to Kilograms

| Pounds | = | Kilograms | Pounds | = | Kilograms |
|--------|---|-----------|--------|---|-----------|
| 100 | | 45 | 155 | | 70 |
| 105 | | 48 | 160 | | 73 |
| 110 | | 50 | 165 | | 75 |
| 115 | | 52 | 170 | | 77 |
| 120 | | 54 | 175 | | 80 |
| 125 | | 56 | 180 | | 82 |
| 130 | | 59 | 185 | | 84 |
| 135 | | 61 | 190 | | 86 |
| 140 | | 64 | 195 | | 89 |
| 145 | | 66 | 200 | | 91 |
| 150 | | 68 | 205 | | 93 |

Because BMR is calculated as a function of kilogram weight, to estimate the calories you need, first convert your current body weight into kilograms by dividing the number of pounds you weigh by 2.2. For example, a man weighing 175 pounds weighs 80 kilograms.

The BMR factors used in the following examples are 1.0 for men and .9 for women.

| Man | | Woman |
|---|---|---|
| 80 | Weight in kilograms | 70 |
| × 1.0 | × BMR factor | × .9 |
| = 80 | = Calories needed per hour | = 63 |
| × 24 | × Hours in 1 day | × 24 |
| = 1,920 | = Calories needed per day for BMR | = 1,512 |

To calculate your own BMR, use the same formula:

| Men | | Women |
|---|---|---|
| ____ | Your weight in kilograms | ____ |
| × 1.0 | × BMR factor | × .9 |
| = ____ | = Calories needed per hour | = ____ |
| × 24 | × Hours in 1 day | × 24 |
| = ____ | = Calories needed per day for BMR | = ____ |

## Physical Energy Expenditure

Because people do more than simply stay at rest during waking hours, their bodies require additional calories for physical activities — and the more active they are, the more calories they need to consume.

Physical energy expenditure (PEE) has the greatest impact of any other variable on total caloric requirements. Whereas the average sedentary person usually expends only 300 to 800 calories a day in physical activity, athletes in training or workers engaged in heavy manual labor may expend as many as 3,000 calories.

Physical energy expenditure needs are estimated as a factor of basal metabolism below, while degrees of physical activity are expressed as percentages of the basal metabolic requirement.

| Physical Activity Level | Factor |
|---|---|
| Sedentary most of the time | 15 percent |
| Sedentary job; regular exercise | 20 percent |

| | |
|---|---|
| Physically active job; no regular exercise | 20 percent |
| Physically active job; regular exercise | 25 percent |

If a man has a sedentary job, for example, but exercises on a regular basis, his physical activity factor is 20 percent. A woman who has a physically active job and also exercises has a PEE factor of 25 percent.

*Physical Energy Expenditure Formula.* Using the same couple as above as examples, the formula for PEE is easily illustrated:

| Man | | Woman |
|---|---|---|
| 1,680 | BMR calories needed | 1,512 |
| × .20 | × Activity level | × .25 |
| 336 | = Daily calories needed for PEE | 378 |

Note that even though the woman's BMR requires fewer calories than does the man's, she has a greater need for additional calories because of her higher rate of physical activity.

To determine the calories you need for physical activity, use the following calculation:

| Men | | Women |
|---|---|---|
| _____ | My BMR calories needed | _____ |
| × _____ | × My activity level (from chart) | × _____ |
| = _____ | Daily calories needed for my PEE | = _____ |

## Digestive Metabolism

The third area to be measured is the number of calories required for the body to perform its essential digestive functions. This need, called digestive metabolism, is a factor of total BMR and PEE calories. A multiplier of 10 percent is used for both men and women. The woman in this example would calculate her digestive calories as follows:

| | |
|---|---|
| BMR calories | 1,512 |
| Physical energy expenditure (PEE) calories | + 378 |
| Subtotal | 1,890 |
| Digestion factor | × .10 |
| Daily calories needed for digestive functions | 189 |

Thus the woman needs 189 additional calories each day in order to give her body sufficient energy to digest foods and nutrients.

To calculate your digestive metabolism:

| | |
|---|---|
| My BMR calories | _____ |
| My physical energy expenditure calories | + _____ |
| Subtotal | |
| Digestion factor | × .10 |
| Daily calories needed for my digestive functions | _____ |

## TOTAL METABOLIC NEEDS

Totaling the caloric requirements of each area (BMR, PEE, and digestion) to a single number represents the daily calories needed to maintain a certain weight. To determine the calories necessary to meet your total current metabolic need, use the following formula:

| | |
|---|---|
| My BMR requirements | _____ |
| My PEE requirements | + _____ |
| My digestive requirements | + _____ |
| Daily caloric requirements | = _____ |

Use this same procedure to calculate the total daily calories required to maintain your ideal weight.

This chapter has described how people can easily determine their current body weight, frame size, waist-to-hip ratio, body mass index, body fat, ideal body weight, basal metabolic rate, physical energy expenditure, digestive metabolism, and total daily caloric requirements, all of which can be listed on the physical status worksheet provided. Used in conjunction with the self-administered nutritional assessment detailed in Chapter 3, readers are now in a position to determine their dietary goals in terms of such criteria as total weight loss, balancing insulin levels, preserving lean body mass, or preventing a medical problem for which they are genetically predisposed, as covered in the next chapter, Defining Your Diet Goals.

# 4

---

# Defining Your Diet Goals

**M**any diet books boldly promise that one eating plan is appropriate for all people and they typically guarantee identical results to everyone regardless of lifestyle, medical status, or need. In effect, such books suggest that people in quest of nutritional well-being and slimmer bodies all eat, think, and react to all foods alike. They fail to consider the fact that diets can only succeed if they accommodate an individual's personal nutritional and physical fitness status.

For example, to use a medical analogy, two people might suffer from the same disorder and be given different prescriptions because their bodies react differently to the same chemicals. Diets are also prescriptions — precise combinations of chemical nutrients — and ideally should be individualized as are prescription medications. This is especially true for weight loss because as Chapters 5 through 9 explain, people vary substantially in *where* and *how fast* they gain or lose weight. Each dieter also has distinct eating habits, lifestyles, and attitudes toward food that also influence the kind of diet that suits them best.

This book suggests that no single eating plan or diet can serve everyone's needs. Because every person's body is unique, each person ought to choose personal diet goals which accommodate their nutritional (Chapter 2) and physical fitness (Chapter 3) status. Diets which do not take into account the unique biochemistry of your body as well as your personal medical condition and lifestyle will deliver only short-term results.

This chapter presents a brief survey of possible "diet goals" as well as "target diets" which are analyzed in considerable detail in later chapters. We have used the excellent four-step model developed by Dr. George Blackburn which appears in *Weighing the Options: Criteria for Evaluating Weight-Management Programs.*

- Step 1: Individuals analyze their nutritional (Chapter 2) and physical fitness status (Chapter 3), and with their physician identify their risk factors for developing chronic disease.
- Step 2: Individuals adopt nutritional and lifestyle programs recommended by diets reviewed in this book which reduce or eliminate the risk of developing morbid diseases. In some cases this will require screening by the patient's primary care physician.
- Step 3: If a person's condition does not respond to diet therapy, he should be referred to his primary care physician for further monitoring and supervision.
- Step 4: Intensive therapies such as extremely restrictive diet, medication, surgery (if necessary), and psychotherapy may be necessary and appropriate.

## DIET GOAL 1: WEIGHT GAIN

Gaining weight might seem an odd diet goal, yet many Americans are severely underweight or malnourished, and do not consume daily amounts of essential nutrients. These persons are often poor, but also include people with addictions and eating disorders such as anorexia nervosa (AN) and bulimia nervosa (BN).

Individuals with anorexia nervosa are usually young females of normal or slightly above normal weight who start on an "innocent" diet and eventually begin suppressing hunger sensations to the point of self-starvation. They may subsist on as few as 250 calories a day. The physiological symptoms can include semistarvation, a notably lowered basal metabolic rate, and reduced gonadotropin production, which results in cessation of menses in some females. Specific dietary inadequacies can eventually lead to nutritional deficiencies and osteoporosis.

The causes of anorexia nervosa are primarily psychological, although some people with the disorder may have a genetic predisposition that can be triggered by psychological factors. The reason psychological factors are suspected is because the vast majority of anorexics are white North American women between the ages of 13 and 22. Many of these women are starting to menstruate or have just graduated from high school. The widespread pressure on these women to diet and stay thin just as they enter society may contribute to anorexia.

Treatment for anorexia typically involves reducing the patient's fears of a normal body weight by encouraging them to gradually regain their natural body weight. Group support and medication play an important role in subsequently reducing their anxiety about eating. Some nutrient supplements and nasogastric or intravenous feeding also have proven successful. Nutritional supplements alone are usually insufficient, however, because the underlying psychological causes must be treated as well.

Diets for anorexics should reflect nutrient needs and identify energy allowances that take into account the degree of starvation. For these patients, relatively small, gradual increases are usually made in caloric level of the diet during treatment. It is very important, however, that meal plans always consider individual needs.

### Target Diet 1: Weight Gain for Anorexics

1. Restore satisfactory nutritional state, preferably through the patient's own efforts.
2. Restore adequate weight and normal eating patterns.
3. If necessary, patients should be given intravenous feedings to restore fluids and electrolytes.
4. Oral intake should be supported by peripheral parenteral nutrition if the patient's nutritional status is precarious.
5. Patients should immediately set goal weights, individualized on their understanding of their growth patterns and growth need.
6. Care must be taken not to reinforce compulsive rituals and preoccupation with food that often cause anorexia in the first place.

An increasing number of young Americans, particularly females, consume large amounts of food and then vomit. This disorder is called bulimia nervosa. Bulimia usually begins in conjunction with a diet and, once the binge-purge cycle begins, victims cannot stop themselves from either eating excessive amounts or vomiting. The average meal for a normal nonbulimic person contains approximately 1,000 calories. People with bulimia may eat from 5,000 to as many as 50,000 calories in one extended meal and then vomit once the binge is over. Some bulimics may be underweight and a few may be obese, but most tend to maintain a fairly normal weight. In some bulimic women, the menstrual cycle becomes irregular and the rate of sexual intercourse usually declines.

There are two potentially fatal aspects of bulimia. If people dramatically increase their body weight in a short amount of time, they may develop heart problems and high blood pressure. In addition, vomiting for extended periods of time can cause chloride and potassium deficiencies which often lead to heart arrhythmias and heart damage. Usually most bulimics have very low self-esteem and are often depressed.

Some bulimic patients have been successfully treated with behavioral modification programs. Patients with severe cases, however, sometimes require intensive treatment, either in a hospital or an inpatient unit. Medication may also be useful in certain circumstances, including antidepressants, but there is to date no antibulimia drug per se.

The holistic approach to bulimia recognizes that while genetic and physiological factors may contribute to the disorder, any successful elimination of the problem must involve rebuilding the patient's self-esteem. Small doses of natural or synthetic serotonin have proven helpful in preventing bulimics from binge eating. Hopefully, further study will lead to more successful treatments.

Other psychological approaches may also prove effective. For example, bulimic patients often mistakenly think that vomiting helps them lose weight quickly. In fact, however, vomiting does not immediately cause weight loss because calories are retained in the gastrointestinal tract even after vomiting. Bulimic patients in several studies have been shown to eat slower than control groups, and also take significantly longer to start eating. If bulimic patients are placed in support groups which stress exercise and intervene before they initiate binge eating, it may be possible to eventually cure their disorder.

According to an article by Lucas and Huse, "Behavioral Disorders Affecting Food Intake: Anorexia Nervosa and Bulimia Nervosa" in *Modern Nutrition in Health and Disease,* underweight patients with anorexia and bulimia usually do not need to consume above-average quantities of food. The initial use of small quantities meets the psychological needs of the patient, who is fearful of gaining weight rapidly and of becoming fat. Eating large quantities and high caloric snacks can actually be countertherapeutic. Treatment usually involves several phases, which include obtaining a detailed diet history; determining the calorie content of the initial diet; designing an appropriate diet plan; planning gradual progression in the diet; considering weight gain expectations; and designing a diet plan for weight maintenance.

**Target Diet 1: Weight Gain for Bulimics**
1. Determine actual caloric expenditure by measuring oxygen consumption.

2. Patient should be counseled by a physician about a diet that provides an appropriate nutrient composition and caloric content.

3. The initial and prerogative diets should be designed to include foods from each of the basic food groups, with portions being increased as caloric increase is made. Food should provide all vitamins and mineral needs and supplements are not usually necessary.

4. A varied diet should be emphasized which reflects the patient's likes and dislikes.

5. Weighing foods helps ensure that adequate portions are being consumed and gives bulimics greater confidence that overeating will not occur.

6. Individualized meal plans should ensure that a wide variety of foods are included in three meals and snacks.

7. The bulk content of meals should not be excessive in the initial stages because of the filling and discomfort that is often experienced.

8. Gradually increase weekly intake by 200 calories during the early stages of the diet, with greater increases when the patient becomes more comfortable with eating.

In general, both anorexics and bulimics must avoid fasting, skipping meals, and eating inadequate amounts at meals, as they often contribute to recurrence of binges. Keeping food records is also extremely helpful and should include a notation of the times of the binges, the kinds of foods eaten, and the occurrence of vomiting and laxative and/or diuretic abuse.

## DIET GOAL 2: WEIGHT MAINTENANCE

Dieters whose goals include gaining or losing weight to a prescribed level must then maintain their weight at the prescribed level, usually identified as their ideal body weight (IBW). As discussed in Chapter 3, maintaining an IBW is achieved by matching the number of calories consumed with the number burned in physical exertion. Weight maintenance diets are usually designed when IBW has been attained. The caloric level of this diet is best determined by the basal calories for the person's height, age, sex, and goal weight, with the addition of an appropriate increment of physical activity. Ideally a goal weight that is physiologically appropriate should be set, using previous growth history as a guide. Weight maintenance dieters follow a diet composed of essential lowfat nutrient-dense foods consistent with energy expenditure.

### Target Diet 2: Maintaining Current Weight

1. Limit consumption of foods relatively high in calories, fats, and sugars and minimize alcohol consumption.
2. Increase energy expenditure through regular and sustained physical activity.

## DIET GOAL 3: WEIGHT LOSS: 1 POUND/WEEK

The majority of people who go on a weight-loss diet do so for cosmetic reasons. A weight-loss plan that has proved successful for many people is to reduce the number of calories ingested each day and increase the number of calories expended each day, for a net deficit of 500 calories per day. This program will produce a loss of one pound a week.

The energy equivalent of one pound of body fat is 3,500 calories. To lose one pound a month, it is necessary to adopt a diet and physical activity plan which produces a net daily deficit of 120 calories. By walking three times a week or restricting sugar-rich foods such as soft drinks and desserts, most people can easily eliminate 300 calories a week. Nevertheless, to achieve permanent weight loss and energy balance at a desired weight, they must change long-term eating behaviors and levels of physical activity. Successful weight loss and permanent weight control always require substantial lifestyle changes.

### Target Diet 3: Weight Loss: 500 Calories/Week

1. Eat less fat and fatty foods, especially unsaturated fat.
2. Eat less sugar and sweets.
3. Limit alcohol to one drink per day.
4. Eat a lowfat breakfast with whole-grain cereals.
5. Eat smaller portions, avoid seconds, and limit snacking and heavy meals.
6. Increase physical activity.

## DIET GOAL 4: WEIGHT LOSS: 30 PERCENT OF BODY WEIGHT

People who are more than 30 percent over their IBW are usually defined as "obese." Obesity, however, is not a single disorder, but rather a heterogeneous group of disorders that are associated with varying types and degrees of risk for morbidity and mortality. Obesity, for example, increases the risk for high blood pressure, stroke, and high blood cholesterol levels associated with coronary heart disease (Chapter 17). Safe weight-loss diets have been shown to reduce high blood pressure and high blood cholesterol.

Although evidence suggests a genetic component to the tendency of many people to become overweight, caloric intake and energy expenditure play a key role. Sustained and long-term efforts to reduce body weight can best be achieved as a result of improving energy balance by reducing energy consumption and raising energy expenditure through physical activity and exercise.

### Target Diet 4: Low Calorie Diet (LCD)
1. Restrict caloric intake to 1,200 calories/day.
2. Take dietary supplements if necessary.
3. Restrict fats to 7 to 10 percent and increase fiber to decrease hunger.
4. Increase carbohydrate intake to more than 55 percent of total calories primarily by increasing complex carbohydrates (vegetables, fruits, grain, and legumes).
5. Completely restrict alcohol, sugar, and high fat foods.
6. Establish a three-meal per day pattern and gradually increase physical activity.

## DIET GOAL 5: WEIGHT LOSS: 100 PERCENT OF BODY WEIGHT

Morbidly obese people are defined as being 100 pounds or 100 percent above their "desirable weight." People with long-standing (more than three years) morbid obesity complicated by medical problems may require surgery. According to *Weighing the Options,* however, diet can effectively treat most cases of morbid obesity if used in conjunction with exercise and other conjunctive therapies.

### Target Diet 5: Very Low Calorie Diet (VLCD). (See Chapter 5)
1. Dieters consume 800 calories or less per day.
2. This diet should only be used to ameliorate other life-threatening conditions and should be administered under the supervision of a physician.

## DIET GOAL 6: WEIGHT LOSS: INACTIVE THYROID

An inefficient thyroid gland (hypothyroidism) can be the cause of sluggish metabolic rates, and correcting this problem can often lead to weight loss. Some chronically overweight persons with underactive thyroid glands benefit from a combined therapy of thyroid medication and diets which raise their basal metabolism. They should be tested for thyroxine and take supplements that help raise their metabolic rate. Excessive or unnecessary thyroid medication for any length of time, however, can result in rapid or irregular heartbeats, nervousness, insomnia, muscle weakness, bone loss, and loss of lean body mass.

### Target Diet 6: Weight Loss by Correcting Thyroid Imbalances

1. If possible, correct the thyroid imbalance with moderate doses of iodine or the amino acid tyrosine, a raw material for thyroid hormone, along with B vitamins, zinc, and copper.
2. Thyroid extracts may necessary in some cases.
3. Temporary medications should be monitored by a physician and can restore thyroid functioning.

## DIET GOAL 7: WEIGHT LOSS: STABILIZING INSULIN LEVELS

Many cases of obesity are due to an imbalance of the hormone insulin. Factors such as genetic predisposition, food allergies, eating habits, and stress may interfere with glucose and carbohydrate utilization, resulting in a condition known as glucose intolerance. Excessive sugar consumption (refined carbohydrates) may also contribute to glucose intolerance and obesity.

High insulin levels are often observed in overweight and obese persons. Apparently the insulin receptors on their body cells are blocked from doing their function. This prevents insulin from stimulating the transfer of glucose to the cells to give them energy, which explains why so many overweight people feel tired so often. To make matters worse, since the insulin is not converting the glucose to energy, more glucose is then stored in fat cells.

Excess insulin in overweight people can lead to other problems, including increased fat and water retention; sleep disorders caused by insulin interference with neurotransmitters; the production of more LDL (bad cholesterol) by the liver due to insulin stimulation; interference with the thyroid hormone thyroxin, thereby aggravating low metabolism; decreased cell wall permeability, which can cause an increase in cell size; and hypoglycemia, hunger, and a further craving for simple carbohydrates.

Dr. Michelle Pouliot of Torrington, Connecticut, believes that insulin imbalances occur frequently in women who have 20 or fewer pounds to lose. Many women in this range, she suggests, have a history of yo-yo dieting and their bodies are very resistant to weight loss. With these women she attempts to decrease fat intake to 30 grams daily and to increase exercise. For some women that is enough to get them losing weight and for others, not at all. Dr. Pouliot stabilizes her patients with various herbs and nutrients including ephedra and yohimbe, which encourage the burning of fat. She also puts her women dieters on plans designed to rebalance their insulin levels and that limit their meals to three a day, although carbohydrates are unlimited. Two meals cannot contain more than four grams of carbohydrates each. She also encourages her dieters to exercise every other day.

### Target Diet 7: Stabilizing Insulin Levels

1. Reduce body fat by curbing fat intake but not by undereating, which will only arouse your body's defenses.
2. Allow for moderate, not drastically restricted, amounts of foods.
3. Avoid eating large amounts of food in one sitting; binging stimulates alpha fat cells to multiply.
4. Eat three regular meals or more frequent smaller ones throughout the day.
5. Use diet menus. Consume recommended sizes and portions until this way of eating becomes second nature.
6. Combine smart dieting, group support, and a vigorous exercise that works the heart and lungs and the large muscle groups. Exercise preserves and increases muscle tissue, stimulates body-trimming beta and brown fat cells, and increases the basal metabolic rate.

## DIET GOAL 8: WOMEN'S SPECIALTY DIETS

The hormonal processes women undergo during menstruation deplete them of essential nutrients such as calcium, zinc, and iron. Women also have slower basal metabolic rates, as well as a greater number of fat cells and less muscle mass. Chapter 10 presents three specialty diets for women based on these considerations.

### Target Diet 8: Gittleman's Diet for Women

1. Consume 30 to 40 percent of daily calories as carbohydrate (50–55 percent if heavy exerciser).
2. Consume 30 percent of daily calories as fat; consume 1 to 2 tablespoons of purified, unrefined, expeller-pressed raw or virgin oils

daily to help prevent cardiovascular disorders, binge eating, to normalize appetite, and to stabilize weight.

3. Consume 25 to 35 grams daily of fat-soluble fibers from oats, legumes, sweet potatoes, and fresh fruits and a wide range of vegetables, fruits, protein, nonfat milk, and complex carbohydrates.

4. Include lean meats, eggs, and calcium-rich foods such as green leafy vegetables.

5. Increase essential and healthy oils, food sources such as dark deep-sea fish and oils such as safflower, sesame, olive, or canola.

**Target Diet 8: Somer's Diet for Women**

1. Consume 50 to 55 percent of daily calories as complex carbohydrates such as whole-grain breads and cereals, potatoes, and legumes each day.

2. Limit consumption of protein to 10 percent of daily calories; restrict consumption of extra-lean meat, poultry, and seafood to no more than six ounces a day or two three-ounce servings.

3. Consume at least three to four calcium-rich foods daily, including nonfat milk or yogurt, lowfat cheeses, dark green leafy vegetables, tofu, or canned salmon with the bones.

4. When daily calorie intake drops below 2,000, take a moderate-dose vitamin/mineral supplement that provides 100 to 300 percent of the U.S. RDA for vitamins A (preferably beta-carotene), E, C, B1, B2, niacin, B6, B12, folic acid, pantothenic acid and biotin, calcium, copper, iron, magnesium, zinc, chromium, manganese, and selenium.

## DIET GOAL 9: PROVIDE OPTIMUM NUTRITION FOR CHILDREN

Several national studies show that American children consume substantially less than the recommended daily amounts of vitamin A, B12, folate and C, iron, zinc, and calcium. This problem is compounded by the fact that 60 to 80 percent of American schoolchildren are now estimated to exceed the RDAs for daily protein, total fat, saturated fat, cholesterol, and sodium. As a result, an increasing number of American children are overweight or obese.

Nevertheless, nutritional experts have not reached consensus on one diet which is beneficial for all children of different ages. Chapter 11 provides two different diet protocols, summarized below.

**Target Diet 9: Children's Nutrition Research Center's Diet (Chapter 11)**
1. Eat a variety of foods which provide the more than 40 essential nutrients required for growth and health maintenance.
2. Consume 55 percent of daily calories as carbohydrate, 10 to 15 percent as protein.
3. Maintain a healthy weight.
4. Choose a diet low in fat, saturated fat, and cholesterol.
5. Consume at least 1,200 milligrams of calcium daily.
6. Use sugars, salt, and sodium in moderation.
7. Do not drink alcoholic beverages.
8. Consume 10 grams of fiber every day.

**Target Diet 9: Feed Your Kids Bright Diet (Chapter 11)**
1. Consume foods daily from 11 food groups: fish, meats, dairy products, grains, legumes, nuts and seeds, vegetables, fats, sweets, herbs, condiments, and flavorings.
2. Children ages 3 to 5 need to consume higher amounts of fats and cholesterol than currently recommended in the RDAs.
3. Children should consume as much as 30 percent of calories daily in complete proteins.
4. Children should consume less than the currently recommended level of 55 percent carbohydrate because this can cause protein deprivation, fat deprivation, and vitamin and mineral deficiencies.

## DIET GOAL 10: MAXIMUM NUTRITION FOR THE ELDERLY

Elderly persons must be especially conscientious about what they eat if they wish to forestall the symptoms of aging. With advancing years, it becomes more and more difficult for even the most conscientious to consume and digest nutrient-dense foods. Social isolation, limited resources, lack of education regarding nutrition, lack of family support, loss of significant others or care givers, and the decreased mobility that results from sociophysical disabilities or from social isolation can all lessen the availability of nutritious foods.

In many cases elderly persons require more calories to maintain their body cell mass. If they have inadvertently decreased their caloric intake, it often takes them longer to subsequently restore body cell mass. Sometimes it also takes more time to regain body fat mass.

**Target Diet 10: Walford Anti-Aging Diet (Chapter 12):**
1. To reduce the risk of coronary heart disease, arteriosclerosis, hypertension, cancer, and osteoporosis diverticulosis, consume 1,500 to 2,000 calories per day. They should come mostly from nutrient-dense foods.
2. Consume 75 to 80 percent of daily calories as complex carbohydrates; consume 40 to 60 grams of fiber daily; consume 65 to 70 protein grams per day.
3. Consume the RDA of all essential nutrients and increased amounts of vitamins A (25,000 IUs), E (300 IUs), C (500 milligrams), selenium (100 micrograms), magnesium (1 gram), and Coenzyme Q12 (20 milligrams).
4. Consume generous amounts of natural fiber and fluid intake (64 ounces per day).

**Target Diet 10: Somer and Feltin's Diet for the Elderly**
1. Consume a minimum of 1,800 calories daily.
2. Consume 55 percent of calories as complex carbohydrates; 30 percent fat; 12 to 15 percent protein.
3. Consume optimal amounts of essential vitamins and minerals in excess of RDAs as necessary.

## DIET GOAL 11: BALANCED VEGETARIAN REGIMEN

Meat eaters have a higher risk of developing heart disease, diabetes, colon cancer, and hypertension. To reduce the risk of developing these disorders as well as obesity, diabetes, and diverticulosis, some readers may wish to adopt a vegetarian diet containing more fiber, vitamins, and minerals and less fat and cholesterol than meat diets.

There are many reasons to adopt a more plant-based diet. First, important antioxidant nutrients including vitamins C, E, beta-carotene, and many cancer-fighting substances are found in fruits, vegetables, and grains. These antioxidant nutrients are considered the best protection against age- and environmental-related diseases, from dandruff and bad breath to cataracts and cancer. The high fiber content of plant foods helps keep the digestive tract clean by absorbing and eliminating many potentially dangerous toxins. Plant foods also tend to have a lower toxicity than animal foods to begin with, because they are lower on the food chain, and as such have had less exposure to accumulating toxins.

**Target Diet 11: Kushi and Null's Macrobiotic Diet (Chapter 13)**

1. Consume 50 to 60 percent whole-grain cereals, 20 to 25 percent fresh vegetables, 5 to 10 percent beans and bean products, and 5 to 10 percent soups.
2. Occasional supplemental foods include fish and seafood (less fatty varieties), seasonal fruits (cooked, dried, and fresh), nuts and seeds, natural nonaromatic and nonstimulant beverages, and natural processed seasonings and condiments.
3. Minimize consumption of refined carbohydrates and unrefined fats.
4. Consume the RDAs for all essential vitamins and minerals in fresh, whole foods.
5. Eat a wide variety of foods and rotate foods (especially breakfast oats and brans) periodically.

**Target Diet 11: Mayo Clinic Vegetarian Diet (Chapter 13)**

1. Consume nutrient-dense combinations of foods that provide complete proteins.
2. Maintain caloric intake sufficient to meet energy needs.
3. Consume two of the following essential four food groups in every meal:

   *Group A:* Whole grains and cereals: wheat, rye, barley, corn, millet, oats, rice, buckwheat, triticale, and bulgur.

   *Group B:* Legumes: peanuts, peas, mung beans, broad beans, black-eyed peas, lentils, lima beans, soybeans, black beans, kidney beans, garbanzos, chick peas, and navy beans.

   *Group C:* Nuts and seeds: cashews, pistachios, walnuts, brazil nuts, almonds, pecans, pumpkin seeds, squash seeds, sunflower seeds, sesame seeds, filberts, and pine nuts.

   *Group D:* Vegetables: potatoes, dark green vegetables, other vegetables.

## DIET GOAL 12: INCREASE ATHLETIC PERFORMANCE

Many athletes do not eat correctly, and their diets are often low in vitamin C, B1, B6, calcium, iron, magnesium, and zinc. A high-carbohydrate ("carbo loading") diet is recommended for high-intensity, high-endurance events.

**Target Diet 12: Burke and Nieman's High-Carbohydrate Athletic Performance Diet (Chapter 14)**

1. Eat a variety of foods.
2. Consume 50 to 60 percent of total calories as complex carbohydrates; higher levels should be set for endurance athletes and those undertaking lengthy daily training sessions.
3. Total dietary fat intake should represent less than 30 percent of total calories, with saturated fat contributing less than 10 percent. Cholesterol intake should be below 300 milligrams a day.
4. Use sugars, salt, and sodium in moderation.
5. Regularly restore both fluid and electrolyte levels with a sports drink after strenuous exercise or a little salt at the next meal. Avoid salt tablets.
6. Maintain day-to-day fluid balance during training and replace any fluid losses.
7. Limit alcoholic beverages to no more than two drinks a day (men) or no more than one drink a day (women).

**Target Diet 12: Dr. Barry Sears's Zone Sports Diet (Chapter 9)**

1. Consume 40 percent carbohydrates, 30 percent fat, 30 percent protein at every meal and snack.
2. Consume the majority of carbohydrates as complex carbohydrates.
3. Consume preferably monounsaturated fats (found in olive oil, canola oil, macadamia nuts, and avocados).
4. Eliminate arachidonic acid fats such as egg yolks, organ meats, and fatty red meat; restrict fats found in animal protein and whole fat dairy products.
5. Avoid caffeine because it stimulates insulin production.

## DIET GOAL 13: REDUCE OSTEOPOROSIS

Twenty-four million Americans (80 percent of them women) suffer from osteoporosis, a progressive condition in which bones lose mass and become extremely brittle and prone to injury under the slightest amount of stress. Adolescent girls and adult women who wish to prevent osteoporosis through diet should increase their consumption of foods high in calcium, including lowfat dairy products. Inadequate dietary calcium consumption in the first three of four decades of life may be associated with increased risk for osteoporosis in later life (see Chapter 15). Chronically low calcium intake, especially during adolescence and early adulthood, may compromise development of peak bone mass. For elderly women, estrogen replacement therapy under medical supervision is the most effective means to reduce the rate of bone loss and risk for fractures.

### Target Diet 13: Osteoporosis Diet (Chapter 15)

1. Increase intakes of dietary calcium-rich foods such as grain products, lowfat dairy products, canned fish, and vegetables.
2. Increase consumption of vitamin D (100 to 400 units).
3. Avoid diets that exceed 35 grams of fiber per day or contain excessive protein.
4. Avoid smoking and excess use of alcohol (that is, consume no more than 1 to 2 drinks per day).
5. Women should discuss natural estrogen therapy with their physician.
6. Consume the RDAs for all essential nutrients and take a multivitamin mineral supplement, if necessary, that includes 5 to 50 milligrams vitamin B6, 5 milligrams folic acid, 1,000 milligrams vitamin C, 100 to 500 micrograms of vitamin E, 400 to 1,200 milligrams of calcium, 200 to 600 milligrams of magnesium, 10 to 30 milligrams zinc, 1 to 2 milligrams copper, 5 to 20 milligrams manganese, 1 to 3 milligrams boron, and .5 to 3 milligrams strontium.

## DIET GOAL 14: REDUCE ARTHRITIC INFLAMMATION

One of every two Americans has a 50 percent chance of suffering from some form of arthritis by the age of 50. Specific diets have not been shown yet to prevent arthritis, although three diets outlined in Chapter 16 suggest that nutritional regimens can reduce inflammation and flareups. Primary dietary therapy involves the achievement of normal body weight; excess weight means increased stress on weight-bearing joints affected with osteoarthritis.

### Target Diet 14: Arthritis Diet (Chapter 16)

1. Consume 60 to 70 percent of daily calories from complex carbohydrates.
2. Consume 25 to 35 grams of fiber daily either as food or from fiber supplements.
3. Consume 10 to 15 percent of total daily caloric intake as lowfat protein with the primary sources being fish, poultry, vegetables, and dairy products.

4. Reduce saturated animal fat intake and minimize polyunsaturated oil intake, specifically arachidonic and linoleic acids (which produce antagonistic prostaglandins).

5. Change protein sources from high-fat meats to lowfat fish, poultry, skim milk and other lowfat dairy products, and beans and vegetables.

6. Persons with rheumatoid arthritis may benefit from eliminating all foods which contain solanum alkaloids, especially the nightshade plants such as tomatoes, white potatoes, eggplant, peppers, and tobacco.

7. Reduce consumption of processed and canned foods, along with caffeine, sugar, and simple carbohydrate foods that are immediately converted into sugar upon digestion.

8. Balance nutrients and use vitamin and mineral supplements to ensure up to 100 percent of the RDA for all essential nutrients.

## DIET GOAL 15: PREVENT CORONARY ARTERY DISEASE

High blood cholesterol levels increase the risk for heart attacks, stroke, and high blood pressure. The reason for this is that when the blood carries too much cholesterol, the cholesterol may attach itself to artery walls, restricting or plugging the vessel. If arteries feeding the heart become clogged, a heart attack can occur. And if an artery going to the brain becomes clogged, the person may suffer a stroke.

### Target Diet 15: The American Heart Association (AHA) Diet (Chapter 17)

1. Limit total fat intake to less than 20 percent of calories.
2. Limit saturated fat intake to less than 20 percent of calories.
3. Limit polyunsaturated fat to less than 10 percent of calories.
4. Limit cholesterol intake to less than 300 mg/day.
5. Consume at least 50 percent of calories as carbohydrates.
6. Protein intake should provide the remainder of the calories.
7. Sodium intake should not exceed three grams/day.
8. Limit alcoholic consumption to 1 to 2 fluid ounces per day.

### Target Diet 15: Reversing Coronary Artery Disease (Chapter 17)

1. Limit total fat intake to less than 10 percent of calories.
2. Completely eliminate intake of cholesterol.

3. Eliminate foods high in saturated fat, including avocados, olives, coconut, cocoa products, nuts, and seeds.
4. Increase fiber consumption to 35 grams daily.
5. Limit alcohol consumption to two ounces per day.
6. Eliminate all oils and animal products except nonfat milk and yogurt.
7. Substitute egg whites for all foods requiring eggs.
8. Eliminate caffeine, other stimulants, and MSG.
9. Use salt and sugar in moderation.

## DIET GOAL 16: STABILIZE DIABETES

Diabetes mellitus is one of the three most serious diseases in the United States, following heart disease and cancer in causing total annual deaths. Its incidence is estimated to have increased tenfold in the past forty-five years, and it currently affects more than 14 million Americans. In addition, it is currently the number-one killer of women in the United States.

### Target Diet 16: Diabetes (Chapter 18)
1. If obese, follow a low-calorie diet to reduce weight, then a caloric-controlled diet to maintain a desirable weight.
2. Limit simple carbohydrates to 10 to 15 percent of total calories.
3. Use less sugar, including white sugar, brown sugar, raw sugar, honey, and syrups.
4. Select fresh fruits or fruit canned without sugar, or use light syrup rather than heavy syrup.
5. Read food labels to avoid products with sucrose, glucose, maltose, dextrose, lactose, fructose, or syrup.
6. Eliminate candy, soft drinks, ice cream, cakes, cookies. Keep the timing of the meals and the composition of the diet consistent from day to day, with the carbohydrate content evenly divided from meal to meal.
7. Plan a bedtime snack to prevent nocturnal hypoglycemia; mid-morning and mid-afternoon snacks, if needed, to match the food intake to the peak insulin action.
8. Depending upon the insulin regimen, plan for food to be taken to correct hypoglycemic episodes.
9. Plan for food and fluids to be taken for periods of increased physical activity or during illness.

## DIET GOAL 17: ELIMINATE FOOD ALLERGIES

More than 35 million Americans are allergic to some types of foods. Allergies can be disabling and life-threatening for certain chemically sensitive people. Although most allergies are incurable, they are manageable if the allergens are identified and eliminated from the diet.

### Target Diet 17: Food Allergy Elimination (Chapter 19)
1. Set up a four-day rotation plan and test all foods for allergic reactions.
2. Eliminate allergenic foods for six weeks, and then retest to determine if you have regained tolerance.
3. Consume RDAs for all essential nutrients, preferably in fresh, organic substitute foods purchased at organic food stores.
4. If necessary, take a vitamin mineral supplement that has vitamins C, B3, B6, zinc, magnesium, calcium, GTF chromium, evening primrose oil, and MaxEPA.
5. Upon advice of a physician or nutritionist, correct effects of hypochloridia with hydrochloric acid capsules and pancreatic digestive enzyme supplements.

## DIET GOAL 18: REDUCE HYPERTENSION (HIGH BLOOD PRESSURE)

Hypertension (excessive and sustained blood pressure against the walls of the arteries) is the most common stress-related disorder in the U.S. and a major cause of death. Approximately 60 million Americans suffer from hypertension (or high blood pressure), and half of them do not even know they have the condition. Nutritional causes of hypertension include excessive salt, sugar, licorice, coffee, and alcohol intake.

Readers who think they might be suffering from hypertension will benefit by comparing the diets described in Chapter 20, as dietary considerations are now known to play a significant role in both causing and subsequently lowering high blood pressure.

### Target Diet 18: Reduce Hypertension (Chapter 20)
1. Lose weight if overweight.
2. Limit alcohol intake to one ounce daily.
3. Reduce sodium intake to less than 100 milligrams per day.

4. Use freshly grated citrus peel as a salt substitute.
5. Adjust the seasoning in recipes to use more nonsalt spices.
6. Experiment with dry white wines in cooking sauces and soups as a salt substitute.
7. Spice soups and salads with vinegar, hot pepper, or sodium chloride/potassium chloride salt brands, such as Litesalt.
8. Use low-sodium baking powder.
9. Rinse salted canned foods to remove the sodium added as a preservative.
10. Maintain adequate dietary potassium, calcium, and magnesium intake.
11. Stop smoking and reduce dietary saturated fat and cholesterol intake.

## DIET GOAL 19: REVERSE HYPOGLYCEMIA

Most patients who complain of continual fatigue usually have low blood sugar levels, a condition termed "hypoglycemia." While the condition is not life-threatening, it can lead to diabetes, Addison's disease, cancer, heart disease, and brain dysfunction (due to reduced supplies of glucose to the brain). The only way to treat this condition is with diet.

### Target Diet 19: Hypoglycemia Reversal Diet (Chapter 21)
1. Consume 50 to 60 percent of daily calories as carbohydrates.
2. Consume 40 to 50 grams of complex carbohydrates at every meal to stabilize blood sugar levels (those engaging in strenuous exercise may need to consume more).
3. Consume higher amounts of whole-grain breads and cereals, seeds, nuts, fruits, vegetables, fermented dairy products, high-fiber foods, lean meats, and fish.
4. Avoid caffeine, alcohol, and tobacco. Refined sugars and sugar products are normally restricted.
5. Upon the advice of a physician or dietitian, take a multiple vitamin mineral supplement which includes vitamins A, D, C, B complex, E, magnesium, calcium, potassium citrate, lecithin, and kelp.
6. Upon the advice of a naturopath or herbalist, take supplements of juniper cedar berries, licorice root, Mexican wild yam, golden seal, and lobelia.

## DIET GOAL 20: ALLEVIATE IRRITABLE BOWEL SYNDROME (IBS)

As many as 24 percent of Americans experience some of the symptoms of irritable bowel syndrome, including abdominal pain, excessive gas, bloating, indigestion, constipation, and diarrhea. IBS is not life-threatening, does not appear to progress to other serious diseases, and can be treated with the diets discussed in Chapter 22.

**Target Diet 20: IBS Reversal Diet (Chapter 22)**
1. Keep a food diary to identify "trigger" foods and food intolerances.
2. Avoid offending foods as needed, including milk and dairy products, gas-forming foods and beverages, foods that contain high amounts of fructose and raffinose, or dietetic foods that contain sorbitol.
3. Eat regular, small, frequent lowfat meals.
4. Gradually increase dietary fiber to approximately 15 to 25 grams per day.
5. Limit caffeine and alcohol intake.
6. Exercise regularly and practice stress reduction techniques.
7. Drink 8 or more cups of water or fluid per day.

## DIET GOAL 21: CONTROL MULTIPLE SCLEROSIS (MS)

People with MS have severe impairments of their nervous system which often leave them paralyzed. Several special diets can help alleviate some of the symptoms, and persons will need to experiment with food groups to determine which do or do not cause flareup symptoms.

**Target Diet 21: Stabilize MS Diet (Chapter 23)**
1. Restrict saturated fat intake to no more than 10 grams per day.
2. Restrict intake of polyunsaturated oils to 40 to 50 grams per day (margarine, shortening, and hydrogenated oils are not allowed).
3. Normal amounts of protein are recommended.
4. Fish should be eaten three or more times a week.
5. Fresh whole foods should be emphasized and animal foods (with the exception of fish) should be reduced, if not completely eliminated.

The following suggestions may prove helpful in assisting you to choose and maintain your diet objectives:

1. Determine a starting point by filling out the nutritional and physical fitness assessment forms.

2. Identify safe and realistic goals based on your current nutritional intake and recommended body mass index for your age.

3. Determine the number of daily calories you need to maintain your present and/or ideal weight. Depending on your goals, you may choose any one of the weight-loss programs described in Chapters 5 through 9.

4. Do not set yourself up for failure by trying to improve your lifestyle if you are distracted by other major problems. It takes a substantial amount of mental and physical energy to change your eating habits.

5. Make a commitment: if your goal is weight loss, decide to lose weight because you want to, not to please someone else. You must be internally motivated to stay on any diet because diets always involve lifestyle changes and sacrifice; you must do it for yourself, not for someone else. If you are having marital or financial problems, or if you are unhappy with the major aspects of your life, you may be less likely to follow through on your good intentions. Your timing of when you start to implement your goals is therefore critical.

6. Set weekly or monthly goals that allow you to monitor your successes, and reward yourself appropriately.

7. While you restrict certain unhealthy foods on your particular diet, learn to replace them with more nutritious natural whole foods.

8. Stay active. With few exceptions, all of the target diets discussed in this book include an exercise program.

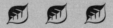

## DIET GOAL 22: REDUCE CANCER RISK

An overall increase in intake of foods high in fiber may decrease the risk for colon cancer. Other diet components associated with decreased cancer risk are whole-grain cereal products containing complex carbohydrates and fiber; dark green and deep yellow vegetables, cabbage and broccoli, dried beans and peas, and fruits.

**Target 22: Reduce Cancer Risk (Chapter 24)**

1. Maintain a desirable body weight.
2. Eat a varied diet that includes vegetables and fruits.
3. Increase consumption of complex carbohydrates to 55 percent; carbohydrate-rich foods, especially vegetables and fruits, have a cancer-protective effect.
4. Eat more high-fiber foods, such as whole-grain cereals, legumes, vegetables, and fruits.
5. Reduce total fat intake to less than 30 percent of calories.
6. Limit consumption of alcoholic beverages.
7. Limit consumption of salt-cured and nitrite-preserved foods.

## SUGGESTIONS FOR IMPLEMENTING YOUR GOALS

Whether you are considering dieting to lose weight or to maximize other goals, you must first be clear about your current nutritional status and your diet objectives. The best diets are those designed in consultation with a physician or dietitian which take into account the biochemical uniqueness of the patient and may combine several goals.

Nutritional needs are different for each person. In order to choose the most appropriate diet, you'll need to have assessed your nutritional and physical status. Once you have reached initial conclusions about your own biochemical makeup, a nutritionist can then help you develop one of the target diets outlined in this chapter.

# Part Two

# 5

## Medically Supervised Diet Programs: Very-Low-Calorie-Diet Programs

Five years ago, talk-show host Oprah Winfrey weighed more than 200 pounds. Her obesity put her at medical risk for developing diabetes, heart disease, and several forms of cancer. "My weight," she said recently, "was an apology to the world." Ms. Winfrey needed to lose as much as 70 pounds, and decided to enroll in the OPTIFAST Very-Low-Calorie-Diet (VLCD) program, the oldest of the six VLCD programs analyzed in this chapter.

VLCDs are physician-supervised modified fasting weight-loss programs that provide less than 800 calories per day, and usually substitute liquid formula for solid foods. Most are based in hospitals or clinics, and are staffed by a multidisciplinary team of physicians, behavioral therapists, dietitians, exercise physiologists, and nurses. Medical supervision is essential because extreme diets such as VLCDs can cause a variety of medical complications, including heart, liver, and kidney problems. For this reason, pregnant women, the elderly, and dieters with cancer, insulin-dependent diabetes, or psychiatric problems are normally discouraged from enrolling in a VLCD program. On average, women who participate in a VLCD program lose 2 to 3 pounds a week during the initial weight-loss phase, while men lose 4 to 5 pounds a week.

The recommended or required foods, daily calorie levels, level of medical supervision, and importance of exercise in a VLCD vary substantially. All VLCD programs are required by the Food and Drug Administration to report the average weight lost and dropout rates, and to discuss the risk of gallbladder disease with potential clients. All VLCD diet formula must contain at least 10 grams of fat per day (15 percent of calories in an 800 calories diet). The FDA also requires that every VLCD program provide a minimum of 70 grams of protein daily, as well as the RDAs for essential vitamins, potassium, magnesium, phosphate, and sodium.

For many readers considering enrolling in a VLCD program, cost will also be an important factor. Total costs for the six programs analyzed vary substantially, depending on whether they are hospital-, program-, or physician-based; the length of each program; the total number of group meetings; the total number of individual sessions with physicians; the degree of one-on-one nutritional counseling; and the cost and amounts of supplements and prepackaged food required. For comparison purposes, the average cost and length of each VLCD program are shown below.

**Total Cost of VLCD Programs**

| | |
|---|---|
| HMR | $2,250 |
| Weigh to Live | $400–$450 |
| OPTITRIM | $1,300–$1,800 |
| OPTIFAST | $2,800–$3,200 |
| Medifast | $1,880 |

## MEDICAL INSURANCE COVERAGE

The HMR, Medifast, and OPTIFAST programs state that their fees can be partially covered by some health insurance policies. Most policies require that a referring physician provide a written prescription for weight loss in order for dieters to be reimbursed. Readers are advised to check with their insurance carrier to determine which, if any, components of the VLCD programs in which they are interested will be covered by their existing policy.

## HEALTH MANAGEMENT RESOURCES (HMR)

59 Temple Place, Suite 704
Boston, Massachusetts 02111
(617) 357-9876
Year founded: 1983
Cost: $2,380
Average length of program: 15 months, which includes weight loss and maintenance

Of the six VLCDs analyzed in this chapter, dieters enrolled in the HMR program lose the most weight — an average of 52 pounds after twenty weeks. And 56 percent maintain this weight loss for at least two years. HMR, which is partially reimbursable through health insurance, offers three flavors of liquid supplements during the weight-loss phase, which can last a minimum of twelve weeks. Dieters can subsequently prepare their own meals according to individual caloric needs. All participants in the program receive an HMR Risk Factor Profile both before and after weight loss, which assesses sixteen medical and lifestyle risk factors, identifies specific areas for improvement, and reinforces new, healthier eating habits. The HMR formulas are among the highest in carbohydrates and the lowest in fat, reducing possible ketogenic side effects such as depleted energy. Behavior modification is stressed throughout the duration of the medically supervised program.

## Locations

HMR's more than two hundred sites nationwide are located in hospitals, physician group practices, and private medical practices. While staffs vary in size, each site provides at least one physician, a nurse, and a health educator trained in the HMR program. Registered dietitians are also available at some locations.

## Eligibility

Applicants for the medically supervised HMR program must be at least 20 percent (or approximately 40 pounds) over their ideal body weight. HMR also has a moderately restricted program for anyone less than 20 percent above their ideal body weight. All applicants are screened to determine medical eligibility prior to beginning the program and at periodic intervals. While a physician's referral is recommended, it is not required.

## Cost

HMR program prices vary, depending on the site, the diet chosen, and the level of supervision required. The average cost for three months of weight loss is approximately $420 per month, which includes foods, liquid supplements, weekly meetings, medical tests, and visits. The cost for maintenance totals $90 a month. Total cost, therefore, for three months of weight loss and twelve months of maintenance is $2,800. Many participants receive insurance reimbursements to pay for a portion of the program.

## HMR Phase I

The objective of Phase 1, Weight Loss, is to help dieters reach their goal weight. It lasts for a minimum of twelve weeks, and the average weight loss is two to five pounds per week.

During this initial phase, dieters — depending on desired weight loss and the discretion of their physician — are given a powdered supplement (to which water is added) that totals between 520 and 800 calories a day. (Dieters can also use a combination of supplements and prepackaged HMR entrees for a total of 800 to 1,300 calories per day. This is called the HMR Moderate Program.) The powder (available in chocolate, vanilla, and chicken soup flavors) can be mixed cold or heated, and even used in coffee or other hot beverages. An HMR recipe book is also provided to create additional variations and to diminish the tedium of this type of dieting. The supplements are accompanied by two vitamin and mineral tablets daily. Clients are also advised to consume two quarts of liquid per day, including coffee, tea, water, and diet sodas, in addition to the diet supplement.

HMR monitors the dieter's health on a weekly basis and periodically performs blood chemistry tests. Medically supervised patients undergo an EKG after every 25 to 50 pounds of weight loss. Throughout Phase 1, weekly mandatory educational meetings are held which stress fat reduction, increasing the consumption of fruits and vegetables and increasing amounts of physical activity. Dieters also meet weekly with a health educator.

## HMR Phase 2

Phase 2, Transition, lasts four to six weeks and focuses on helping dieters transition to eating real foods as they decrease the use of liquid supplements and increase food calories.

Dieters and staff work together to formulate a realistic, practical eating plan which gradually increases solid foods, including fruits and vegetables. This is a crucial transition phase in all VLCD programs because at this point the temptation to return to old eating habits is greatest.

Throughout Phase 2, dieters meet weekly with the supervising physician and health educator to discuss and update their eating plan, while continuing to attend classes.

## HMR Phase 3

Phase 3, Maintenance, focuses on helping dieters become fully independent and able to prepare their own meals according to their individual caloric needs. Phase 3, a required part of the HMR program, lasts a minimum of twelve months and additional maintenance programming is available.

Dieters work with their health educator to prepare menu plans, which are customized according to their body weight, amount of exercise, and eating habits. The HMR Calorie System teaches the caloric content of all foods and helps dieters make intelligent dietary choices based on their own needs. During this phase, no food is forbidden to minimize any sense of deprivation, although three "essentials" are stressed: at least 2,000 calories of physical activity a week; no more than 25 to 30 percent of total calories from fat; and 35 weekly servings of fruits and/or vegetables.

Dieters are weighed weekly, and are required to attend sixty-minute closed-group classes with other maintenance members. Classes are led by a health educator, or "coach," who discusses diet strategies and helps participants practice new weight management skills until they are incorporated into their lifestyle. HMR dieters also analyze exercise/energy expenditure charts to help increase and maintain high levels of physical activity.

## Nutritional Analysis

HMR offers three liquid supplements: a 520-calorie formula (called HMR 500), an 800-calorie formula, and a 520-calorie lactose-free formula for dieters with lactose intolerance. The HMR formulas are compared below with the Recommended Dietary Allowances (RDAs) for average Americans who are not dieting.

| HMR 500 (chocolate): | | RDAs (for comparison) |
|---|---|---|
| Carbohydrates | 60 percent | 55 to 65 percent |
| Protein | 38 percent | 10 to 15 percent |
| Fat | 1 percent | Less than 30 percent |
| Sodium | 780 milligrams | |
| Fiber | 4 grams | |

| HMR 800: | | RDAs (for comparison) |
|---|---|---|
| Carbohydrates | 49 percent | 55 to 65 percent |
| Protein | 40 percent | 10 to 15 percent |

| Fat | 11 percent | Less than 30 percent |
| Sodium | 1,250 milligrams | |
| Fiber | 5 grams | |

| **HMR 500 (vanilla):** | | **RDAs (for comparison)** |
| Carbohydrates | 60 percent | 55 to 65 percent |
| Protein | 38 percent | 10 to 15 percent |
| Fat | 1 percent | Less than 30 percent |
| Sodium | 780 milligrams | |
| Fiber | 1.5 grams | |

| **HMR 800:** | | **RDAs (for comparison)** |
| Carbohydrates | 48 percent | 55 to 65 percent |
| Protein | 40 percent | 10 to 15 percent |
| Fat | 11 percent | Less than 30 percent |
| Sodium | 1,250 milligrams | |
| Fiber | 5 grams | |

The carbohydrate in the HMR formulas is made up of sugars and methylcellulose, which is a good source of fiber and decreases the production of ketones with their accompanying negative side effects. Carbohydrates are necessarily high in the HMR 500 formula in order to balance the extremely lowfat content (1 percent). Carbohydrates are lower in the HMR 800 formula because more energy is provided by fat (11 percent). The protein in both formulas consists of dry nonfat milk and egg white — high-grade, complete protein sources.

Sodium levels in both formulas are significantly lower than what the average nondieting American normally consumes in a day — 3,000 milligrams. Both HMR formulas also provide approximately 100 percent of the RDAs of most essential vitamins and minerals.

Fiber levels are low in both formulas because fiber, especially if insoluble, tends to retain water and maintain weight. Soluble fiber, however, could be increased as it helps slow down the absorption of carbohydrates and keeps blood sugar levels more constant.

| **HMR 70 Plus (lactose-free):** | | **RDAs (for comparison)** |
| Carbohydrates | 46 percent | 55 to 65 percent |
| Protein | 53 percent | 10 to 15 percent |
| Fat | 5 percent | Less than 30 percent |

| Sodium | 920 milligrams |
|--------|----------------|
| Fiber | 6 grams (chocolate) |
| | 1 gram (vanilla) |

The carbohydrate level of HMR 70 Plus is average for this kind of diet. Protein, which is made up of egg white solids, is almost four times the RDAs, while sodium levels are low. Some dieters may need to monitor their sodium levels — symptoms of a deficiency include muscle and stomach cramps, nausea, fatigue, and appetite loss.

## Advantages

The HMR program is well established with an impressive track record: it has treated more than 250,000 patients. It is also extremely convenient — dieters may use other HMR sites while traveling and maintain contact with their home-based health educator by phone. HMR maintains a national data system on participants which monitors the program's effectiveness and enhances quality control. HMR credits the program's success on recognizing that "a weight problem is a health problem," and adopting a "total health approach with strong emphasis on teaching patients the skills and behaviors they need to change the way they live for good."

## Disadvantages

Pregnant and lactating women and acute substance abusers are not permitted to enter the program. Also, some locations may not offer the full multidisciplinary approach needed for optimum weight loss and maintenance, although patients can compensate by contacting outside sources for exercise and additional group support.

## WEIGH TO LIVE (WTL)

2281 205th Street, Suite 105
Torrance, CA 90501
(800) 554-LIVE
(310) 533-0221
Year founded: 1982
Cost: $400–$450
Average length of program: 16 months

While Weigh to Live (WTL) costs less than the other five programs analyzed in this chapter, it is available at only twelve centers in four states, all of which are franchised to hospitals or medical clinics. The program differs from other hospital-based VLCD plans in that dieters can choose from among three variations during the weight-loss phase. This seems to encourage an earlier reliance on nutritional education, and makes travel and dining out much easier than with other similar diets. Each client receives a computerized program that accommodates individual taste preferences and medical needs, including dieters who follow kosher or vegetarian diets or who are lactose-gluten intolerant. An average of 24 pounds is lost during the first sixteen-week phase, followed by four weeks of maintenance and a lifelong "access" program that includes weekly counseling and ongoing support to help dieters maintain their ideal body weight.

### Location

As noted, Weigh to Live maintains eight centers in four states (New York, New Jersey, California, and Hawaii), all of which are franchised to hospitals. Program staff are either physicians with registered dietitians or behavior counselors who are trained in the Weigh to Live philosophy.

### Cost

The cost of the program ranges from $400 to $450 depending on location, including all medical supervision, powdered formula, and four to six weeks of maintenance. This totals as little as $10 per pound of weight lost — the least expensive of the VLCDs. For an additional $20 per month, Weigh to Live members may continue to attend biweekly maintenance classes. The cost of the Weigh to Be (WTB) program, as described below, ranges from $200 to $250, depending on location, and includes group sessions, computerized "MenuMax" meals, and a year-long maintenance program. The fee for ongoing maintenance varies from $100 to $150 annually.

### Eligibility

The Weigh to Live Med System program is designed for people who are 30 percent over their ideal body weight and are at medical risk. Participants with medical problems such as a heart condition or diabetes must be referred by a physician. A second program, Weigh to Be, was introduced in 1995 for those who want to achieve weight loss but are not at medical risk.

Dieters are automatically enrolled in either of the programs based on their medical condition and the amount of weight they need to lose. Both the Weigh to Live Med System and the Weigh to Be program consist of three phases.

## WTL Phase 1

Phase 1, Weight Control, is designed to help dieters reach their desired weight goal. This initial phase lasts approximately twelve weeks for Med System participants and eight weeks for those following the WTB plan, who tend to lose two to three pounds a week.

Participants may choose one of three programs: the liquid formula diet (a powdered supplement available in vanilla or chocolate, served cold); the MenuMax plan, which uses regular foods; or a combination of the two. If the first option is selected, the formula contains 650 calories for the Weigh to Live Med System dieters and 800 calories for Weigh to Be participants. If the MenuMax plan is preferred, dieters meet with a health professional who (utilizing the company's "Weigh to Be personalized computer") helps determine a specific food calorie plan, shopping lists, and recipes. Those opting for a combination plan are provided a computer-generated, customized calorie level, and can choose either supermarket foods or WTL's liquid formula for all meals.

Weekly meetings, both one-on-one and in a group setting, are held to monitor progress and help encourage behavior modification. Phase 1 is supervised by either a physician or a health professional who provides clients with an individualized exercise program during the fourth week. Brisk walking, stationary bike riding, and swimming are encouraged to facilitate the transition from normally sedentary lifestyles, and activity levels are monitored.

## WTL Phase 2

The objective of Phase 2, Maintenance, is to establish a precise calorie level for each client that will make it possible to stay at the desired weight level. Phase 2 lasts for four weeks, during which time levels of protein and carbohydrate in the daily diet are changed in order to accommodate maintenance rather than weight loss.

Dieters are given meal programs, possibly including some of the liquid formula, individualized to their taste preferences and specific caloric needs.

Counseling by a health professional continues to be provided weekly, and dieters attend group meetings. Group support meetings are mandatory to ensure that the original reasons the dieters became overweight (stress, anxiety, boredom, compulsions) are adequately addressed at this important transitional stage.

## WTL Phase 3

The goal of Phase 3, Access, is to help dieters maintain weight loss by providing an ongoing, lifelong support plan.

Dieters who qualify for individualized food plans eat only real foods which they prepare after consulting with the program's dietitian. The emphasis in this phase is on teaching WTL or WTB clients to understand the importance of eating the right foods in the right amounts and maintaining healthy eating habits. When returning to real foods, for example, dieters are counseled to eat slowly, as it takes approximately twenty minutes for the brain to "turn off" the hunger button and let the body know that it has eaten enough to satisfy the appetite.

Counseling is provided to help dieters maintain their ideal weight, which they establish in consultation with a counselor. This counseling is not mandatory and dieters are not required to either meet with or be examined by a physician. Weekly maintenance classes are available for $20 per month.

## Nutritional Analysis

Weigh to Live offers two different formulas, which provide calories as follows:

| Formula I 650: | | RDAs (for comparison) |
|---|---|---|
| Carbohydrates | 39 percent | 55 to 65 percent |
| Protein | 48 percent | 10 to 15 percent |
| Fat | 13 percent | Less than 30 percent |
| Sodium | 1,000 milligrams | |
| Fiber | 0 | |

| Formula I +800: | | RDAs (for comparison) |
|---|---|---|
| Carbohydrates | 56 percent | 55 to 65 percent |
| Protein | 30 percent | 10 to 15 percent |

| | | |
|---|---|---|
| Fat | 14 percent | Less than 30 percent |
| Sodium | 1,000 milligrams | |
| Fiber | 0 | |

The carbohydrate percentage in Formula I +800 is within the range of the RDAs for average nondieting Americans, while the percentage in the Formula I 650 is below it. Carbohydrates are a better source of energy than fat because very little of complex carbohydrates are converted into body fat. Protein is significantly higher than the RDAs in both formulas and helps preserve lean muscle mass. Several recent studies suggest that people on a VLCD program should consume at least 70 grams of protein a day in order to preserve lean muscle tissue. Sodium and fat levels conform to U.S. dietary recommendations.

Both formulas contain more fat than other VLCD programs, and Dr. Dean Ornish's "heart reversal" diet (10 percent) has helped some patients lose as much as 70 pounds. Sodium levels in both formulas are safe, although dieters with heart irregularities must monitor their levels carefully. Both formulas provide 100 percent of the RDAs of essential vitamins and minerals. There is no fiber in this formula and dieters may experience some bowel irregularity as a result, even though the formula is liquid. Soluble fiber could safely be added, as it will help increase the excretion of any cholesterol in the bile.

## Advantages

The Weigh to Live program is the least expensive of those analyzed in this chapter, and offers dieters three variations. Dieters choose the one best suited to their individual taste preferences and medical needs. The program is also flexible, offering the Weigh to Live Med System for people who are severely overweight and Weigh to Be for people who are moderately overweight. Dieters on the MenuMax plan can travel and dine out and are responsible for monitoring their calories.

Weigh to Live has just completed a ten-year study of dieters who maintained their weight loss. According to program cofounder Dr. Annette Dalman, the study shows that the most important factor for dieters who maintained long-term weight loss was their determination to choose a positive, healthy lifestyle. The liquid food formulas, group meetings, and program exercise regimen were contributing factors. The computer analysis of daily food menus and meetings with physicians were also helpful.

The successful dieter, however, took the encouragement and information and "operationalized" them.

## Disadvantages

The program is offered in only twelve locations, making it unavailable to most people. Phase 1, Weight Control, lasts up to sixteen weeks. However, studies by Dr. George L. Blackburn of the Harvard Medical School suggest that the body cannot effectively lose weight for more than twelve consecutive weeks — and anyone trying to do so for a longer period of time is apt to encounter frustration. Also, the behavioral modification portion of the program consists of open meetings, which some analysts have suggested may diminish the support and bonding that characterize closed-group sessions. Dr. Dalman, however, suggests that closed meetings encouraged the wrong kind of bonding. WTL contends that members of closed groups tend to reinforce each other and dieters are not as challenged to meet their goals. WTL's open meetings are led by cotherapists — former dieters trained to lead groups.

## OPTITRIM

> 5320 West 23rd Street
> Minneapolis, MN 55440
> (800) 999-9978
> Year founded: 1988
> Cost: Ranges from $250 to $1,000 based on medical supervision needed
> Average length of program: Varies from 8 to 18 weeks

The OPTITRIM program is a clinic-based weight management program that features a low-calorie diet made up of powdered supplements and self-prepared or packaged meals. After initial weight loss, patients are gradually transitioned to a diet containing predominately self-prepared foods.

## Location

Up to fifty centers in the United States currently offer the OPTITRIM program.

## Cost

Program costs vary from $250 to $1,000, depending on location, the length of the program, and the level of medical monitoring offered at each location.

## Eligibility

OPTITRIM is designed for people who have moderate amounts of weight to lose (less than 40 pounds), and who are not at high risk for medical problems. Potential clients must complete a medical/behavioral questionnaire and undergo a medical examination that includes a blood chemistry analysis prior to participation.

## Nutritional Program

Patients follow a diet between 950 and 1,200 calories based on individual nutritional assessment. A combination of OPTITRIM supplement nutritional bars and self-prepared or prepackaged meals are included in the plan based on the dieter's needs and calorie level.

## Staff Support

Dieters are seen weekly and receive periodic medical checkups and laboratory analyses based on their medical needs. Dieters also participate in weekly group or individual counseling sessions designed to provide participants with the information they need to make the right food choices for the rest of their lives. Physicians, nurses, registered dietitians, and psychologists are an integral part of the program.

## Nutritional Analysis

The OPTITRIM calories per day break down as follows:

**OPTITRIM Formula (233 calories per packet)**

|  |  | **Grams per Packet** |
|---|---|---|
| Carbohydrates | 50 percent | 29 grams |
| Protein | 29 percent | 17 grams |
| Fat | 19 percent | 5 grams |
| Sodium | 370 milligrams (per packet) | |

## Advantages

OPTITRIM is a medically monitored VLCD program that customizes therapy to meet individual patient needs. It includes an extensive behavioral modification program that focuses on long-term lifestyle changes. Close contact with nurses, physicians, dietitians, and psychologists is emphasized. Extended maintenance programs are provided at some locations.

## Disadvantages

Some people find that Optitrim's mandatory group support classes cause a conflict with work or vacation schedules. Extensive travel is discouraged, although because the foods are shelf-stable, some travel is feasible. OPTITRIM requires a strong commitment on the patient's part for time and participation in weekly counseling sessions and medical testing. The program is not designed for those with large amounts of weight to lose or those with multiple medical problems requiring close supervision.

## OPTIFAST

5320 West 23rd Street
Minneapolis, MN 55440
(800) 999-9978
Year founded: 1976
Cost: $1,500 to $3,000 (depending on location and insurance reimbursement)
Average length of program: 25 weeks

OPTIFAST is a medically supervised clinical weight management program that averages twenty-five weeks in duration. During the initial twelve-week phase, dieters limit themselves to about 800 calories per day by taking a high-quality powder supplement enriched with vitamins and minerals. By the end of the eighteenth week, the use of powdered supplement is gradually decreased and clients consume regular foods based upon an individualized plan created with the help of a registered dietitian. Weekly group meetings with a health professional are scheduled for twenty-six weeks, and each dieter is given a personalized exercise program to help develop a more active lifestyle. The average weight loss is approximately 20 percent of starting weight, and on average 60 percent of those who start the program complete it.

## Locations

OPTIFAST is offered at more than 200 centers in the U.S., including OPTIFAST clinics, participating hospitals (on an outpatient basis), and private group physician practices.

## Cost

Program costs range from $250 to $500 per month, with the entire program (including the powdered meals) totaling approximately $1,500 to $3,000, depending on location. This approximates $40 per pound lost. Several insurance programs may cover a portion of the program's cost, such as laboratory fees and physician visits, if the referring physician provides a written prescription for weight loss.

## Eligibility

Dieters must be at least 30 percent above their ideal body weight or at least 50 pounds overweight. Before admission to the program, all patients must undergo medical screening to identify any health problems which may preclude program participation and to assist the physician with individualizing the level of medical monitoring throughout the program.

## Staff Support

Throughout the program clients receive periodic medical examinations, including blood tests and urinalyses. Close contact with physicians, nurses, and registered dietitians is maintained, and weekly group sessions are led by dietitians or psychologists. These group sessions focus on behavioral change and lifestyle modification necessary to maintain long-term weight loss.

## Nutritional Analysis

The caloric levels (420 for women, 800 for men) are broken down as follows:

**OPTIFAST 800 (5 packets per day for a total of 800 calories)**

|  | % of Nutrient | Grams Per Day |
| --- | --- | --- |
| Carbohydrates | 50 percent | 100 grams |
| Protein | 35 percent | 70 grams |

| Fat | 15 percent | 13 grams |
|-----|-----------|----------|
| Sodium | 1,150 milligrams | |
| Fiber | 0 | |

## Advantages

The OPTIFAST program features one of the most comprehensive behavioral modification components, with weekly meetings continuing from the first through the twenty-sixth week. Group leaders are behavioral counselors, registered dietitians, or exercise physiologists. Each clinic also offers an extended maintenance program which is strongly encouraged. The program offers close contact with health professionals and is most beneficial for patients with health problems.

## Disadvantages

OPTIFAST requires a strong commitment on the patient's part to continue weekly sessions, weigh-ins, medical tests, and other monitoring. Since special diet products are an integral part of the program and medical supervision is essential, eating out may be somewhat difficult during the early part of the program. Patients can travel and may remain in the program as long as they maintain their weight loss and as long as they are not at medical risk. This program is not designed for those who have less than 50 pounds of weight to lose.

## MEDIFAST

11435 Cronhill Drive
P.O. Box 370
Owings Mill, MD 21117-0370
(800) 638-7867
Year founded: 1983
Cost: $1,880
Average length of program: 34 weeks

By far the most accessible of all VLCD programs with more than eight thousand locations in the United States, Medifast credits its success to its practicality, relative affordability, and emphasis on one-on-one counseling. Medifast is primarily doctor-based, rather than hospital-based, and dieters can enroll in the program and buy all their supplements directly from a participating physician. During the initial weight-loss phase, dieters consume powdered supplements that total 440 calories a day. These supplement shakes may be augmented with replacement items such as creamy soups, supplement bars, hot cocoa, instant soups, or crackers. The second phase gradually reintroduces solid foods and eventually completely eliminates supplements. The total program, including twelve weeks of maintenance, lasts thirty-four weeks. It includes weekly one-hour classes led by a registered dietitian and monthly open forums conducted by a behavioral psychologist. Medifast recommends brisk walking (one mile at 3.5 mph or greater, with gradual increases) as the best transitional exercise for dieters who have previously been sedentary. Clients lose an average of 3 to 5 pounds per week. According to Medifast, 65 percent of those who finish the program remain within four pounds of their goal weight after one year.

## Locations

There are more than eight thousand Medifast locations in the United States, primarily in physician's offices, but also at 120 hospitals on an outpatient basis. Each location has a physician on staff, while the larger ones also have a registered dietitian and behavioral counselor.

## Cost

Medifast locations charge $65 to $85 per week, except for the maintenance phase, which averages $19 per week. The total cost for the 34-week program is $1,880, excluding blood test expenses. According to Medifast, most insurance companies now cover office visits and medical tests.

## Eligibility

Patients admitted to the Medifast program do not have to be referred by a physician, but must be at least 20 percent above their ideal body weight as determined by the Medifast staff. Modified programs are available for people with less weight to lose. Patients attend a one-day orientation during which they undergo a medical evaluation, including an EKG, blood and urine analyses, blood pressure reading, weigh-in, and possibly a computerized body-fat analysis.

## Medifast Phase 1

Phase 1, Weight Reduction, lasts an average of sixteen weeks, although the physician may extend it if dieters have not achieved their ideal body weight.

Participants consume five powdered supplements per day, mixed with six to eight ounces of liquid. The supplements are based on a natural protein formula enriched with micronutrients in five flavors (strawberry, orange, chocolate, vanilla, and mocha). The formula is available in three varieties: Medifast 55, Medifast 70, and Medifast Plus. Medifast 55 contains 55 grams of protein and is prescribed for women who are 30 percent or more above their ideal body weight. Medifast 70 contains 70 grams of protein and is used by men who are 30 percent or more above their ideal body weight. Men or women who are only 20 to 30 pounds above their ideal body weight, adolescents, and those who weigh more than 350 pounds take Medifast Plus, which contains 96 grams of protein and is consumed along with one 480-calorie food meal per day. An alternate plan for Medifast 55 and 70 dieters includes five daily supplements plus one meal of three to four ounces of lean meat and two cups of salad vegetables, which brings the total to 650 calories.

During the first phase, dieters meet biweekly with their physician and are weighed and examined once a week. They also undergo the first phase of Medifast's behavioral modification program, called Lifestyles 1, which addresses behavioral modification issues such as self-esteem, compulsiveness, and stress management. Regular attendance at the one-hour weekly classes is not mandatory.

## Medifast Phase 2

Phase 2, Refeeding (or Realimentation), lasts four to six weeks and gradually reintroduces solid foods while reducing the amount of supplement consumed.

The following is a sample refeeding schedule during Phase 2. After the sixth week, the supplements are completely eliminated:

Week one:     Five packets of powdered supplement daily and 4 ounces of lean protein.

Week two:     Add 1 cup of salad vegetables.

| Week three: | Add 1/2 cup of cooked vegetables. |
| Week four: | Reduce powdered supplement to 4 packets per day, and add 1 fruit. |
| Week five: | Add 1 cup of nonfat milk. |
| Week six: | Add 1 bread or cereal serving. |

Where appropriate, the supervising physician may allow modifications for vegetarian or kosher dieters and those with special food preferences or allergies. An extra packet of powdered supplement is often prescribed for people who are experiencing lightheadedness.

## Medifast Phase 3

Phase 3, Maintenance, lasts twelve weeks and is designed to encourage clients to plan their own menus which maintain the dieter's ideal body weight.

A Medifast physician consults with the client and helps develop a diet that takes into account body weight, food preferences, lifestyle, and exercise regimen.

During the second phase of the behavioral modification program, Lifestyles 2, clients learn to apply the skills they learned during Lifestyles 1 to real-life situations such as restaurant dining and cooking at home. However, not all locations offer Lifestyles 2.

## Nutritional Analysis

| Medifast 55 (five packets = 440 calories): | | RDAs (for comparison) |
|---|---|---|
| Carbohydrates | 41 percent | 55 to 65 percent |
| Protein | 51 percent | 10 to 15 percent |
| Fat | 8 percent | Less than 30 percent |
| Sodium | 1,000 milligrams | |
| Fiber | 4 grams | |

| Medifast 70 (five packets = 460 calories): | | RDAs (for comparison) |
|---|---|---|
| Carbohydrates | 34 percent | 55 to 65 percent |
| Protein | 60 percent | 10 to 15 percent |
| Fat | 6 percent | Less than 30 percent |
| Sodium | 1,000 milligrams | |
| Fiber | 4 grams | |

| Medifast Plus (four packets = 370 calories): | | RDAs (for comparison) |
|---|---|---|
| Carbohydrates | 60 percent | 55 to 65 percent |
| Protein | 35 percent | 10 to 15 percent |
| Fat | 5 percent | Less than 30 percent |
| Sodium | 1,000 milligrams | |

Fat levels in all three formulas are extremely low. The protein level in Medifast 55 and 70 is adequate at 55 and 70 grams respectively, while protein is high in Medifast Plus (96 grams). The sodium level in each formula is three times less than what average nondieting Americans consume per day. The daily fiber in the original Medifast 55 and 70 formulas, as well as the Medifast Plus, is low and could alter bowel function. To address this deficiency, Medifast has now introduced reformulated supplements that contain 15 grams of fiber daily. The amount of potassium has also been increased.

The original formulas, partially egg-based and containing nonfat dry milk, were also high in lactose. The new formulas are very low in lactose, consisting of soy protein isolate, sweet dairy whey, and milk protein isolate. The new formulas also contain no eggs and satisfy all protein requirements.

Medifast also now offers a mocha option to all its formulas. It also makes its formulas available in creamy soups (cream of chicken, cream of tomato, and cream of broccoli) and cholesterol-free instant soup mixes (tomato, chicken, and beef). The line includes two new supplement bars, chocolate supreme and honey nougat, which contain 12 grams of protein and one gram of fiber per serving. A hot cocoa supplement is also featured, as well as multigrain crackers which contain no fat or cholesterol. Regardless of the program they are on (55, 70, or Plus), all clients are required to consume a minimum of three supplement shakes daily. The remaining one or two supplements may be substituted with one of the replacement items.

Because of the low caloric levels in all three Medifast formulas, vitamin and mineral supplements are used to bring dieters' levels up to 100 percent or more of the RDAs.

## Advantages

One-on-one counseling is provided throughout the Medifast program, and the staff is well trained and carefully monitors clients' medical status, and any difficulties they have in adhering to the diet. Also, the supplements come in a greater variety of flavors than any of the VLCDs — including supplement bars and crackers — which helps mitigate the boredom experienced during the initial weight-loss phase.

## Disadvantages

Because Medifast is offered primarily through private physicians, it provides minimal staff support. For example, it does not require nutritional counseling or support groups except where these services are provided in a hospital setting.

## RECENT RESEARCH

Harvard obesity specialist George L. Blackburn, in an article in the October 1, 1993, issue of the *Annals of Internal Medicine,* cites several studies that indicate that VLCDs are the most effective and safest method for obese dieters to lose weight and maintain weight loss. He points out that obesity has been increasingly linked with several metabolic disorders including syndrome X and its individual components (hyperinsulinemia, dyslipidemia, hypertension, and hyperuricemia), and that its treatment must include not only calorie-restricted diets, when appropriate, but other medical interventions as well. Medical supervision of a VLCD program by a physician is mandatory due to the risk of semistarvation (fatigue, weakness, and lightheadedness) and related changes in vital signs (blood pressure, heart rate, and respiratory rate). Obese patients also often have obesity-related medical complications such as hypertension or diabetes, which require physician monitoring for appropriate adjustment of medication.

According to Blackburn, a physician can not only help obese persons lose weight, but also implement behavioral changes. He cautions that research is needed to define the medical criteria to determine when a dieter should be treated under psychiatric supervision, to identify persons at high risk for disability, morbidity, and death, and to determine what role adjunct treatments such as weight control drugs and gastric surgery should play. He emphasizes that stricter guidelines should be established for VLCD medically supervised programs, including indication for electrocardiograph, frequency of electrolyte monitoring, and required blood tests.

## RISK OF GALLSTONES

Overweight people develop gallstones at a higher rate than individuals of normal weight. The most common symptoms of gallbladder disease include cramping pain in the right upper abdomen, nausea, and fever. The pain may also be present in the back or shoulder.

The occurrence of gallstones in individuals 30 percent or more over desirable body weight (50 pounds or more overweight) not undergoing current treatment for obesity is estimated to be 1 in 100 annually, and for individuals who are 20 to 30 percent overweight, about 1 in 200 annually. One danger is that it is possible to have gallstones and not know it. Studies of individuals entering a weight-loss program have documented that one of 10 enrollees had "silent" gallstones at the onset.

Several recent studies cited in *Weighing the Options* report that very lowfat diets (less than 10 percent of calories) and rapid weight loss increase the incidence of gallstone formation and gallbladder inflammation. One study further suggested that the increased level of cholesterol in the bile was the cause of gallstones or "sludge" (a possible forerunner of stones) that developed in their gallbladders during the course of weight loss.

Individuals enrolling in a VLCD weight-loss program with one or more of the risk factors should discuss with their physician the need to test for gallstones, and whether they should take drugs containing bile salts which can aid in preventing gallstones.

## GLUCOSE, INSULIN RATIONS, AND SYNDROME X

Some obese people have a condition called insulin resistance which may contribute to Syndrome X, a set of symptoms linked with diabetes and heart disease. Insulin, a hormone that is secreted when a person eats, helps convert sugar (glucose), transferring it to the muscle cells, where it is used

| RISK FACTORS FOR GALLSTONES | |
|---|---|
| Age group | The risk increases with age, especially after the age of 30. |
| Blood lipid levels | The risk increases with the presence of iriglyceride levels and/or low HDL levels. |
| Cigarette smoking | Smoking doubles the risk. |
| Estrogens | Taking estrogen as female hormone replacement doubles the risk. |
| Recent abdominal surgery | Abdominal surgery within the last one to two years increases the risk. |

as fuel for muscle activity. In people with insulin resistance, the cells resist insulin's efforts to transport sugar into the bloodstream. One result is that more calories from blood sugar (glucose) are stored as fat instead of being burned as energy by muscles and tissues.

Most VLCDs attempt to normalize fasting glucose to insulin (G/I) ratios by lowering blood sugar levels in the blood. Dr. Rena Wing, in an article in the *Journal of the American Dietetic Association*, notes that VLCDs (400 calories daily) were more effective in normalizing G/I ratios than low-calorie diets (1,000 calories per day). She suggests that both weight loss and calorie restriction on a VLCD help decrease blood sugar levels.

## EXERCISE

Oprah Winfrey recently stated that she no longer believes in "crash diet" programs such as OPTIFAST because she subsequently regained the initial weight she had lost. She now believes that exercise is equally important as diet, and since March 1993, she has jogged eight to ten miles a day. Winfrey's experience suggests that exercise plays a crucial role in maintaining weight loss after a person has lost a substantial amount of weight.

All six VLCD programs analyzed in this chapter encourage their dieters to exercise moderately. Several encourage clients to exercise twice a day, once in the morning and once in the evening. The intervals during which a VLCD dieter is reintroduced to solid foods and begins exercise are very important. Eating three modest solid food meals daily (with two small snacks) evenly distributes the amount of energy available to the body throughout the day. If dieters phase their exercise between these three modest meals, they maximize the burning of calories.

### Incorporation of Exercise into VLCD Programs

| Program | Recommended? | Mandatory? | Individualized? |
|---|---|---|---|
| HMR | Yes | No | No |
| Weigh to Live | Yes | No | Yes |
| OPTITRIM | Yes | No | No |
| OPTIFAST | Yes | No | Yes |
| Medifast | Yes | No | Yes |

One important aspect of exercise is that it appears to encourage people to continue to eat less. Ninety-four dieters (65 females and 29 males) in one study by Phinny (1992) were exposed to different exercises while undergoing a twelve-week VLCD program. After twelve weeks, only 8 percent had dropped out of the diet program. Weight loss over the twelve weeks was directly related to participating in the exercise regime. A 24-week follow-up analysis showed a significantly better weight maintenance for patients who continued exercising.

In summary, exercise is important because:

1. It becomes a positive, healthy behavior serving as a replacement for the problem behavior.
2. It can be employed as a coping strategy to overcome difficult or tempting dietary situations.
3. It becomes a constructive means for managing stress, tension, and other negative emotional states that often lead to overeating.
4. It improves mood and a person's self-esteem.
5. It enables a person to consume a greater number of calories than otherwise would be possible.

## OTHER MEDICAL BENEFITS OF VLCD PROGRAMS

Weight loss is one of several important medical benefits of VLCDs. OP-TIFAST conducted a study of 517 of its dieters, for example, and found that successful dieters who lost weight also lowered their blood pressure and cholesterol levels. A similar study published by HMR, "The Total Health Approach to Sustained Weight Loss for Your High-Risk Patients," concluded that dieters who completed its program improved their glycemic control, lowered their blood pressure and cholesterol levels, and increased their longevity. Independent studies of similar VLCDs have indicated that average successful dieters reduce their blood pressure by 5 to 15 percent, their total cholesterol levels by 15 percent, their low-density lipoprotein-cholesterol by 5 to 20 percent, and their triglycerides by 15 to 20 percent.

# 6

## Commercial Weight-Loss Diet Programs

While Sybil Ferguson, Jean Nidetch, Jenny and Sid Craig, and Harold Katz are not exactly household names to most Americans, the commercial programs they founded — Diet Center, Weight Watchers International, Jenny Craig, and Nutri/System — have helped millions of people who could not lose weight on their own do so safely in a group environment which provides education, support, and encouragement.

Although the four programs differ in terms of eligibility, cost, duration, and approach, they share a belief that dieters will tend to be more successful in weight-loss efforts if they focus on making healthy lifestyle changes rather than focusing solely on meal planning. For this reason, all four offer portion-controlled, private-label food items that follow strict guidelines for fat, sodium, and nutrient content. In addition, these programs discourage rapid weight loss — counseling that one to two pounds a week is optimal — and provide a maintenance phase once clients reach their target weight that reinforces basic nutrition, exercise, and behavioral skills as food choices are expanded.

According to Spielman and Blackburn, the variation in cost per kilogram of active weight lost over a twelve-week period of each program appears below:

## Commercial Weight-Loss Diet Programs, Cost per Kilogram of Active Weight Loss (Twelve Weeks)

| Program | 80 kg (137% IBW f) (127% IBW m) | 91 kg (157% IBW f) (146% IBW m) | 114 kg (197% IBW f) (182% IBW m) | 136 kg (236% IBW f) (219% IBW m) | Extra costs (purchased outside clinic) |
|---|---|---|---|---|---|
| Diet Center | $9.00 | $8.00 | $10.00 | $12.50 | Most foods and beverages |
| Jenny Craig | $23.00 | $20.50 | $16.50 | $13.50 | Fresh produce, beverages |
| Nutri/System | $19.00 | $16.50 | $14.50 | $12.00 | Fresh produce, beverages |
| Weight Watchers | $2.50 | $2.00 | $2.00 | $1.50 | All foods and beverages |

## DIET CENTER

Diet Center was started by Sybil Ferguson. She had repeatedly lost and gained weight, much of it from crash dieting, until discovering (when scheduled for surgery) that she was malnourished. Ferguson, in consultation with her personal physician, designed her own weight-loss program and subsequently lost more than 50 pounds. Wanting to share her success with others, she founded Diet Center, Inc., in 1970. Currently, 650 Diet Center franchises exist in the U.S., Canada, Bermuda, Guam, and South America. The organization claims that at any one time approximately 19,500 people are enrolled in its various programs.

### Eligibility

Diet Center's Exclusively You Weight Management Program is designed for individuals 18 years of age and older; those who are anorectic, bulimic, or underweight are ineligible. People who have more than 50 pounds to lose, or who suffer from cancer, diabetes, emphysema, or gallbladder, heart, or kidney disease must obtain their physician's signature to ensure their condition does not contraindicate weight loss. Finally, while pregnant or lactating women may not be counseled for weight loss, they may with physician permission embark on a program for healthy eating.

## How to Join

All new clients, in meeting with a Diet Center counselor, first have their body fat analyzed by a computer. This is repeated every four to six weeks thereafter. It is this ratio of lean muscle mass to body fat — rather than the total number of pounds the client weighs — that forms the basis of the subsequently set goals. As a company spokesperson explains, Diet Center is not a formal food program per se (and, for example, offers the option of buying foods at the supermarket rather than purchasing Diet Center brand products), and is "moving away from the scale" in terms of reduction goals. Key to the program's success, she feels, is that clients help develop their own individualized program and target goals.

## Cost

Costs are variable, ranging from approximately $35 to $50 per week. The one-year maintenance is a one-time flat fee ranging from $50 to $200. Some centers charge additional one-time fees for all body composition analyses and adjustments in diet and exercise goals, as well as a registration fee.

## Basic Nutritional Approach

Diet Center's program follows the Food Guide Pyramid adopted by the U.S. federal government in 1992 (and paralleled by Canada's Food Guide to Healthy Eating), which recommends eating a diet high in complex carbohydrates and low in fat, sodium, and sugar. Diet Center discourages rapid weight loss and counsels its clients that after the first week, weight loss should not exceed two pounds per week.

The Exclusively You programs focus on reducing body fat instead of achieving a predetermined "ideal" number on the scale. A food-exchange system enables people to follow any Exclusively You program and incorporate the foods they enjoy into a balanced eating style. Counselors teach people how to make healthier buying decisions at the supermarket and adopt a lowfat cooking style that accommodates any Exclusively You program.

Clients are encouraged but not required to supplement their supermarket purchases with portion-controlled Diet Center brand foods that follow strict guidelines for fat, sodium, and nutrient content. These brand products also carry food-exchange equivalencies for all Exclusively You programs on their labels.

### Four-Phase Approach

Exclusively You consists of four phases:

Phase 1, Conditioning, lasts two days and is designed to help clients make the transition from their current eating habits to more healthy ones.

Phase 2, Reducing, lasts until clients reach their desired weight and ratio of lean to fat mass. (Diet Center emphasizes body composition, not pounds, as a measure of health and counsels that lean mass should not make up more than 25 percent of weight loss.) Clients select a variety of foods based on the Diet Center exchange system, from the starch, vegetable, fruit, protein, dairy, and fat/oil groups.

Phase 3, Stabilization, lasts six weeks and helps clients manage increasing their caloric intake while maintaining weight lost during the second phase.

Phase 4, Maintenance, lasts one year, during which time basic nutrition, exercise, and behavior skills are reinforced and dieters focus on weight maintenance as food choices are expanded.

### One-on-One Counseling

Diet Center's personal weight-loss trainers educate, guide, and support clients through one-on-one counseling sessions to help them achieve their individual weight-loss goals. These nonprofessional counselors, typically program graduates trained and certified by Diet Center, are linked to in-house registered dietitians through a toll-free telephone service. In addition, they receive ongoing counselor training through regularly scheduled workshops, monthly nutrition education publications, and videotapes.

While some franchises have established a link with local physicians, medical supervision is not normally offered.

### Special Programs

In addition to their standard reducing program, Diet Center also offers special plans for vegetarians, women over 45 years of age, and dieters with a lactose intolerance.

*The Vegetarian Program.* The Vegetarian Program provides a healthy eating guide for people who prefer to limit or eliminate their meat intake while working to lose or maintain their weight. It takes into account personal preferences of vegans (who strictly limit their diet to plant proteins only), ovovegetarians (who include eggs in their diet), lactovegetarians (who eat dairy products), and ovolactovegetarians (who incorporate both dairy products and eggs).

People following any of these customized eating plans are advised to receive regular counseling, follow their individualized exercise plan, carefully weigh and measure foods, and eat only the foods outlined by Diet Center. They also are advised to take a daily vitamin and mineral supplement. Diet Center estimates that 10 to 15 percent of its clients are currently following the vegetarian program.

*WomanStyle Program.* Diet Center offers a nutritional program specifically for women before, during, and after menopause called WomanStyle. It identifies six different phases of menopause, as well as hormonal changes common to each, and prescribes specific dietary regimens accordingly.

For example, the WomanStyle diet reduces protein amounts from animal sources to lean sources only; eliminates egg yolks to reduce dietary cholesterol; includes daily amounts of legumes to ensure high protein intake; and incorporates whole grains, fruits, and vegetables daily to increase fiber intake and reduce the risk of cardiovascular disease and breast cancer.

The diet further requires two servings from the dairy group and 800 milligrams of supplemental calcium citrate daily to enhance calcium absorption; and requires eight glasses of water a day to reduce the risk of urinary tract infections and skin dryness. It also prohibits alcoholic beverages to prevent depletion of calcium from the bones, and limits caffeine intake to one caffeinated beverage daily.

Finally, WomanStyle strongly encourages clients to maintain a program of aerobic exercise and strength-training to protect against cardiovascular disease and osteoporosis, improve blood cholesterol levels, and aid in digestion.

*Lactose Intolerance Program.* Diet Center also offers a special program that enables people who cannot digest lactose to omit or limit dairy products from their healthy eating style without compromising nutritional status.

## Alcohol

Because alcohol is the second most calorie-dense nutrient after fat, it is severely restricted on all Diet Center programs. Women are specifically encouraged to avoid alcohol because they are more sensitive to the impact of alcohol on blood pressure.

## Exercise

Diet Center recommends that all clients (especially those on the Woman-Style program) become involved in a consistent, lifelong program of exercise. As its literature emphasizes, regular exercise expends calories, and experts often cite it as critical for maintenance of weight loss.

## Behavior Modification

Diet Center claims that the emphasis of weight-loss efforts should be placed on long-term lifestyle change to support maintenance of the loss. It endorses this concept through an ongoing behavior management program called Exclusively Me that is designed to support the company's weight-management component. Diet Center counselors guide their clients through its completion.

Providing clients with an activity book (filled with tools and tips) and audiotapes, Exclusively Me actively involves people in designing personal solutions to losing and maintaining their weight that conform to their values and lifestyle. It also helps develop skills, such as preparing for high-risk situations and setting goals, and teaches strategies to positively deal with stressful circumstances.

## One-Year Maintenance Program

Upon attaining a healthy body composition, counselors custom design a computer-generated maintenance program that includes individualized diet and exercise recommendations. Clients gradually taper off their visits to Diet Center, while maintenance counseling reinforces the behavior management skills they have learned and focuses on overcoming maintenance obstacles (such as preventing relapses and avoiding self-sabotage situations).

Contact: Diet Center, 921 Penn. Avenue, Suite 500, Pittsburgh, PA 15222. (800) 333-2581; fax: (412) 338-8743.

## WEIGHT WATCHERS INTERNATIONAL

Weight Watchers International (WW) was founded in the early 1960s by Jean Nidetch, a 214-pound housewife from Queens, New York, who wore a size-44 dress and had become discouraged by years of fad dieting. She began inviting overweight friends over to her house each week for mutual support and sharing and, as they all lost weight together, realized that dieting alone is not a solution for long-term weight management.

Based on the key concepts of changing habits and getting encouragement from people in a similar situation, the company rapidly began to expand as former members who had successfully completed the program and undergone extensive training opened franchises throughout the U.S. and abroad. Weight Watchers became a wholly owned subsidiary of H. J. Heinz Company in 1978 for a purchase price of $72 million.

Since its inception, the company claims to have taught more than 25 million members how to lose weight. Currently, approximately one million people attend one of 29,000 weekly meetings in 24 countries. The majority — 600,000 people attending 15,000 weekly meetings — are in the U.S.

### Eligibility

Individuals who wish to join WW must be at least five pounds above the minimum weight for their height and age. Those who are taking medications, being treated for an illness, have an eating disorder, or are following a therapeutic diet to treat a disease are encouraged to consult with their physician before joining. A physician's written approval is required for pregnant and lactating women and children less than 10 years old.

### How to Join

Weight Watchers does not require members to sign any contracts upon joining. A registration fee (which is sometimes waived during promotions) and weekly fee are paid at the first meeting attended. From that point on, WW is a pay-as-you-go system with no continuing obligations. Members simply pay a weekly fee (which entitles them to unlimited meetings for that week) until they choose to discontinue their memberships.

Upon registration, members receive a stamped Membership Book in which weight (taken confidentially) and attendance are recorded each week. Only WW members can attend meetings, although guests are permitted on special occasions.

If they are unable to attend their usual weekly meeting, members may attend a meeting anywhere in the world by simply presenting a valid Membership Book and paying the weekly fee.

No personalized counseling is provided except in select markets.

## Cost

Weekly fees, payment methods, and promotional offers vary, although the average cost to join WW ranges from $14 to $17, while weekly membership fees average $10 to $14. Monthly meetings are free for Lifetime Members who have completed the WW maintenance plan and maintained their weight goal within two pounds. The prices of prepackaged foods also vary. Personal Cuisine averages $70 weekly, while Fat & Fiber Plan foods average between $3.00 and $3.50 per entree.

## Basic Nutritional Approach

The Weight Watchers program is based on the premise that to lose weight safely and sensibly, people must learn to eat more nutritiously, increase their level of physical activity, and successfully handle the challenges encountered in the process of behavior modification.

WW claims that its program was developed under the guidance and direction of obesity specialists including nutritionists, psychologists, and exercise physiologists, and that its food plans comply with the nutritional recommendations of many major health organizations in the U.S. and Canada. High in complex carbohydrates, moderate in protein, and low in fat, the food plans also encourage dieters to eat a wide variety of foods in amounts appropriate for healthy weight loss.

Over the years, Weight Watchers has increasingly encouraged members to customize their diet program. As head nutritionist Linda Kirili states: "Weight Watchers provides the map. Our dieters choose the road they want to take. I think what distinguishes our program is that we are flexible and we give dieters choices."

The WW program is designed to promote a gradual weight loss of up to two pounds per week (after the first three weeks when water loss may be a factor). Long-term participation is encouraged so members can attain and maintain their weight-loss goals.

## Three Food Plan Options

Weight Watchers offers three food plans: the classic Selection Plan, the Fat & Fiber Plan, and the Superstart Plan. Members can follow any of these plans based on their own personal needs and preferences, and also switch from one to another.

The Selection plan is a highly structured food exchange system in which people make certain selections from each food group and, in so doing, limit their calories and learn how to create healthy food habits. The Fat & Fiber Plan sets a maximum daily intake of fat grams and a minimum daily intake of fiber grams. By giving more control over which foods and how much food members eat, they learn to plan their meals and lose weight at their own pace. The Superstart Plan, which offers more rapid initial weight loss, is the most structured of the three because it prescribes precise amounts of specific foods which dieters must eat for all meals and snacks.

## Weight Watchers at Work Program

The Weight Watchers at Work program provides "on-site" weight-loss programs at major corporations for employees who attend meetings held either before work, during lunch hours, or after work. More than 1,800 companies in the United States, including many of the Fortune 500, now offer this option.

## Lifetime Membership

When members reach their goal weight, follow the WW maintenance plan for six consecutive weeks, and are no more than two pounds above their goal weight at the end of that period, they achieve Lifetime Membership status. This gives them the privilege of attending monthly meetings free of charge, as long as they stay within two pounds of their goal weight, to reinforce the weight control skills they have learned.

## Exercise

Weight Watchers contends that increased physical activity — over and above the normal routine — is an important component of weight management. Its Activity Plan, which is designed to enhance weight loss and help improve overall fitness and health, follows the recommendations of the Center for Disease Control and Prevention and the American College of Sports Medicine for physical activity. The three-tiered approach includes toning, stretching, and calorie-burning activities, as well as tips for exercising safely.

## Behavioral Modification

The Behavioral Support Plan offered by Weight Watchers is designed to teach members how to meet and overcome the personal challenges encountered at various stages of the weight-loss process. At the weekly meetings, discussions are held on such topics as staying motivated, managing stress, controlling emotional eating, and dealing with plateaus and setbacks.

## Group Support System

Weight Watchers considers its Group Support System the cornerstone or hallmark of its program, and offers this support through weekly meetings that are interactive and encourage hands-on learning through group activities and discussions. For example, meetings might include videos featuring nutrition and exercise experts, or strategy discussions with members who have learned how to lose and maintain their weight. The Group Support System continues throughout the maintenance period of the WW program when members learn how to stay within their goal weight range.

## Weight Watchers Product Line

Many mainstream consumers who may not be aware of the WW franchise program may nevertheless recognize the broad line of reduced-calorie, portion-controlled entrees, breakfasts, snacks, and desserts manufactured by the Weight Watchers Food Company, also an affiliate of H. J. Heinz, available in supermarkets nationwide. These items, designed to fit into the WW food plan, are part of the products and services offered under the WW trademark that also include cookbooks, exercise tapes, and a national magazine.

   Contact: Weight Watchers International, 500 North Broadway, Jericho, New York 11753. (516) 939-0400.

## JENNY CRAIG

The Jenny Craig weight-loss chain, which was founded in Australia by Jenny and Sid Craig, has expanded to more than 730 centers worldwide, 600 of which are in the United States. The Jenny Craig Personal Weight Management Program, according to company literature, offers a comprehensive approach to weight management, with an emphasis on safety and long-term weight maintenance. Clients learn to manage their weight by focusing on proper nutrition, exercise, and behavior change. These elements, combined with the desire of clients to achieve and maintain an attractive, healthy body, provide the basis for success.

### Eligibility

Jenny Craig does not accept people who are underweight, pregnant, suffering from celiac disease, diabetic (if they inject more than twice daily or are under 18 years of age), allergic to ubiquitous ingredients in the company's food products, or below the age of 13. People who have one or more of 18 specific medical conditions must obtain a doctor's written permission before enrolling. Regardless of their health condition, clients are encouraged to communicate with their personal physician throughout the duration of the program.

### How to Join

To join, prospective clients visit a local center where in consultation with a Jenny Craig counselor they are given a computer analysis of their current body weight and set up a reasonable weight-loss schedule — the goal being to lose an average of one to two pounds a week or 1 percent of their current body weight.

### Cost

Program fees vary by market, and can range from $99 to $299 depending on the options chosen (including inclusion of home audio- and videocassettes). Jenny Craig cuisine costs average $70 weekly, or $3.50 per meal.

### Weekly Consultations

Individual, mandatory weekly consultations are performed by Jenny Craig staff, who have been trained to implement the program as developed by health care professionals. The consultant's major responsibilities are to review Lifestyle Logs with clients, provide support and encouragement, and help clients solve individual challenges.

Corporate dietitians are also available to address individual client questions and concerns at no extra charge.

## Adolescent Program

Healthy children 13 to 17 years of age may enroll in the Jenny Craig Adolescent Program with parental permission. This 12-month program is based on the same nutritional, psychological, and exercise principles as the adult program, but includes a special menu plan and supporting educational materials designed specifically for the young client (e.g., a parental-managed reward system and strategies for managing peer pressure and handling popular snacks and fast foods).

## Basic Nutritional Approach

During the first half of weight loss, menu plans feature Jenny Craig cuisine, which includes shelf-stable and frozen, individually packaged entrées and snacks. In addition, menu plans include fresh fruits, vegetables, whole grains, and lowfat dairy products. Clients are also encouraged to drink eight 8-ounce glasses of water each day. The underlying rationale is that by following preplanned menus that include preportioned food, clients can focus attention on their eating behaviors.

When clients have attained half of their desired weight loss, they decrease their reliance on Jenny Craig foods, using them only five days a week. During the other two days, they plan their own nutritious, lowfat menus using a modified food exchange system. When clients reach their desired body weight, they gradually make the transition to seven days of self-planned menus.

In addition to regular meal plans (which are low in fat, sodium, and cholesterol), Jenny Craig registered dieticians have designed menu plans for diabetic, hypoglycemic, kosher, and breast-feeding clients, as well as for ovolactovegetarians and people who prefer not to eat red meat.

The Jenny Craig diet ranges from 1,000 to 2,600 calories daily, based on client needs. Meal plans are interchangeable, provided that exchanges are of equivalent caloric levels.

## Vitamin and Mineral Supplements

Jenny Craig offers its own vitamin and mineral supplement, CompleVite, to complement the menu plans. The supplement is not intended to replace healthful food, but rather to ensure that the RDAs for vitamins, minerals, and trace elements are met.

## Exercise

Jenny Craig considers exercise as essential to weight management success, and encourages clients to gradually become more physically active (based on their own baseline fitness level) on a regular basis. It provides guidebooks and other materials to help clients develop a safe, personalized exercise program, and advises them to participate in cardiorespiratory activities 3 to 5 times a week for 20 to 60 minutes at 50 to 80 percent of maximum heart rate. People are further advised to perform resistance activities two to three times a week. Walking is highly recommended for those who have been physically inactive, and the company provides audiocassettes and booklets to guide them in a stepped approach to building fitness. Clients are strongly encouraged to keep a daily record of their physical activity along with a daily food diary that is reviewed by their weight-loss counselor.

## Behavioral Modification

According to company literature, lifestyle modification is the cornerstone of the Jenny Craig program. By following a series of guidebooks, clients learn cognitive behavioral techniques for relapse prevention and problem management to help them achieve lasting lifestyle changes. Each of the major lifestyle factors that is integral to weight management — eating style, emotional eating, social situations, nutrition, and physical activity — is addressed.

In addition, individual consultations and interactive group classes help clients personalize and apply the information, while providing motivation and peer exchange. According to a company spokesperson, "All of the literature shows group support is very important for weight loss. That is the purpose of our classes."

## Maintenance

The twelve-month Lifestyle Maintenance Program, which begins when clients achieve their desired weight, is based on twelve guidebooks that address relevant issues such as dealing with a new body size, enjoying greater freedom with food choices, and maintaining the motivation to exercise.

Contact: Jenny Craig, 445 Marine View Avenue, Suite 300, Del Mar, CA 92014-3950. (619) 259-7000; fax: (619) 259-2812.

# NUTRI/SYSTEM

The present Nutri/System diet program was founded in the early 1970s by Harold Katz, a Philadelphia businessman who wanted to help his mother lose weight, in consultation with a physician and several nutritionists. Katz sold the company in 1986, and the current management group assumed ownership in 1994. Nutri/System currently has six hundred centers nationwide, most of which are franchised.

## Eligibility

Individuals who are pregnant, less than fourteen years old, underweight, or anorectic are not eligible to join, while written permission from a physician is required for lactating women and people with a variety of conditions, including diabetes (if insulin shots are required), heart disease (that limits normal activity), and kidney disease.

## How to Join

Those joining the program are not required to undergo a medical examination, although Nutri/System recommends that they consult their personal physician beforehand. After prospective clients attend an introductory meeting and undergo a free preliminary consultation, a general health assessment is administered (and entered into the company's proprietary computer system) to determine their eligibility (i.e., lack of medical risk) and any special dietary needs (such as reduced sodium or protein, or sugar or lactose intolerance).

After joining, clients undergo a second assessment to ascertain, based on their age, sex, and weight, their resting energy expenditure. From these calculations, Nutri/System designs a customized menu plan based on dieters' specific medical conditions and ideal goal weight (based on a one-to two-pound weekly weight loss). Nutri/System clients are weighed once a week, although this is not mandatory.

## Cost

The cost of Nutri/System programs varies because franchisees control their own pricing. According to Dr. Joseph J. DiBartolomeo, vice president of Scientific Affairs, the minimum cost to achieve goal weight is typically $99. Nutri/System also offers two full-service programs: the Assurance Weight Loss Plan and the Premier Weight Loss Plan (which gives purchasers the option of rejoining in the future for a preset fee). Both full-service programs include a Johnson & Johnson–developed "Real Solutions" wellness plan, maintenance materials, and a rebate (dieters get 50 percent of their money back if they maintain their goal weight for a year), and range in price from $249 to $399, depending on the geographical region.

A six-product line of vitamin and mineral supplements, an at-home cholesterol test, motivational audiocassettes, and exercise audio/videocassettes are not included in these costs, nor are the company's prepackaged meals, which average $49 a week.

## Medical Supervision

Although Nutri/System does not provide medical supervision at its local centers, registered dietitians are available through a toll-free number to address clients' questions. Its overall program is developed at the corporate level by staff dietitians, health educators, and doctors in consultation with a scientific advisory board. Weekly guidance is provided to clients by counselors with education and experience in psychology, nutrition, counseling, and health-related fields.

## Basic Nutritional Approach

The Nutri/System diet is built around its own private-label, prepackaged food items, referred to as the Nutri/System Menu Plan. There are more than 340 entrées, snacks, beverages, desserts, and fat-free salad dressings to choose from, many of which are individually portioned and portable for convenience.

Specifically designed to help achieve successful weight loss, the Nutri/System Menu Plan contains on a daily basis less than 100 milligrams of cholesterol, 58 percent of calories from carbohydrates (primarily complex carbohydrates), 2,000 milligrams of sodium, and 20 percent of calories from fat (compared to 42 percent in the typical American diet).

In addition to selecting foods each day from the Nutri/System Menu Plan while losing weight, dieters have the flexibility of choosing a certain amount of vegetables, fruits and fruit juices, condiments, and diet beverages. They are also counseled to drink a minimum of eight 8-ounce glasses of water a day and to take a vitamin and mineral supplement.

## Maintenance

Once clients reach their goal weight, as set when joining Nutri/System's program, they undergo a one-year maintenance program. During this period, reliance on company foods is gradually reduced to a minimum of two days per week.

## Real Solutions Program

Clients choosing either Nutri/System's Assurance or Premier Weight Loss Plan are entitled to the Real Solutions program, developed by Johnson & Johnson, to help people lose weight and develop healthier lifestyle habits.

This twelve-week program includes a personalized computer profile, information and motivational materials, and one-on-one counseling. Each week focuses on a particular area of health, including nutrition, exercise, stress management, blood pressure, cholesterol, salt, sugar, eating out, and home meal preparation, and how it contributes to weight loss. In addition, weekly goals are set that tie in with the area of focus, such as fitting more walking into the dieter's routine, adding fiber, reducing a risk factor that may cause high blood pressure, and finding a lower sodium alternative.

Contact: Nutri/System, 410 Horsham Road, Horsham, PA 19044. (215) 442-5411.

# 7

## Weight-Loss Support Groups

The two weight-loss organizations discussed in this chapter — Overeaters Anonymous (OA) and Take Off Pounds Sensibly (TOPS) — were founded for the sole purpose of helping people with eating disorders and/or weight problems. Key to their success, as articulated by a TOPS member, is that "We are a support group. We help each other help ourselves."

Unlike the commercial organizations described in Chapter 6, OA and TOPS, which collectively boast 330,000 current members in 47 countries, are both nonprofit. In addition, neither furnishes or recommends specific food plans, products, or diets, but rather promotes a sensible approach to weight control.

The primary method by which OA and TOPS members achieve their weight-loss goals is weekly group meetings that offer fellowship with, and encouragement from, people who also want to achieve control over eating patterns, their weight, and their lives in general.

### OVEREATERS ANONYMOUS

Overeaters Anonymous was started by three women in Los Angeles in 1960 to help them overcome their eating problems, despite failed attempts in the past. The program they created was — and continues to be — patterned after Alcoholics Anonymous. Today, OA is a worldwide fellowship of men and women from all walks of life who meet in order to help solve a common problem — compulsive overeating. OA claims to have more than 120,000 members in approximately 10,500 local chapters in 47 countries.

## Eligibility

There are no requirements for membership except the desire to stop eating compulsively.

## Cost

OA has no dues or fees for membership and is entirely self-supporting through contributions, events, and publications. Its international monthly journal, *Lifeline*, costs $12.99 a year. The nonprofit organization does not solicit or accept outside contributions, and most groups "pass the bucket" at meetings to cover expenses. No membership lists are maintained.

## Basic Nutritional Approach

The concept of abstinence (or the action of refraining from compulsive eating) is the basis of OA's program of recovery. By admitting an inability to control compulsive overeating in the past, and abandoning the idea that all people need to be able to eat normally is "a little willpower," it becomes possible for members to abstain from overeating — one day at a time.

For weight loss, OA does not furnish food plans or diets, counseling services, hospitalization, or treatment, nor does the organization participate or conduct research and training in the field of eating disorders. Any medically approved eating plan is acceptable.

And in contrast to other diets based on calorie counting or ones that permit and even encourage eating between meals by substituting low-calorie foods, OA simply limits food to three moderate meals a day with nothing in between except nonnutritive beverages. (Exceptions are made for medically prescribed eating regimens.)

## Group Support

OA believes that food and weight are only symptoms of deeper psychological problems and that most people use food as the alcoholic uses alcohol and the drug addict uses drugs. While a diet can help people lose weight, according to OA, it often intensifies the compulsion to overeat.

For this reason, OA offers the structure of a group environment that members can consistently rely on for unconditional acceptance and support. In their closed, weekly group meetings, members, by sharing their experiences in an atmosphere of respect and confidence, are given an opportunity to identify with others who have the same problem.

## Three Levels of Recovery

In OA, people recognize that they have a threefold illness — physical, emotional, and spiritual. They learn that they must strive for recovery on all three levels if they hope to maintain their weight loss and achieve a more satisfying way of life.

*Physical Recovery.* Compulsive overeating is viewed by OA as an illness that often manifests itself physically. Most dieters who enroll in OA have alternated for years between excessive eating and starvation diets and, as a result, have been steadily destroying their health.

*Emotional Recovery.* OA believes that many people overeat compulsively because they feel isolated and are unable to communicate their feelings fully and honestly. OA helps people understand that what they are doing is insulating themselves from reality and escaping through food.

In addition, OA has found that the longer a person has abused food, the greater the tendency to meet any disturbing situation or tensions with a food response. This circularity is what makes diet programs that focus on restricting foods fail, and why OA claims that its psychological/emotional approach has proven successful.

*Spiritual Recovery.* OA believes that the spiritual component of its program is particularly important because compulsive overeaters are unable to stop their self-destructive behavior. In OA, members admit that they are powerless over food and that a power greater than themselves can help them if they allow it. This greater power can range in interpretation from the concept of God to the OA group itself.

## Developing an Eating Plan

Some OA members find that following an eating plan simplifies their lives and frees them from on-the-spot decision making or facing food choices throughout the day. An effective plan might include specific foods and portions, and the elimination of known binge foods or foods compulsively craved. For others, an eating plan might be as simple as having a set number of moderate meals a day, or weighing and measuring all portions. Before choosing a specific eating plan, OA suggests that members consult a qualified professional.

## The Eight Tools of Recovery

OA has developed eight tools to help members toward their goal of recovery, although not everyone uses them all.

- Abstinence. As previously defined, abstinence is the action of refraining from eating compulsively. Upon recovery, the symptom of compulsive eating is removed on a daily basis.
- Sponsorship. Sponsors, who follow the tenets of the OA program to the best of their ability, help other members recover on all three levels — physical, emotional, and spiritual — by sharing their own experiences. A member may work with more than one sponsor and change sponsors at will.
- Meetings. Meetings are defined as gatherings of two or more compulsive overeaters who come together to share their personal experiences and the strength and hope OA has given them.
- Telephone network. OA encourages members to call their sponsors and each other on a regular basis (even daily) to avoid feelings of isolation, to ask for help, and to extend help to others.
- Writing. OA contends that by putting their thoughts and feelings down on paper, members can better understand their actions and reactions and see situations more clearly.
- Literature. Many OA members have found that reading and studying the organization's literature, including *Lifeline*, its monthly journal, gives them insight into their problem of eating compulsively and strength to deal with their problems.
- Anonymity. This principle ensures that only OA members have the right to make their membership known within their community. It also means that whatever they share at meetings will be held in respect and confidence, and that all members are equal.
- Service. Service is a key aspect of OA, springing from a belief that members begin to heal (i.e., abstain from compulsive overeating) when they reach out and serve others. The most fundamental form of service is carrying the message to other compulsive overeaters. This can range from getting to meetings to putting out literature or talking to newcomers.

### Suggested Actions to Promote Personal Abstinence

OA's suggestions to help members promote their abstinence are intended to instill conscious, healthful daily eating habits.

- Remember H.A.L.T. It is suggested that members not get too hungry, angry, lonely, or tired. They should particularly avoid skipping meals, which may tempt them to overeat later, justifying it as "making up for" that missed meal.
- Enjoy your meals. OA contends that abstinence releases the pain and guilt accumulated over many years of overeating. Members are encouraged to relax and to take the time to enjoy their meals.
- Be conscious of the amount of food eaten. Some members purposefully do not take second helpings at meals, because overeating often begins with "just a little bit more."
- Follow a predetermined weighing plan. Many members have found that weighing monthly is advisable. Frequent weighing or refusal to weigh can put too much emphasis on physical recovery alone.

### The Twelve Steps

Although OA has no religious requirement, affiliation, or orientation, its twelve-step program of recovery — similar to that of Alcoholics Anonymous — is considered spiritual because it deals with inner change. The twelve steps are intended to guide members to individual recovery.

### 1992 OA Membership Survey Results

In its 1992 membership survey, nearly 1,700 OA members in the U.S. answered a variety of questions that were subsequently analyzed by the Gallup Organization. These are some of the results:

- 45 percent of respondents said they began eating compulsively before the age of 12.
- When asked what they liked most about participating in OA, 51 percent listed fellowship, sharing of experiences/group discussion of feelings/hearing about others' experiences, support, understanding/caring/loving people, and acceptance.
- The average amount that respondents were overweight when joining OA was 68.1 pounds.

- The average amount of weight respondents lost after joining OA was 40.8 pounds.
- Of the 30 percent of respondents who reported reaching a comfortable weight, the average maintenance time was 3.97 years.
- 93 percent of respondents reported improved emotional/mental health since joining OA.
- 94 percent of respondents reported a "higher" or "much higher" level of self-esteem since joining OA.

Contact: World Service Office, 6075 Zenith Court, Rio Rancho, NM 87124. (505) 891-2662; fax: (505) 891-4320.

## TAKE OFF POUNDS SENSIBLY (TOPS)

TOPS is a nonprofit organization founded in 1948 by Esther S. Manz, an overweight housewife, in the kitchen of her Milwaukee home. TOPS defines its purpose as threefold: to aid the overweight in attaining and maintaining their physician-prescribed weight goals through group support and fellowship; to promote a sensible approach to weight control; and to encourage undertaking a dietary regimen only after consultation with one's personal physician.

TOPS claims to have almost 310,000 members in 11,700 chapters in 20 countries, mostly the U.S. and Canada. Members include men, women, and children.

### Eligibility

According to TOPS, anyone who sincerely wishes to cure their problem of overeating can join the organization. The only requirement is attending a weekly meeting (the first of which is free with no obligation to join) and filling out a simple application form with the assistance of a TOPS member.

### Cost

Membership fees total $16 annually for the first two years ($20 in Canada) and $14 annually thereafter ($18 in Canada). The fees cover the cost of *Top News,* a monthly magazine on health and nutrition that features inspirational stories, recipes, and coverage of TOPS chapter activities around the world. Local dues are set by each chapter (which can consist of as few as four members) to cover expenses, and are normally less than $5 a month.

## Basic Nutritional Approach

Like OA, TOPS is nonprofit and noncommercial, and does not accept advertising in its monthly membership magazine. TOPS also does not sell, promote, or endorse any weight-loss products, nor does it recommend specific diets, or restrict or eliminate certain foods. It does, however, promote a sensible approach to weight control (incorporating, for example, food planning, limiting portion sizes, and eating less sugar and fat) and recommends that members consult with their personal physicians to determine a realistic weight-loss goal and timetable, as well as an exercise plan (which are then submitted in writing).

TOPS also publishes *A Nutritional Monograph for Taking Pounds Off Sensibly* that contains a detailed exchange system for meal planning, as well as practical advice on such topics as eating patterns, exercise, fast foods, and fiber. Also featured are menus for dieters consuming 1,200, 1,500, and 1,800 calories daily ranging from breakfasts to salads and soups, entrees, and desserts. (However, TOPS members are not required to buy the book or follow its suggestions.)

## Weekly Meetings

TOPS weekly meetings function as the primary method by which members achieve their weight-loss goals, and are characterized by a spirit of competition in losing and keeping off weight. All meetings start with a mandatory and confidential weigh-in. Records are kept, with weight "losers" becoming eligible for awards and prizes. They are honored at chapter, area, and state levels; the greatest weight losses are recognized at the annual international conference.

Members also trade information on lowfat recipes, and sometimes listen to advice from a guest speaker, such as a dietitian, about a variety of health-related weight-management topics — including self-esteem. In keeping with the organization's nonendorsement policy, speakers are forbidden to promote products of any kind.

A recent meeting in Wisconsin, for example, addressed "closet anxiety," the fear of having to decide what to wear. As the leader of the chapter explained, "People need to look nice while they are losing weight, and not wait until they've reached their goals. You end up wearing the same old thing and worrying about how you look. You have to reward yourself for the little things."

As another TOPS member in St. Petersburg, Florida, articulated, when asked to explain the importance of the weekly meetings, "We are a support group. We help each other help ourselves."

While programs vary from chapter to chapter (with volunteer leaders elected from the membership to direct and organize activities for one year), all in some way provide members with positive reinforcement and motivation in adhering to their individual food and exercise plans.

## Exercise

While TOPS does not require that members undertake a specific exercise regime, exercise — particularly walking — is highly recommended as an adjunct to weight loss.

## Behavioral Modification

TOPS relies on group support, lively meetings, and materials to positively encourage dieters to lose weight and maintain their weight loss. Members who maintain their goal weight loss for three months are honored as KOPS (Keep Off Pounds Sensibly) members. And because staying at goal weight can also be challenging, TOPS meetings provide information and support for members at this level as well.

## Medical Research

TOPS's financial support of medically oriented activities began in 1966 with the funding of an obesity and metabolic research program at the Medical College of Wisconsin in Milwaukee. To date, according to TOPS, $4.5 million from TOPS earnings (over and above operating expenses) and members' contributions have helped fund these research efforts. Findings from the program have been published in more than 140 papers in medical journals. TOPS members are currently taking part in a landmark research project examining the role of genetics in obesity.

Contact: TOPS International Headquarters, 4575 South Fifth Street, P.O. Box 07360, Milwaukee, WI 53207-0360. (800) 932-8677.

# 8

---

# Over-the-Counter
# Botanical Diet Programs

According to *Alternative Medicine: The Definitive Guide,* several herbs or botanical formulas have proven effective in weight loss, including (-) hydroxycitric acid (HCA) and ephedra, commonly known as mahuang. This chapter reviews two over-the-counter (OTC) weight-loss programs. CitraMax All Natural-Diet Plan contains HCA extracted from *Garcinia cambogia,* a tropical fruit; and Thermogenics Plus uses ephedra, aspirin, and caffeine. Both appear to depress the appetite, reduce food consumption, and accelerate the body's metabolic rate (the speed at which it burns nutrients, especially fat). Both should be used under the supervision of a physician or herbalist to minimize the risk of side effects.

## CITRIMAX ALL-NATURAL DIET PLAN

The CitriMax All-Natural Diet Plan, currently marketed by the Inter-Health Company, emphasizes moderate fat and alcohol consumption, increased intake of fiber and fluids, and regular exercise. The dietary supplement upon which it is based is an "all-natural plant extract rich in (-) hydroxycitric acid." This extract, originally formulated by Dr. John M. Lowenstein of the Department of Biochemistry at Brandeis University, is derived from *Garcinia cambogia* (also known as brindall berry), a plant native to southern Asia, primarily India. There it is used as a spice (in preparing curries and condiments, for example), a food preservative, and a digestive aid. It is also considered effective in making meals more filling.

According to InterHealth literature, while CitriMax serves as an appetite suppressant, it does not do so by stimulating the central nervous system, which can cause side effects such as insomnia, nervousness, depression, hypertension, and an accelerated heart rate. Rather, as its name implies, CitriMax HCA is closely related in structure to the citric acid found in fruits such as oranges, lemons, and limes. By increasing the body's capacity to store glycogen, thereby enhancing the body's satiety signal to the brain, HCA curbs appetite and reduces food intake.

InterHealth further claims that the HCA contained in CitriMax reduces fatty acid synthesis by approximately 40 to 70 percent for 8 to 12 hours following a meal. As a result, less LDL cholesterol and triglycerides are produced and stored.

## Eligibility

InterHealth cautions that individuals under medical supervision should seek the advice of their physician prior to starting any weight-loss or exercise program. In addition, CitriMax should not be used with diets supplying less than 1,000 calories per day without medical supervision.

## Basic Nutritional Approach

The CitriMax All-Natural Diet Plan combines store-bought foods with its HCA-based herbal formula that the formulators recommend be taken in doses of between 250 and 1,000 milligrams three times daily, 30 to 60 minutes before meals. (CitriMax contains 50 percent HCA. Thus 500 milligrams of CitriMax equals 250 milligrams of HCA.)

InterHealth provides the following guidelines to safely and effectively lose excess pounds and maintain an ideal weight:

- Limit calories and eat nutrient-rich foods high in lowfat proteins and complex carbohydrates to maintain lean muscle tissue, increase energy, and encourage maximum fat loss.
- Add fiber to your diet to help reach satiety or "fullness" more quickly. Fiber also helps to improve regularity and carry off undigested fats and cholesterol. Lightly cooked vegetables and whole grains are an excellent source of fiber.
- Eat five to six times a day, including lowfat meals and between-meal snacks. More frequent eating of moderate-size meals and healthy snacks stimulates metabolism and helps burn calories during the digestive process.
- Drink 8 to 10 eight-ounce glasses of water each day. Water rids the body of waste products and reduces water retention.

- Keep fat intake as low as possible. Thirty percent of total calories is an absolute maximum; 10 to 25 percent is preferable for weight loss.
- If alcohol is consumed, limit intake to one or two drinks per day.
- Chew your food thoroughly for a maximum feeling of satiety, as well as for better digestion.
- Take a good multiple vitamin/mineral supplement daily to ensure complete nutrition.

## Sample Menu Plan

CitriMax also provides a sample three-day menu plan based on the Exchange Lists for Meal Planning developed by the American Diabetes Association and the American Dietetic Association. Each day's menu plan totals 1,250 calories. The sample menu for Day 1 includes:

### Day 1

**Breakfast:** One slice of toast, one cup of nonfat yogurt, and one-half cup of fruit.

**Midmorning snack:** Three graham crackers and one-half cup of orange, apple, grapefruit, or pineapple juice.

**Lunch:** One-half cup of water-packed tuna, one large sliced tomato, green salad with one tablespoon of salad dressing, and four crackers.

**Midafternoon snack:** One large apple.

**Dinner:** Eight medium lemon-broiled scallops or shrimp, one-half cup of steamed broccoli, and one medium baked potato with one teaspoon of butter or margarine.

**Dessert:** Two fat-free cookies with one cup of nonfat milk.

## Exercise

The CitriMax Diet Plan advises people to get 20 to 30 minutes of light aerobic exercise daily, such as medium-paced walking, which trains the body for greater metabolic efficiency and fat burning.

## THERMOGENICS PLUS WEIGHT-LOSS PROGRAM

One popular botanical weight-loss product, marketed in capsule form and manufactured by Silver Sage, is called ThermoGenics Plus. Its ingredients include mahuang (standardized to 8 percent alkaloids), bissey nut (standardized to xanthine, calculated as caffeine), vitamin C, Siberian ginseng, aspirin, willow bark, wintergreen, cayenne, pantothenic acid, ginger root, zinc, manganese, and selenium.

## Eligibility

Pregnant and lactating women, or women planning to become pregnant, are cautioned not to take ThermoGenics Plus. In addition, people using MAO inhibitors, and those with high blood pressure, a history of cardiovascular or thyroid disease, prostrate problems, or diabetes (or people using medications for any of these conditions) are advised to take this or any similar product only under the supervision of their physician. People sensitive to aspirin or stimulants such as caffeine or aspirin are warned to avoid it as well.

## Basic Nutritional Approach

The ThermoGenics Plus plan is designed to reactivate the body's natural fat-burning process. Its formulators recommend taking one capsule at breakfast with 8 to 10 ounces of water the first and second days. On the third day, dieters are advised to take one capsule in the morning and one at noon with a full glass of water. On the fourth day, people should take two capsules in the morning and one at noon with water. Three capsules per day is the maximum dosage, with dieters advised to only take the capsules five days at a time, followed by two days off. Also, to avoid restlessness, people should not take ThermoGenics Plus after 3 P.M.

## Dietary Guidelines

To become more healthy while burning fat, ThermoGenics Plus advises people to eat at least three meals each day and to not under any circumstances skip meals. The formulators suggest it is better to consume five or six small meals a day, if possible, because this will provide constant fuel and energy to the body and help maintain the dieter's metabolic rate. People are also advised to drink four to eight glasses of water a day, which is essential to burn fat, and to minimize or eliminate the amount of caffeine-containing beverages consumed while taking ThermoGenics Plus.

## Recommended Foods

It is recommended that people following the ThermoGenics Plus weight management plan keep fat calories at 30 percent or less of total daily intake. Recommended foods include lean turkey or chicken breast, fish or very lean red meat, vegetables, fruits, baked potatoes (with limited butter or other high-fat toppings), pasta, and rice.

## Eliminated Foods

ThermoGenics Plus suggests eliminating high-carbohydrate foods before bedtime, and avoiding fried foods and the addition of oil to foods.

## Exercise

ThermoGenics Plus states that exercise is beneficial to maintaining basic health, and recommends aerobic exercises such as walking, cycling, or jogging for 20 to 30 minutes at least three times a week. The formulators advocate maintaining a consistent pace (rather than overdoing exercise) and suggest that people allow their body temperature to cool at least two hours after exercising before consuming ThermoGenics Plus. The capsules should also not be taken for at least three hours before exercising.

## RECENT RESEARCH

The two major types of over-the-counter botanical formula described in this chapter — lipogenic and thermogenic — appear to help people, especially obese persons, lose weight and maintain their weight loss. More research is needed, however, to conclude that either lipogenic or thermogenic formulas effectively accelerate the burning of white or brown adipose tissue (fat). It should also be noted that HCA and ECA formulas have not completed clinical testing required by the FDA for approval.

There is indirect evidence that ephedra-based formulas may be effective, however. Ephedra contains botanical ephedrine, a stimulant that suppresses the appetite. Synthetic ephedrine, a laboratory-produced stimulant resembling botanical ephedrine, has proven extremely effective for weight loss in several clinical studies. P. A. Daly and colleagues at Harvard Medical School (as described in the February 1993 issue of the *International Journal of Obesity and Related Metabolic Disorders*), studied the safety and efficacy of a mixture of 75 to 150 milligrams of ephedrine, 150 milligrams of caffeine, and 330 milligrams of aspirin. The ephedrine-caffeine-aspirin (ECA) formula was divided into premeal doses and given to 11 of 24 obese individuals, all of whom continued to consume their normal diets in a randomized, double-blind trial. The group that took the ECA formula lost three times as much weight over the course of the eight-week trial as those who took a placebo.

After the trial concluded, one participant subsequently lost more than 120 pounds over a thirteen-month period using a combination of the ECA formula and a self-imposed, calorie-restricted diet.

The researchers concluded that "in all studies, no significant changes in heart rate, blood pressure, blood glucose, insulin, and cholesterol levels were observed, and no differences in the frequency of side effects were found. ECA in these doses is thus well tolerated in otherwise healthy obese subjects, supports modest, sustained weight loss even without prescribed caloric restriction, and may be more effective in conjunction with restriction of energy intake."

## EC and Lean Muscle Mass

While EC (ephedrine-caffeine) and ECA formulas have been shown to be effective in weight loss, some researchers were concerned that much of the weight lost was lean body mass. S. Toubro and colleagues, of the Research Department of Human Nutrition, Royal Veterinary and Agricultural University, Copenhagen, Denmark, report in the February 1993 issue of the *International Journal of Obesity and Related Metabolic Disorders* that, in fact, EC has lean-body-mass conserving properties. In a randomized, placebo-controlled, double-blind, eight-week study of obese subjects, they found that a combination of ephedrine (20 milligrams) and caffeine (200 milligrams) "is effective in improving and maintaining weight loss, and further has lean body mass saving properties. The side effects are minor and transient and no withdrawal symptoms have been found."

## EC and HDL Cholesterol

Another group of researchers from the Royal Veterinary and Agricultural University subsequently studied the effect of the same EC formula on HDL cholesterol and plasma triglyceride levels. They reported in the May 1994 issue of the *International Journal of Obesity and Related Metabolic*

*Disorders* that thirty-two obese women were given either the EC formula or a placebo three times a day for eight weeks.

While no effect was seen on plasma triglyceride concentration in the placebo group, a decrease was observed in those taking the EC formula. Further, HDL cholesterol concentration was decreased in the placebo group, while the EC formula did not decrease HDL levels. The researchers concluded that "EC combinations abolish the decline in HDL cholesterol during active weight loss due to the beta-agonistic properties of ephedrine."

## PRESCRIPTION WEIGHT-LOSS DRUGS

Several other prescription drugs have also proven effective in weight-loss experiments in the U.S. and Europe. These drugs, either approved or in development for treating obesity, appear to decrease energy intake, increase energy expenditure or thermogenesis, stimulate lipolysis, or decrease fat and other macronutrient absorption. Current FDA regulations, however, prevent their widespread use in the U.S.

The safety and effectiveness of one prescription drug, dexfenfluramine (DF), was compared with an EC formula in a research trial conducted by L. Breum and colleagues at the Royal Veterinary and Agricultural University in Denmark. The trial was reported in the February 1994 issue of the *International Journal of Obesity and Related Metabolic Disorders.*

In the double-blind, 15-week study of 81 subjects who were 20 to 80 percent overweight, 43 received 15 milligrams of DF twice daily while 38 received 20 milligrams of ephedrine/200 milligrams of caffeine three times daily.

Those who took the EC formula had a greater mean weight loss, losing approximately 20 pounds, while the DF group lost an average of approximately 15 pounds. Systolic and diastolic blood pressures were similarly reduced in each group, while both reported side effects. Central nervous system side effects, especially agitation, were more pronounced in the EC group, whereas gastrointestinal symptoms were more frequent in the DF group.

As noted, more clinical research is needed to confirm the safety and effectiveness of HCA and ephedra-based weight-loss products. Pending FDA approval, these products should be used with caution, carefully monitored on a day-by-day basis, and used as only one component of a comprehensive weight-reduction program that includes attention to diet, exercise, and behavioral modification. Furthermore, dieters contemplating the use of a botanical formula should consult with their health care provider to determine if they have any medical conditions that put them at risk.

# 9

## Popular Book Diet Programs

Judging from the number of books and magazine articles extolling various revolutionary weight-loss programs, dieting would appear to be the American national pastime. Surveys indicate that among adults in the United States, 50 to 70 percent of women and 25 to 40 percent of men are on reducing diets. About the same percentages hold for teenagers.

We asked this book's Medical Advisory Board to recommend for review current popular diet books not discussed in other chapters. The Board's suggestions included *The McDougall Program for Maximum Weight Loss* by Dr. John McDougall; *The Carbohydrate Addict's Diet* by Dr. Richard and Rachel Heller; *Enter the Zone* by Dr. Barry Sears; Covert Bailey's *The Fit or Fat Target Diet*; Dr. William and Sonja Connors' *The New American Diet*; *Outsmarting the Female Fat Cell* by Debra Waterhouse; and *Stop the Insanity* by Susan Powter. One cookbook was highly recommended, *In the Kitchen with Rosie* by Oprah Winfrey and Rosie Daley. It is briefly reviewed at the end of the chapter. A list of other exemplary cookbooks appears in the References and Resources section.

### THE MCDOUGALL PROGRAM FOR MAXIMUM WEIGHT LOSS

Dr. John McDougall, a northern California physician, has conducted diet and weight-loss clinics since 1983. His diet program appears in *The McDougall Program for Maximum Weight Loss*.

#### Basic Nutritional Approach

In Chapter 1, "Never Be Hungry Again," McDougall states that his low-cholesterol diet is "for people who have a single overriding priority: to get rid of unattractive excess weight and keep it off permanently." He details a study he conducted of 574 people who attended his live-in program at St. Helena Hospital and Health Center in Napa Valley, California. In eleven days, overweight men (weighing more than 200 pounds) lose on the average 8.3 pounds while women who weighed over 150 pounds lost an average of 4.4 pounds. Based on his study, McDougall suggests that dieters who follow his program "can expect to lose between 6 and 15 pounds a month" and experience "greater vitality, mental clarity, and self-esteem."

## Recommended Foods

McDougall's diet is rich in complex carbohydrates and fiber, low in protein and fat, and free of animal foods. Recommended foods include:

- all whole grains and whole-grain cereals: brown rice, corn, oatmeal, barley, millet and wheat berries, packaged grain cereals, puffed grains, and other healthful cereals
- acorn, butternut, buttercup, pumpkin, and zucchini varieties of squash
- root vegetables such as carrots, potatoes, sweet potatoes, and yams
- legumes such as peas, split peas, black-eyed peas, string beans, chickpeas, lentils, adzuki beans, navy, pinto, and black beans
- green and yellow vegetables including collard greens, broccoli, kale, mustard greens, cabbage, lettuce, watercress, celery, cauliflower, carrots, and asparagus
- fruits, especially apples, bananas, berries, grapefruit, oranges, peaches, and pears (limited to two servings per day)

## Restricted or Eliminated Foods

While stressing the importance of fruits, vegetables, and nonsalt and non-sugar spices in his diet, McDougall eliminates the following foods:

- all oils, including olive, safflower, peanut, and corn oil
- all red meats, including beef, pork, and lamb, which are rich in fat, cholesterol, and other harmful substances
- all poultry and fish, which have the same amounts of cholesterol as red meat
- all eggs (high in fat and cholesterol)
- all dried fruit and fruit juices high in sugar

- all processed flour products, such as non-whole-grain breads, bagels, and pretzels, which are often composed of grain fragments and small particles that increase absorption and retard weight loss
- all dairy products, including milk, yogurt, and cheese, all of which are high in fat and cholesterol
- nuts, seeds, avocados, olives, and soybean products, including tofu, soy cheese, and soy milk. Soybean products are high in fat unless they have been specially processed. (Lowfat varieties also are not recommended by McDougall.)

Essentially, McDougall recommends a high-carbohydrate, high-fiber, lowfat all-vegetarian diet because this nutritional combination makes insulin work more efficiently and decreases the amount of insulin needed by the body. Fat foods, on the other hand, he suggests "dramatically increase insulin production." Refined foods such as white bread, white pastas, and white rice, for example, move rapidly into the blood and cause a surge of insulin production. Sugar produces an even greater exaggerated insulin response.

According to McDougall, the following factors elevate insulin levels: obesity, high-fat foods, sugar-refined foods, infrequent meals, physical inactivity, diabetes, some prescription pills, and insulin injections. To stabilize insulin levels, McDougall's diet advises dieters to 1) eat until satisfied; 2) graze: eat small, frequent meals; 3) allow time for digestion; 4) chew foods thoroughly; and 5) restrict variety — make a meal of only one starch, one vegetable, or one fruit. McDougall cites several studies that show that people consume more calories in a meal consisting of a variety of foods.

McDougall's diet encourages the consumption of large quantities of nutrient-rich foods plentiful in proteins, carbohydrates, essential fats, vitamins, and minerals. He suggests that 11 of the 13 vitamins are made by plants and his diet is rich in foods which supply these 11 essential vitamins. Vitamin B12 is only available in meats, soy, and grains, and thus dieters who follow his all-vegetable diet should take a vitamin B12 supplement.

To motivate dieters to change their behavior long enough to realize how good they feel on his diet, McDougall outlines in the chapter "Establishing a Healthy Way of Life" a series of behavioral steps to help his dieters overcome their fear of failure.

The final component of McDougall's diet plan is a rigorous exercise program. He recommends aerobic exercise and weight training. He suggests getting up a half hour earlier each day or skipping a TV program to do his exercise program. Any aerobic exercise will work — he specifically recommends walking, bicycling, tennis, swimming, water aerobics, or weight training at home — and dieters are urged to exercise four times a week.

## THE CARBOHYDRATE ADDICT'S DIET

Dr. McDougall, like the authors of several others reviewed in this book, argues that a high carbohydrate (55 to 70 percent) diet is best for preventing chronic disease and losing weight. Interestingly, several diet books have directly challenged this theory.

Dr. Richard and Rachel Heller, cofounders of the Carbohydrate Addict's Center at Mt. Sinai Medical Center in New York City, believe that certain people are genetically predisposed to become "carbohydrate addicts" — that is, the more carbohydrates, the more they crave — and this addiction makes weight loss virtually impossible. Their low-carbohydrate diet, which permits one carbohydrate meal a day, appears in *The Carbohydrate Addict's Diet*.

The Hellers were both overweight and experimented with many different diets. "Personally and professionally," they write, "we discovered that any weight-loss diet that prescribes three or more small meals each day containing anything more than minor amounts of carbohydrates will fail with the carbohydrate addict. Such a diet will trigger the insulin response and signal the carbohydrate addict to eat once again."

In 1983, as they explain, they founded the Center for Weight and Eating Control to test a low-carbohydrate diet with 6,000 members of Overeaters Anonymous and more than 800 members of Weight Watchers. They designed a dynamic eating plan that allows dieters to eat daily Complementary Meals and Reward Meals in combinations that help them to greatly reduce their hunger for carbohydrates while they lose weight and permanently maintain the weight loss.

Each week dieters on the Hellers' program follow an eating plan based on the amount of weight they lost that week and the amount of weight they want to lose in the upcoming week. Their diet takes into account all factors that influence a person's response to dieting, including age, gender, metabolic rate, and activity level.

The Hellers' Carbohydrate Addict's Diet provides five plans (entry plan and plans A, B, C, and D) that consist of various combinations of

Complementary Meals and Reward Meals. Each plan has a different effect on a person's weight loss.

Clients beginning the Carbohydrate Addict's Diet follow the entry plan for two weeks. They weigh themselves every day and record their weight. At the end of two weeks, dieters are usually able to see obvious weight-loss results. They then choose plan A, B, C, or D to follow in the coming week in order to meet their weight-loss or weight-maintenance goal. Each week the diet guide helps them select the most appropriate diet plan based on how much weight they have lost.

## Basic Guidelines

According to the Hellers, basic guidelines for dieters include:

1. Eat complementary meals daily. When dieters keep the fiber intake high, fat low, and carbohydrate intake low during their Complementary Meals, their body responds by producing and releasing less insulin. Less insulin means less hunger, fewer cravings, and a feeling of satisfaction. Best of all, lower insulin levels stimulate the body to metabolize (burn) storage fat.

2. Eat a Reward Meal every day. Dieters are permitted to eat one Reward meal once per day. All foods are allowed, although the Hellers suggest that it should be nourishing and well balanced. Eating a high-carbohydrate meal once a day actually helps to keep carbohydrate insulin levels normal.

3. Complete the Reward Meal within one hour. The important thing is timing. According to the Hellers, the second phase of insulin release occurs approximately 1 1/2 hours after the dieter begins eating. This release comes from a reading made by the body as to how much carbohydrate the dieter has eaten at that meal. Dieters may eat whatever they desire in whatever quantity they wish, but they must complete the Reward Meal within one hour.

4. Consume all alcoholic beverages during the Reward Meal. The Heller diet permits alcoholic beverages such as beer, wine, and cocktails as long as they are enjoyed during the Reward Meal.

5. Do not snack between meals. According to the Hellers, even small quantities of carbohydrates, such as a piece of fruit, can stimulate insulin release and reverse the whole metabolic process that is emptying the fat cells. Thus, they stress that on their diet *nothing* can be eaten between regularly scheduled meals.

The Hellers state that in most cases obesity is caused by eating the wrong foods in the wrong amounts at the wrong time. This imbalance produces unstable amounts of insulin in the blood. Although they concede that obesity may be caused by a number of different disorders, insulin imbalances are almost always involved. They explain that when a normal person consumes carbohydrates for a prolonged period of time, additional insulin is released in proportion to the amount of carbohydrates eaten at that particular time. In the average healthy person, just enough insulin is released to help deliver the carbohydrate energy (in the form of the blood sugar glucose) to the liver and to muscle or fat cells throughout the body. As the cells take in glucose, the level of insulin in the blood drops. This drop causes the release of the brain chemical serotonin, which produces a feeling of satisfaction and reduces hunger.

Obviously, the balance of carbohydrates and insulin is critical. Consuming high amounts should stimulate insulin levels to decline and appetite *should* be quelled. But, according to the Hellers, within a few minutes of eating carbohydrates, the carbohydrate addict's body releases far more insulin than is necessary. This overabundance interferes with the normal absorption of glucose, and one result is that excess insulin remains in the bloodstream. Because insulin levels do not decline, brain levels of serotonin do not increase, and carbohydrate addicts remain hungry, craving more food. Some addicts, for example, report that they feel like eating again several hours after consuming a very large meal. If they later attempt to satisfy their hunger by eating more carbohydrates, their next insulin release will be even greater and the sense of satisfaction decreased. The repetition of this cycle forms the physical basis of what the Hellers call "carbohydrate addiction."

In general, the Heller diet allows clients to eat two high-fiber, lowfat, low-carbohydrate meals daily and to confine their carbohydrate-rich foods to one daily sitting that makes up the third meal. In this way, they believe the fundamental mechanism causing excessive hunger, recurring cravings, and weight gain is corrected because insulin release is dramatically reduced as serotonin levels are simultaneously increased. The addict feels satisfied and stays satisfied for many hours. Weight drops off naturally, fat deposits decrease, and the addictive cycle is broken.

In summary, the Hellers state, "We have found that by consuming only one carbohydrate-rich meal per day, the carbohydrate addict experienced less intense hunger and fewer cravings as well as significantly greater weight loss." They explain that this appears to be caused by: 1) a lowered insulin production and/or release; 2) an increase in carbohydrate receptor sites due to the decrease in insulin, with an accompanying increase in the rate at which insulin is removed from the blood. Thus, if carbohydrate addicts change the number of times they consume carbohydrates each day, they can reduce the intensity and recurrence of hunger and cravings and increase their body's tendency to lose weight.

The Hellers claim that more than 80 percent of their clients successfully lose weight and maintain their weight loss on this diet. They believe they discovered an important treatment for weight loss through their research, which proves that it is not only the *amount* of carbohydrates consumed that matters but the *frequency* with which they are consumed during the course of a day. They are currently pursuing other avenues of research involving triglyceride levels and cholesterol levels in relation to frequency of carbohydrate intake.

## THE ZONE SPORTS DIET

The three sports performance diets reviewed in Chapter 14 suggest that carbohydrates should be the main ingredient (60 to 70 percent of calories) of the diets of competitive athletes. Most sports nutritionists believe that carbohydrates should be the major fuel supply for endurance athletes, especially those in high-intensity sports. Protein enjoys the next most favored status due to its role as a muscle builder. The third major dietary element, fat, has the notoriety of a villain.

Nevertheless, Barry Sears, an endocrinologist, advocates a relatively low carbohydrate diet for athletes: 40 percent carbohydrate, 30 percent protein, and 30 percent fat. What is more, Sears claims his diet produces weight loss. Sears's diet, which appears in *Enter the Zone,* is designed for weight loss, improving competitive sports performance, and preventing chronic disease.

While a researcher at MIT, Sears developed cancer drugs that could be delivered in foods. He discovered that certain fatty acids associated with natural lipids formed the building blocks of "eicosanoids." "Eicosanoids," he writes, "are involved in virtually everything the body does," and he conjectures that many chronic diseases such as heart disease, diabetes, arthritis, and cancer might be the result of imbalances among the eicosanoid hormones. Virtually every disease state "can be viewed at the molecular level as the body simply making bad eicosanoids and fewer good ones."

Optimal health requires a balance of good and bad eicosanoids —

**135**

what Sears calls "the zone." He argues that if dieters stay in the zone, they reduce the risk of chronic disease conditions such as obesity, heart disease, cancer, diabetes, depression, and alcoholism. Each disease, he cautions, has a genetic potential for expression, although eating to stay in the zone dramatically decreases the likelihood that these genes will be expressed. "The further you are from the zone," he writes, "the more likely these genes will be expressed. In the zone you'll have greater access to stored body fat (instead of stored carbohydrate) for energy. You'll also benefit from greater mental concentration, which will not only help you be more productive, but it will improve your physical performance as well. If you follow a 'zone-favorable' diet, you will go to the zone faster and stay there for the rest of your life."

According to Sears, a "zone-favorable" diet is a diet in which the balance of macronutrients (protein, carbohydrate, and fat) is tightly controlled for every meal and snack throughout the day. As noted, Sears's diet provides 40 percent carbohydrates, 30 percent fat, and 30 percent protein. It is relatively high in fat because Sears believes fat is the chemical building block for all eicosanoids. Protein and carbohydrate levels are balanced because they control the insulin-glucagon axis, which in turn determines whether the eicosanoids your body makes are "good" or "bad." Sears suggests that if a person consumes a diet too rich in carbohydrate (the 60 to 70 percent carbohydrate diet now recommended by many health-oriented organizations), his or her body will make more "bad" eicosanoids. The reason, he explains, is because overconsuming carbohydrates causes an overproduction of insulin which imbalances blood sugar levels. This prevents the metabolism (burning) of stored body fat and ultimately leads to disease. Excess carbohydrate consumption, Sears contends, like the Hellers, drives a person out of the zone — out of a balanced carbohydrate to fat to protein ratio.

### Sports Performance Diet

Sears states that he had an opportunity to work in 1992 with the Stanford men's swim team coached by Richard Quick and Skip Kenny. At the Olympic trials in Indianapolis, six Stanford swimmers qualified for the Olympic team, not surprisingly to Sears, all of them following a zone-favorable diet. Sears cites a number of athletes who have used the zone diet to win competitions.

The best formula is a 40/30/30 carb/protein/fat diet combined with aerobic exercise, the best form of which, according to Sears, is walking. The higher the intensity of exercise, the more hormonal responses are affected. Specifically, higher-intensity aerobic exercise reduces insulin levels and increases glucagon levels — exactly what the zone-favorable diet does.

## Sears Weight-Loss Diet

A favorable balance of eicosanoids means that you are releasing more stored body fat from the adipose tissue. Thus, when people stay in the zone, they set the conditions for maximal fat release and burn more carbohydrates.

Sears offers the following advice for weight-loss dieters:

1. Eating fat does not make you fat. It is your body's response to excess carbohydrates in your diet that makes you fat. The body has a limited capacity to store excess carbohydrate but it can easily convert excess carbohydrate into excess body fat.
2. It's not hard to lose weight simply by restricting calories. Eating less and losing excess body fat do not automatically go hand in hand. Low-calorie, high-carbohydrate diets generate a series of biochemical signals in the body that take you out of the zone, making it more difficult to access stored body fat for energy. As a result, dieters reach a weight-loss plateau, beyond which they cannot effectively lose additional weight.
3. Diets based on calorie counting and restriction usually fail. People on restrictive diets get tired of feeling hungry and deprived. They stop dieting, put the weight back on (primarily as increased body fat), and then feel bad about themselves for not having enough willpower, discipline, or motivation.
4. Weight loss has little to do with willpower. By adhering to a diet of zone-favorable meals, dieters can eat enough to feel satisfied and still lose fat — without obsessively counting calories or fat grams.
5. Foods can be good or bad: the ratio of macronutrients (protein, carbohydrate, and fat) in the meals is the key to permanent weight loss and optimal health. The important thing is to stay in the zone.

Sears contends that there are other hormonal rewards that derive from exercising in the zone: the "good" eicosanoids help dilate the blood vessels, increasing the transfer of oxygen from the blood to the muscles. Thus, once a person is in the zone (where oxygen transfer is increased), they can stay in aerobic metabolism for longer periods of time even during periods of increased exercise demands. And as they exercise with higher levels of intensity, they begin to create the hormonal changes that are the real fruits of exercise, just as hormonal changes are the real power of nutrition.

The cardinal nutritional rule for staying in the zone, Sears concludes, is to "maintain a beneficial ratio of protein to carbohydrate every time you eat. Every time you open your mouth, you must have the right combination. My diet is contrary to everything the American public has been told about healthy eating. It may seem like a radical approach, but it has thirty years of endocrinology behind it."

## OUTSMARTING THE FEMALE FAT CELL

The Outsmarting the Female Fat Cell weight-control program specifically designed for women was developed by Debra Waterhouse, a nationally known dietitian and weight counselor. Her program is outlined in her best-selling book *Outsmarting the Female Fat Cell.*

Waterhouse states in the first page of her book that hers is a weight-loss plan, not a weight-loss diet. Her book, she states, has two major purposes:

1. To provide an understanding of how female fat cells function
2. To provide the solution to permanently outsmarting female fat cells and achieving a comfortable weight

According to Waterhouse, men and women have approximately 30 billion fat cells which are capable of storing 150-plus pounds of fat. Both men and women have about the same number of cells, although women have more lipogenic enzymes, which means they store fat more easily. And the more fat they store, the bigger their fat cells become. Men have more lipolytic enzymes, which means they release (metabolize) fats easier and faster. As a result, their fat cells are smaller in size.

Waterhouse explains that estrogen, the female sex hormone, appears to activate and multiply lipogenic enzymes, which explains why some women develop more body fat during puberty, pregnancy, and while taking oral contraceptives or undergoing estrogen replacement therapy. Estrogen not only stimulates the lipogenic enzymes to store fat, but it also causes fat to be stored in a woman's buttocks, hips, and thighs.

When men gain weight, it's more likely deposited in the waist area (they have apple-shaped bodies) because of the effects of the male sex hormone, testosterone. Women gain weight first and take it off last in the hips and thighs, and have pear-shaped bodies. Fat cells in the lower body are larger and have more lipogenic-storing enzymes. As a result, women who begin dieting and exercising usually lose fat first from the upper half of their bodies.

Body types also tend to be hereditary. Apple-shaped bodies tend to run in families: their abdominal fat cells tend to be smaller and contain more lipolytic enzymes, which cause more rapid weight loss. Compared to "pears," women with apple-shaped bodies respond more quickly to exercise and positive eating habits.

Having explained these essential fat-storing and burning processes, Waterhouse emphasizes that dieting actually sabotages a woman's attempt to lose weight. Dieting, she writes, "is the female fat cell's best friend" because it *increases* the size of a woman's fat cells, *improves* her body's ability to store fat, and *limits* its ability to burn it. Men's fat cells, on the other hand, react differently to dieting. When men go on a traditional diet, they can more efficiently lose weight and keep it off; as a matter of fact, they are twice as likely to keep excess weight off. Men also have about 40 percent more muscle cells containing calorie-burning structures called mitochondria that convert calories to heat and water. The more muscle cells a person has, the more calories are directed to the muscle cells to be burned and the less to the fat cells to be stored.

According to Waterhouse, when a woman diets:

1. The lipogenic enzymes are increased, which causes her to store more fat. She states that most studies show that low-calorie diets at least double the lipogenic storage enzymes — and women already have more storage enzymes than men, and dieting doubles them.
2. The fat-releasing lipolytic enzymes in women are decreased by 50 percent; women already have fewer lipolytic enzymes than men, and dieting cuts them in half.
3. Her fat cells become bigger, while her muscle cells become smaller and weaker. The less muscle, in turn, slows down her metabolism. The fewer calories she burns, the more fat she will store, and the more weight she will gain. Each time a woman diets, the fat loss is not permanent; her muscle loss, however, may be permanent. Each time she goes off a diet and back to her old eating habits, the

weight she gains back is not muscle but fat. A woman can eventually replenish the lost muscle mass — but only by exercising, not by dieting.

Given these warnings about women dieting, Waterhouse outlines a six-step OFF plan which she says will switch female fat cells off because they are directly opposed to what switches fat cells on:

| Switching fat cells on | Switching fat cells off |
|---|---|
| Inactivity | Aerobicize fat cells |
| Dieting | Stop dieting and start eating |
| Overeating | Feed your body, not your fat cells |
| Skipping meals | Shrink and multiply your meals |
| Nocturnal eating | Become a daytime eater |
| High-fat intake | Fat-proof your diet |

Exercise, according to Waterhouse, is the most important of these steps. To permanently and successfully outsmart female fat cells, regular aerobic exercise and the OFF plan eating strategies constitute the winning combination for making fat cells smaller. Exercise will ensure fat release, and eating habit changes will prevent fat storage. By exercising 45 minutes at a moderate intensity three times a week, dieters will condition their stubborn fat cells to release fat and shrink their fat cells.

Waterhouse stresses two essential points, also emphasized by Susan Powter: in order for women to lose weight, they must *eat and exercise.* Female dieters, however, should not eat before sleeping. And preferably, they should eat six small meals instead of three large meals. Overeating any food, Waterhouse warns, will lead to larger fat cells, but overeating fat will lead to the largest fat cells of all — about 25 percent larger than carbohydrates and proteins. Fat increases fat cell size and also is not the preferred energy source for the body to function most efficiently; carbohydrates are the best source for all of the organs and cells.

Waterhouse argues emphatically that "there really is no good fat." If it is not linked to heart disease, it's linked to cancer. Like other authors in this book, she recommends reducing fat intake to 20 percent to significantly reduce the risk of heart disease and cancer and to reduce weight; and less than 10 percent to reduce the risk of all diseases and to lose weight.

## THE NEW AMERICAN DIET

One of the most comprehensive heart disease diet plans, the New American Diet, developed by Dr. William and Sonja Connor, appears in their book of the same title.

Dr. William Connor, a medical doctor in private practice, began in the early 1960s researching the effects of lowfat diets on reversing coronary heart disease. He was one of the original developers of the lowfat, high-complex carbohydrate diet. In the early 1970s he published pioneering research which showed that reducing dietary fat and blood cholesterol levels by following his New American Diet could prevent, and in some cases, reverse, coronary artery disease. He proved that "significant atherosclerosis and the diseases that follow from it will not occur if blood levels of cholesterol can be maintained at between 160 and 180 milligrams per 100 milligrams or lower over much of the lifetime of the individual." Even in the event, however, that moderate to advanced atherosclerosis has already set in, Connor states that his diet can lower blood concentrations of cholesterol enough to help "prevent further damage and even reverse some of the existing damage over a period of time."

The Connors' book outlines their lowfat, low-cholesterol, high-carbohydrate diet. They suggest that if average Americans would adhere to their diet, more than 1 million could prevent heart disease. The Connors believe that their New American Diet program could save "far more lives because of its additional protective effects against cancer, hypertension, and diabetes." The Connors intensively studied all diseases of over- and underconsumption and deliberately formulated a unified dietary approach that combats them all. Their diet, they claim, "has the best possible combination of all foods and nutrients, given the current state of knowledge on how to prevent atherosclerosis and coronary heart disease, stroke, hypertension (high blood pressure), diabetes mellitus, several forms of cancer, and a number of other disorders. It is, in addition, ideally suited for gradual weight loss and long-term weight maintenance."

Nevertheless, a diet that people reject is not useful. The Connors believe that what sets their New American Diet apart is that it was designed to be acceptable to people of all kinds for their entire lifetimes, not just for a few weeks or months. They tested their diet on 233 families as part of their Family Heart Study, and found that after five years only 10 percent of families and 20 percent of individuals had discontinued the diet.

The specific objectives of the New American Diet are

- cut average cholesterol consumption from 400 to less than 100 milligrams daily;
- reduce fat intake to 20 percent of daily calories;
- decrease saturated fat intake to 5 to 6 percent of daily calories;
- increase carbohydrate intake to 65 percent of daily calories;
- decrease the intake of refined sugars to 10 percent;
- cut salt intake substantially.

The Connor diet consists of three major phases:

**Phase 1: Substitutions**
- avoid egg yolks, butterfat, lard, and organ meats (liver, heart, brains, kidney, gizzards);
- substitute soft margarine for butter; vegetable oils and shortening for lard; skim milk and skim milk products for whole milk and whole-milk products; egg whites for whole eggs;
- trim fat off meat and skin from chicken;
- choose commercial food products lower in cholesterol and fat (lowfat cheeses, egg substitutes, soy meat substitutes, frozen yogurt, etc.);
- modify favorite recipes by using less fat or sugar and vegetable oils instead of butter or lard;
- decrease use of table salt, and use lower sodium salt (Lite Salt).

**Phase II: New Recipes**
- replace meat and cheese with chicken and fish;
- consume meat, chicken, or fish only once a day;
- restrict fat in spreads, salads, cooking, and baking;
- consume more grains, beans, fruits, and vegetables;
- choose lowfat, low-cholesterol foods when eating out;
- reduce consumption of salt.

**Phase III: A New Way of Eating**
- consume meat, cheese, poultry, shellfish, and fish as "condiments" to other foods rather than as main courses;
- eat more beans and grain products as protein sources;
- use only 4 to 7 teaspoons of fat daily as spreads, salad dressing, and in cooking and baking;
- drink 4 to 6 glasses of water daily;

- limit extra meat, regular cheese, chocolate, candy, coconut, and commercially prepared food to special occasions (once a month or less);
- enjoy a wide variety of new foods and food combinations;
- continue to decrease the daily amount of salt consumed.

*The New American Diet* includes sample one-week meal plans for each of the three phases of their diet program. It also provides numerous other meal and recipe suggestions, including many snacks, fast-to-prepare meals, as well as more exotic, gourmet fare. Part 2 includes chapters on weight loss and weight maintenance, eating out, entertaining, holidays, camping trips, pregnancy and breast-feeding, feeding of infants, and vegetarians. It also explains how dieters can test themselves for cholesterol and other blood fats as well as for high blood pressure.

The Connors conclude their book by stating: "The New American Diet embraces the concept of preventive nutrition. The earlier in life it is adopted the better. But it can be started at any age after weaning and still deliver significant, measurable benefits. And this is true whether an individual is healthy or already afflicted by one of these diseases. The diet can help halt the onslaught or, in many cases, even reverse some of the damage of disease, but clearly, its greatest impact is in the prevention of disease."

## THE FIT OR FAT TARGET DIET

Covert Bailey was one of the first diet formulators to stress the integral interrelationship between exercise and weight-loss diets. His research on the importance of a lowfat diet and aerobic exercise weight loss appears in *The Fit or Fat Target Diet,* one of the all-time best-selling diet books, with more than 4 million sold. Through his books and PBS TV series, Bailey has helped millions of Americans lose weight and maintain weight loss.

Bailey states in Chapter 1, "Diets Don't Work," that his Target Diet is not a diet but a *system* for evaluating foods, diets, and menus. In Chapter 3, he states, "To achieve a perfect diet, you need obey only four rules: 1) be sure to eat a balanced diet; 2) select foods that are low in fat; 3) select foods that are low in sugar; and 4) select foods that are high in fiber."

If you follow these rules, he adds, "You needn't worry about cholesterol, saturated fats, vitamins, trace minerals, or most of today's other nutritional concerns. You don't even have to worry about preservatives or other additives in food. In short, observe the four basic rules, and the rest comes without asking."

According to Bailey, balancing the diet is the rule most often neglected, and the most important, because it underlies all of his nutritional considerations. "We must eat a variety of foods in order to be certain that we get the full variety of nutrients. No single food or group of foods contains everything we need. Therefore taking the most level-headed approach, we should eat from a wide selection of foods from four main groups: meats and dairy products, vegetables, grains, and cereals."

Bailey's diet features a tear-out target sheet which can be taped to the refrigerator. To help illustrate his rules of lowfat, low-sugar, high-fiber, inner circles are added to the Four-Food-Group circle, making it into a target. Foods are graded until the best ones (lowest in fat) in that group are in the center of the target and the worst selections are on the periphery. All the foods above the center line (the meats and milks) are graded according to their fat content. According to Bailey, very fat people should eat from the bull's-eye only. The less fat can add the next ring of foods, and the very fit can get away with limited peripheral selections. "If everybody ate from the Target Diet," Bailey writes, "we would bring about 90 percent of the dietary change that is needed. The myriad books on bran, mixing and matching proteins, and vitamin supplements are superfluous."

Bailey emphasizes that his target diet actually provides for most of today's other dietary requirements as well, because it is:

| | |
|---|---|
| Low in fat | Low in saturated fats |
| Low in sugar | Low in cost |
| Low in calories | Highly storable |
| Low in salt | High in fiber |
| Low in additives | High in nutrient density |
| Low in cholesterol | A balanced diet |

Bailey says his diet allows him to eat a lot of food, thus satisfying his desire to "pig out." His diet does not ask him to go hungry. "I am able to eat any foods I happen to enjoy, as long as they are near the center of the target. In fact, once you get used to the target diet, you will have no feeling of denial at all."

Bailey states that everyone needs to consume vitamins and minerals, and whether one needs to take supplements will depend on what they eat. Dieters who consume natural foods on his diet, however, "can get more than enough vitamins and minerals and decrease the empty-calorie fats, sugars, white flour, and alcohol that are making us fat."

> ## FAT
>
> As the title of his book suggests, Bailey believes America's number one enemy is fat — fat in our bodies and fat in our diets. And exercise is the key to fighting it, although its benefits go way beyond simple weight loss. It's not weight that most Americans need to lose, Bailey insists, it's fat. "Fat is almost exclusively burned in muscle. It cannot be melted, dissolved, or magically erased. The only way fat is burned is when it is released from the blood to be carried to muscles. If the muscles don't burn the fat, it returns to be stored again in another fat depot. The only way you are ever going to lose weight on a fat-loss program is if your muscles burn the fat. Following the Target Diet," he adds, "will maximize the body's ability to metabolize fat."

Bailey says most people should be concerned about their percentage of body fat, not their total weight. "You can weigh 250 pounds and be virtually all muscle and bone," he quips, "or weigh 100 pounds and be overfat."

Bailey's book cites new research from England that the exercised body develops cycles in which it actually dissipates calories (burns fat), even in the absence of body movement, possibly through the production of heat. Such cycling, according to the researchers, may persist for two or three days after exercise or even more. These cycles may contribute to other beneficial effects of exercise noted recently by Swedish scientist Per Bjornstrop, who has documented that exercise has a positive effect on obese people even when they are on unrestricted diets. Exercise, according to Bjornstrop, decreases hyperinsulemia, hypertension, and high blood fat levels. Thus, when exercising, even obese people undergo a "metabolic rehabilitation."

Bailey argues that aerobic exercise causes a hypermetabolic state in which the body burns fat more effectively than if on a calorie-restricted diet. Like Waterhouse, he points out that when people diet, they usually lose muscle as well as fat. "It's not total body weight that is important," he argues, "it is total fat weight. For one thing, muscle tissue weighs more than body fat, which means that a person covered with muscle, such as a bodybuilder, could conceivably weigh more than someone who is largely flab. Therefore, losing total weight is the wrong goal. Dieters should instead concentrate on burning fat and building muscle."

Elderly people, especially women, have the most difficult time shedding fat. The reason has to do with their basal metabolic rate and their tendency to try to lose weight by diet alone. People who drastically restrict their caloric intake will lose fat, but also muscle mass.

Bailey concludes by stating he hopes his Fit-or-Fat Target Diet will encourage all Americans to exercise. "I've already affected 2 or 3 million people," he notes, "and I would like to get another 10 million if I can." He cautions that only 10 percent of Americans are exercising. Nevertheless, Bailey is optimistic, because the level used to be 5 percent. "Probably 90 percent of the public knows that they should exercise," he writes. "If you ask people on the street if exercise is as good as it's cracked up to be, most will say yes. All of them know that it helps to control weight, and most people can list a dozen other benefits. Those who used to exercise will tell you that when they did, they felt better, slept better, were less intense, and that they wished they could get started again."

## STOP THE INSANITY

More than 95 percent of people on standard weight-loss diets regain all lost weight within one year. This suggests that 95 percent of all dieters at some time feel they are failures.

Failure — the inability to regain control of weight and eating behavior — is the central theme of Susan Powter's *Stop the Insanity*. After her divorce, Powter says, she fell into a "fat coma" that left her overweight, unfit, and depressed. She tried many starvation and deprivation diets, but none of them worked. "I was a 260-pound housewife," she writes, "feeling desperately out of control, afraid, hurting physically and emotionally, trying every diet out there, and failing."

Powter asserts that she knew her lifestyle was damaging her mentally and physically. She was suffering from depression and hated the way she looked and felt. *Stop the Insanity* is her story about how she broke the cycle of depression, overeating, dieting, and guilt.

The importance of her book is that she has firsthand experience with many weight-loss diets, all of which, she says, *initially* helped her lose weight. She successfully lost weight for good by eating modest amounts of nutritious foods (2,300 calories per day) at regular intervals and exercising.

According to Powter, the turning point in her life came one day when, frustrated with her weight and feeling low in energy, she determined to go outside and just walk. In fact, she only walked back and forth on her driveway for thirty minutes. But that was sufficient, she writes, to get enough oxygen into her lungs that she felt calmer and more energized. Eventually, daily exercise produced enough oxygen to energize her to change her life — and she did. Quite remarkably.

*Stop the Insanity* does not present a weight-loss diet, but rather a weight plan, because, Powter adamantly states several times, "Diets do not work. Stop dieting forever. Dieting is the wrong way to lose weight. Starving yourself is not the way to lose weight. There is no diet on earth that works."

Powter has been criticized for being too judgmental of weight-loss diets in general. Clearly, some weight-loss diets, including calorie restrictive diets, work. Patients can lose weight. But the question is, as Powter, Debra Waterhouse, Covert Bailey, and many others correctly ask: How much weight does one lose safely; for how long; and what type of weight is lost — muscle or fat?

Powter herself lost more than 130 pounds by eating enough nutritious lowfat foods to give her energy each day to exercise. She advises dieters to start by limiting themselves to 30 percent fat in daily calories. She recommends that dieters start by counting the fat grams of "everything you put into your mouth." She explains how to calculate fat grams per serving and stresses the importance of eating a balanced diet. She quotes Covert Bailey's *The New Fit or Fat* and suggests that if dieters eat a balanced diet, they will easily get enough protein and fat.

## Recommended Foods

Powter arranges her balanced diet in what she calls a "high-volume, lowfat, high-quality food pyramid," which consists of

1. *whole grains:* brown rice, bulgur, long grain rice, millet, wild rice, and kasha;
2. *legumes:* beans, peas, and lentils;
3. *vegetables:* green leafy vegetables, spinach, broccoli, asparagus, carrots, zucchini, squash, eggplant, okra, mushrooms, and peppers;
4. *processed grains and starches:* corn tortillas, whole-wheat bread, whole-wheat pita, cereals, bagels, English muffins, and oatmeal;
5. *fruit:* Bananas, oranges, apples, pears, grapes, melon, berries, and plums;
6. *very lean protein options:* fish (except salmon, mackerel, and bluefish), white chicken, white turkey, and egg whites.

She recommends eating foods from each group and stresses the importance of eating high volumes of lowfat foods. She lists whole grains first in her pyramid because they are the foundation of her eating program: "Whole grains give your body the nutrients it needs to be well. They will supply you with the highest-quality fuel your body can get. Low in fat, high in complex carbohydrates, protein, and fiber — that's it. That's how to change the way you look and feel. The easiest and fastest way to change your body is to eat the highest-quality, lowest-fat, highest-volume foods. And you can't get better than whole grains."

Powter's diet is not strictly vegetarian because white chicken, white turkey, and egg whites are permitted in limited amounts. Nevertheless, Powter herself does not eat much meat. "Beef," she states, "is a high-fat, low-volume, saturated-fat food, no matter how the beef industry wants you to look at it. If it's meat you want, white meats are your lean protein options, but remember, Mr. Bean is stronger, better, and leaner and will cause you less heartache (pardon that pun)."

## Exercise Recommendations

Exercise is an integral part of Powter's weight-loss "wellness" program because she believes it is the only way to transform fat-storing cells into fat-releasing cells. Like Waterhouse and Bailey, she explains how exercise causes fat to be transported to muscle cells where it is metabolized (burned). Powter's recommended exercise program thus focuses on changing both fat and muscle physiology. Exercise increases muscle mass and doubles the efficiency of the mitochondria in muscle cells to burn fat. The only way people can permanently lose weight is to constantly minimize the amount of fat they consume and maximize the amount they burn by building muscle.

Because she was herself once overweight, Powter understands how difficult it is for many people to start exercising. Many dieters complain that they don't have the energy to get up and move. Powter explains that dieters must break this cycle: they must consume enough nutritious lowfat foods, preferably grain protein, to have the energy to exercise thirty minutes every day.

She states that a typical exercise workout should include:

- *Aerobics:* moving in oxygen for 30 minutes or more, 5 to 6 times a week. As you become more fit, increase your level of intensity with pace, range of motion, and with the addition of resistance (as with hand-held weights)

- *Strength-training:* moderate weightlifting and calisthenics every other day
- *Flexibility:* stretching
- *Breathing exercise:* at least 100 deep breaths a day

Powter's book has struck a sympathetic chord with many dieters because it teaches a fundamental truth: the fastest, easiest, and safest way to lose weight permanently is to regularly eat high-volume, lowfat foods (mostly grains) *and* exercise. When she was 260 pounds overweight and looking for answers, she says, she had nowhere to turn. "The American Heart Association had the research," she writes, "the four-color posters, the experts, and the controlled study groups, but they didn't reach me. A single, fat, depressed housewife living in Texas didn't understand what they were talking about. I didn't know how to apply what they were saying to my life. It was too complicated." Powter's book can help many overweight Americans who face the problems she faced. The beauty of her book is that it is engagingly funny and uncomplicated.

## OPRAH WINFREY'S COOKBOOK

Whatever the merits of any diet, they still must be translated into daily food plans, menus, and recipes that individuals can enjoy eating day after day. Unfortunately, the word "diet" has come to have a pejorative meaning for many people because it suggests denial, restriction, or limitations. To go on a "diet" usually means to voluntarily put oneself on a starvation regimen of little plates of plainly prepared, sparse, bare vegetables. Not surprisingly, the mind rebels at such a thought.

Nevertheless, the word "diet" can just as easily conjure up images of regal banquets of exotic soups, decorative salads, homemade breads, elegant entrees, and chocolate cheesecakes for dessert. It all depends at whose house you're dining. And who's in the kitchen.

In Oprah Winfrey's case, as she details in her book *In the Kitchen with Rosie,* it was a delightful gourmet chef named Rosie Daley whom Winfrey met while visiting a weight-loss spa. Winfrey loved Daley's lowfat creations so much she begged Daley to move to Chicago to become her personal chef.

*In the Kitchen with Rosie* includes some of Oprah Winfrey's favorite lowfat diet dishes created by Daley. In her introduction, Daley stresses that lowfat meals can be gourmet delights. The secret, she says, is to purchase only fresh foods, cook them without any fat, flavor them with exotic spices, and serve them in elegant, decorative ways. She advises dieters to familiarize themselves with the herbs she uses as substitutes for fat and to read her recipes all the way through before preparing ingredients.

*In the Kitchen with Rosie* is a cookbook and does not provide detailed dietary guidelines or recommendations for an exercise program. Winfrey, however, has stated that she personally has benefited from combining exercise with lowfat dieting. She exercises every day. The value of Winfrey and Daley's beautiful book is the practical way it compresses nutrient-dense, lowfat food recommendations into specific food plans and recipes. It's easy to read, and the food selections are not difficult to prepare. Were more people to read their book, it would be a small wonder if we didn't all become lowfat gourmets. The References and Resources section includes a list of other cookbooks recommended by the Medical Advisory Board.

# Part Three

# 10

## Diets for Women

As professor Henry Higgins lamented in the famed musical *My Fair Lady*, "Why can't a woman be more like a man?" Indisputably, the two sexes differ in significant biological ways — perhaps most notable being the hormonal processes women undergo during menstruation (which depletes them of essential minerals such as calcium, zinc, and iron), lactation, and menopause. In addition, women generally have slower metabolic rates than men, as well as a greater number of fat cells and less muscle mass.

The obvious differences between male and female body chemistries have recently sparked new research into the unique nutritional needs of women, and led to the development of the two diets reviewed in this chapter. The Super Nutrition Diet, designed by Ann L. Gittleman, advises women to increase their intake of calcium-rich foods, add a moderate amount of essential fatty acids, and decrease consumption of high-fiber carbohydrates. Elizabeth Somer's Healthy Woman's Diet is a lowfat, nutrient-dense diet that emphasizes consumption of fruits and vegetables, complex carbohydrates, and calcium-rich foods to maintain optimal health.

### SUPER NUTRITION FOR WOMEN

Ann Louise Gittleman was formerly director of nutrition at the Pritikin Longevity Center in Santa Monica, California. She also served as chief nutritionist of the Pediatric Clinic at Bellevue Hospital, New York, for the USDA's Women, Infants, and Children Food Program. She is a nutritional consultant for preventive medicine and environmental health clinics throughout the U.S., and serves as chairperson of the Department of Nutrition of the American Academy of Nutrition. In her book *Super Nutrition for Women,* Gittleman, who has reviewed more than seven thousand diet histories throughout her career, outlines what she considers is "the first scientifically based dietary program that takes into account a woman's special body chemistry and unique nutritional needs."

## Basic Nutritional Approach

Gittleman believes that popular high-carbohydrate, lowfat diets are designed with men in mind, and that women "are eating themselves into hormonal dysfunction" by following diets that were tested on a man's different body chemistry. She notes that in general, men seem to handle a greater carbohydrate load than women because they tend to have fewer fat cells and more muscle mass, which enables them to burn more carbohydrate calories. However, her female clients do better on a diet containing 30 to 40 percent of calories as carbohydrates — unless they are very physically active in which case they may be able to tolerate 50 to 55 percent.

Specifically, Gittleman recommends:

- Optimize calcium intake through high-quality, calcium-rich foods such as nonfat dairy products, including yogurts, dry curd cottage cheese, and part-skim milk. Other sources include green, leafy vegetables like broccoli, bok choy, kale, collard greens, and sea vegetables such as hijiki (which contains fourteen times the calcium in a glass of milk), wakama, and kombu.
- Eliminate calcium inhibitors such as soft drinks (regular and diet), cocoa, coffee, and tea, which interfere with calcium absorption or increase its excretion.
- Increase blood-building iron by eating at least two servings (three ounces each) of lean beef weekly, along with legumes and green, leafy vegetables. Eating a high vitamin C source, such as citrus fruits, tomatoes, potatoes, green peppers, or strawberries, further enhances iron absorption.
- Consume four eggs a week in the diet (including those used in baking), because they are the richest source of l-cysteine, an amino acid important for skin, hair, and nail health.
- Include two tablespoons of essential fat every day in salad dressings and cooking. All sources of damaged fats, such as commercial vegetable oils, margarine, and vegetable shortening, should be eliminated, and only purified, unrefined, expeller-pressed raw or virgin oils used.
- Avoid simple sugars, sweeteners, and refined carbohydrates, and keep

fruit consumption to three to five portions a day — preferably the fruit itself rather than the juice.

- Vary consumption of complex carbohydrates by choosing more legumes and vegetables such as potatoes, squash, peas, and root vegetables. The overconsumption of grains such as wheat, rye, oats, and barley can inhibit calcium absorption.
- Consume vegetables on a daily basis. Cruciferous vegetables such as Brussels sprouts, cabbage, cauliflower, rutabagas, broccoli, and turnips should be included at least twice a week to help reduce the risk of cancer, while dark green, yellow, or orange vegetables should be consumed three to four times per week for their rich beta-carotene content.
- Eat 25 to 35 grams daily of water-soluble fibers from oats, legumes, sweet potatoes, and other fresh fruits and vegetables to control cholesterol and steady blood sugar levels.
- Avoid excess salt which contributes to high blood pressure. (Average daily intake should not exceed 1,500 milligrams, the equivalent of 3/4 teaspoon.)
- Choose healthy cooking methods such as baking, roasting, broiling, steaming, and poaching. Frying, charcoal grilling, and smoking should be limited because of the harmful chemicals they produce in food.

## Essential Fatty Acids

Despite the popularity of the standard dietary model of the 1970s and 1980s (low in fat and high in complex carbohydrates), Gittleman found that female participants in the Pritikin diet and others like it with whom she worked were tired, cold, retaining fluids, and experiencing menstrual difficulties and recurring yeast infections. In addition, they were hungry most of the time and tried to raise their energy levels with sugar-laden foods and beverages. Despite their lowfat diets, many of these women could not lose weight.

Gittleman contends that a lowfat, high-carbohydrate diet causes problems because it doesn't provide adequate essential fat, and that it emphasizes carbohydrates in the form of excessive grains, which can help remove valuable nutrients such as zinc, calcium, and iron from the body before they are absorbed and used. Instead she argues that adding essential fats to the diet (specifically one to two tablespoons of purified, unrefined, expeller-pressed raw or virgin oils a day) helps prevent cardiovascular disorders and many hair, skin, and nail conditions. Gittleman also claims that eating modest amounts of fat prevents binge eating, and will help normalize a woman's appetite. As a result, her weight will stabilize, and she will more efficiently metabolize calories and maintain weight loss.

## Iron Deficiencies

Women are especially prone to iron deficiencies because they lose an average of two to four tablespoons of blood each month during menstruation, including 15 to 30 milligrams of iron. Contraceptive intrauterine devices (IUDs), by increasing menstrual blood loss, can cause even greater iron depletion, while pregnancy further reduces stores because the mother's blood supplies iron to the fetus. In fact, Gittleman cites Paul Saltman, a biology professor at the University of California, San Diego, who estimates that 30 to 35 percent of American women have low body stores of iron.

At best, only 10 to 30 percent of the iron taken in is absorbed, so Gittleman recommends that women eat more than their bodies need through iron-rich foods such as beef liver (8.8 milligrams per serving), dried or cooked lima beans (5.6 milligrams), spinach (4.7 milligrams), prune juice (10.5 milligrams), and almonds (6.7 milligrams per cup).

She points out that lean red meat contains two and a half times the iron of chicken, while the iron in red meats is 30 percent absorbed. In comparison, the iron in dark green, leafy vegetables is less than 10 percent absorbed, and less than 5 percent in dried yeast. In addition, eating meat with iron-rich vegetables increases the absorption of the vegetable iron.

## Fiber

Gittleman recommends that women consume principally water-soluble nongluten fibers such as oat bran, black-eyed peas, barley, fresh vegetables like carrots and okra, and fresh fruits like apples, prunes, and grapefruit. She further recommends gluten-free grains such as rice, millet, corn, buckwheat, amaranth, quinoa, teff, and spelt. Flours from potatoes, soy, rice, and tapioca can successfully be substituted in cooking.

## Super Female Foods

Because of their abundance of "female" minerals and other nutrients essential to every woman's health, Gittleman has designated the following as "super female foods": blackstrap molasses, brewer's yeast, broccoli, lentils, sea vegetables, sesame seeds, sunflower seeds, and whole brown rice.

## Restricted Foods

Gittleman suggests that women should eliminate vegetable shortenings, processed vegetable oils, and baked goods that contain "unnatural" fats from their diet. Her diet avoids the saturated fats from full-fat cheese and ice cream and hydrogenated fats from commercial vegetable oils, margarine, and shortenings. Gittleman also recommends that women limit or eliminate food inhibitors that affect both calcium and iron absorption, such as caffeine, sugar, and nicotine.

*Sugar.* According to Gittleman, Americans probably eat 30 teaspoons of sugar a day, or close to their weight in sugar each year. That is because everything from cigarettes to peanut butter, mayonnaise, crackers, ketchup, and French fries contains sugar (added in processing or occurring naturally). Not only can overconsumption of sugar create insulin imbalances and excess weight, but it can decrease levels of essential nutrients including chromium, manganese, cobalt, zinc, copper, and magnesium. Sugary foods are also high in calories, which, according to Gittleman, can stimulate the appetite and create cravings.

*Gluten Foods.* Gluten is a naturally occurring water-soluble complex protein contained in grains, grain flours, and modified food starches that are used in almost all processed foods. Excessive amounts are especially difficult for women to absorb and can cause fatigue, persistent intestinal gas, bloating, bowel irregularities, and frequent diarrhea. High levels of gluten in the intestines can also prevent essential proteins, fats, carbohydrates, iron, calcium, folic acid, and vitamins D and K from being properly absorbed. In women, this may mean menstrual irregularities, infertility, osteoporosis, and anemia.

To avoid gluten intolerance, Gittleman presents a detailed list of gluten-rich foods that should be eliminated from the diet. These include: certain alcoholic beverages such as beer, gin, and whiskey; tomato juice; all commercial baked goods; candies such as toffees, fudge, caramel, and marzipan; all cereals containing wheat, barley, rye, or oats; pasta products such as macaroni, noodles, spaghetti, and vermicelli; malted milk, cheese spreads, and dairy products with synthetic creams; all pies and dessert mixes; and commercial salad dressings and mayonnaise.

In addition, foods Gittleman suggests eliminating include pickled fish and frozen breaded fish; all flours containing wheat, barley, rye, and oats;

gravies with thickeners and mixes; all commercial types of ice cream; all commercial meat preparations containing fillings such as sausages, luncheon meats, meat pies, mincemeats, frankfurters, meat pastes, and canned meat; sauces and condiments such as pickles, anchovy sauce, ketchup, and horseradish sauce; snacks such as potato chips and French-fried potatoes; canned, dried, thickened, and creamed soups; spices such as celery salt, chutney, curry powder, and mustard; meat, cheese, and sandwich spreads; and vegetables in sauces, mayonnaise, or cream.

## Vitamin and Mineral Supplements

Gittleman warns that while supplements cannot and should not replace food, most women will benefit from some supplementation. This is because environmental pollutants and medications such as aspirin and birth control pills can deplete nutrients from women's bodies. Food processing and storage time decrease the levels of vitamins and minerals contained in foods. Pregnancy, lactation, and menopause also place demands on a woman's body that even a balanced diet cannot meet.

Gittleman therefore recommends that all women take a multivitamin and mineral supplement that supplies daily requirements of vitamins B3, B6, C, and E, beta-carotene, and the minerals zinc, magnesium, and selenium. Other key "female mineral" supplements she recommends include calcium, phosphorus, and magnesium, as well as the trace elements iron, zinc, copper, iodine, and manganese.

## Smoking

Gittleman cites research by Dr. Evelyn Whitlock, author of *The Calcium Plus Workbook,* that suggests that women who smoke double their risk of osteoporosis, decrease the effectiveness of estrogen, and may experience early menopause. Women who smoke a pack of cigarettes a day, for example, begin menopause an average of two years earlier than nonsmokers.

## Physical Activity

Exercise is particularly important for women, Gittleman notes, because of the fact that they begin losing bone mass as early as age 25 at the rate of one percent per year, which can lead to injury and even death from osteoporosis. Weight-bearing exercise appears to be one element of the formula researchers have determined slows down, if not stops, this loss of bone density and bone mass.

As she points out, bones lose calcium and become porous if they are not used. Conversely, they become stronger with physical stress. In addition, by strengthening the muscles and tendons that protectively surround bone, exercise makes bones less susceptible to injury.

Gittleman recommends jogging, running, walking, tennis, skiing, hiking, jumping rope, or aerobic dancing as good weight-bearing exercises that should be performed at least three times a week for 20 to 60 minutes at a low to medium intensity. She notes that women should choose activities they enjoy (so they are more likely to continue), and that are nontraumatic to bones and muscles. She further counsels including warm-up and cool-down periods of five minutes each, and choosing good equipment such as well-made running shoes.

## THE HEALTHY WOMAN'S DIET

One of the most comprehensive books on female nutrition published to date is Elizabeth Somer's *Nutrition for Women: The Complete Guide,* which summarizes scientific nutrition research from more than two thousand studies on issues pertinent to women's health. Somer is a registered dietitian and editor of *Health Media of America's Nutrition Report,* a monthly summary of the current nutrition and health research from more than six thousand journals. She is the author of *The Essential Guide to Vitamins and Minerals* and *The Nutrition Desk Reference.*

Part 1 of *Nutrition for Women* presents the Healthy Woman's Diet and all the skills necessary for women to adapt their habits to a more healthful eating style, including ten keys for successfully making changes and staying motivated. Part 2 provides the latest research on the role nutrition plays in the many stages of a woman's life, including pregnancy, menopause, and the senior years. Part 3 offers summaries and dietary recommendations based on current research for a wide range of disorders, from AIDS to yeast infections.

### Basic Nutritional Approach

The Healthy Woman's Diet (HWD) is a lowfat, nutrient-dense diet that limits dietary fat intake to less than 30 percent of total calories, saturated fat to less than 10 percent, sugar (which is essentially calories with no redeemable nutrient qualities) to less than 10 percent, cholesterol to less than 300 milligrams per day, and salt to no more than six grams (slightly more than one teaspoon) per day. Between 25 and 35 grams of fiber should be consumed daily.

Specifically, the HWD recommends that women

- consume at least five daily servings of fresh fruits and vegetables, especially dark orange or green vegetables and citrus fruits;
- consume at least six servings of complex carbohydrates such as whole-grain breads and cereals, potatoes, and legumes each day;
- limit consumption of extra-lean meat, poultry, and seafood to no more than six ounces a day, or two three-ounce servings;
- consume at least three to four calcium-rich foods daily, including nonfat milk or yogurt, lowfat cheeses, dark green leafy vegetables, tofu, or canned salmon with the bones;
- consume at least 2,000 calories of the above nutrient-dense foods; select less nutritious foods only after all other nutrient needs for the day have been met;
- include a moderate-dose vitamin/mineral supplement when calorie intake drops below 2,000 calories that provides 100 to 300 percent of the U.S. RDA for the following vitamins and minerals: fat-soluble vitamins A (preferably beta-carotene) and E; water-soluble vitamins C, B1, B2, niacin, B6, B12, folic acid, pantothenic acid and biotin; calcium, copper, iron, magnesium, zinc, chromium, manganese, and selenium;
- balance calorie intake with exercise to maintain a desirable weight; avoid repeated attempts at weight loss;
- limit alcohol consumption to five drinks or less each week (pregnant women or those planning to get pregnant should avoid all alcoholic beverages until after their baby is born);
- drink at least six glasses of water — which Somer terms "the most important and yet often the most likely forgotten nutrient" — a day;
- divide total food intake into four or more small meals and snacks throughout the day.

## Recommended Foods

In her sample shopping list, Somer provides a list of specific lowfat, nutrient-dense foods that she recommends, including

- breads: 100 percent whole-wheat bread, whole-wheat bagels, pita bread and rolls, English muffins, French bread, cornbread, pumpernickel, and corn tortillas;
- crackers and snacks: RyKrisp, Akmak, or other lowfat, whole-wheat crackers, low-salt corn chips, rice cakes, graham crackers, tortilla chips, pretzels, and air-popped popcorn;
- cereals: Nutri-Grain cereal, Grape-Nuts, shredded wheat, puffed wheat and puffed rice, whole-grain hot cereal such as oatmeal, wheat germ, and kasha;
- noodles, rice, and other grains: whole-wheat, spinach, and "enriched" noodles, long-grain or short-grain brown rice, wild rice, millet, cracked wheat or bulgur, barley, tabouli mix, Spanish rice, rice, and wheat pilaf (packets can be omitted for the latter four if sodium is a concern);
- flour: whole-wheat, rye, oat, and unbleached white flours (although less nutritious than the whole-grain varieties);
- fruits: all fresh fruits, canned fruits in their own juices, all 100 percent fruit juices, and canned, bottled, or frozen concentrate;
- vegetables: all fresh or plain frozen vegetables except avocados and olives, all 100 percent vegetable juices, tomato sauce and paste, marinara sauce, salsa, and artichoke hearts canned in water;
- beans and peas: all dried beans and peas, canned cooked dried beans and peas, packaged bean mixes, and peanut butter in small quantities;
- meat, chicken, and fish: Chicken (with skin removed before cooking), extra-lean beef (less than 9 percent fat by weight), extra-lean pork, turkey (with skin removed before cooking), canned tuna packed in water, and all fresh and frozen unprocessed fish;
- milk and eggs: no-fat cheeses, lowfat mozzarella cheese, nonfat or 1 percent fat plain yogurt, milk or buttermilk, nonfat, lowfat or dry curd cottage cheese, lowfat Parmesan cheese, partially skimmed Swiss and ricotta, and one to two eggs weekly (preferably using only the egg white);
- beverages: mineral water, diet soda, tea, and decaffeinated coffee and tea;
- spices and flavorings: garlic powder, selected spices and herbs (including dill), mustard, sugar substitute, clam juice, and pimiento;
- oils and fats: low-calorie margarine and mayonnaise, no-fat salad dressing, safflower oil, dry roasted nuts such as almonds, and sunflower seeds.

- sweets and desserts: jams (preferably all-fruit, no-sugar varieties), angel food cake, sherbet, vanilla wafers, Dole frozen fruit bar and Fruit Ice, and Healthy Choice ice cream.

## Eliminated Foods

Somer recommends that women eliminate the following food additives, either because they have proven harmful or because there is insufficient evidence that they are harmless: artificial colors, BHA and BHT, monosodium glutamate, sodium nitrite and sodium nitrate, sulfites, saccharin, pesticides, bacteria (such as aflatoxin in peanuts and peanut butter, listeria in vegetables and dairy products, and salmonella in eggs and other high-protein foods), caffeine, and sodium chloride and other sodium-containing foods.

## Alcohol

The HWD severely restricts alcohol consumption because it replaces other nutritious foods and thus limits nutrient intake, or is consumed in conjunction with adequate food intake and thus contributes to obesity. Alcohol also increases a woman's requirements for several nutrients, including vitamins B1 and B6, biotin, and niacin, interferes with the body's use of many nutrients such as fat-soluble vitamins, and depletes the body's tissue stores of vitamins A and E and selenium. And, according to Somer, alcohol is suspected of increasing free radical damage to tissues and irritating the digestive tract.

## Smoking

Somer advises all women to stop smoking because tobacco smoke removes vitamin C from the tissues and blood and increases vitamin C requirements to more than 200 milligrams per day (the RDA is 60 milligrams). Levels of vitamin A, beta-carotene, and B6 are lower in smokers than in nonsmokers, and pregnant women who smoke have been observed to have low blood zinc levels. They are more likely than nonsmokers to give birth to zinc-deficient babies who are at high risk for birth defects and disease.

According to Somer, optimal dietary intake of folic acid, the B vitamins, the antioxidant nutrients (vitamin C, beta-carotene, and vitamin E), and certain minerals might help counteract some of the harmful effects of tobacco smoke.

## Physical Activity

Somer claims that women who exercise regularly are healthier than those who are sedentary; are less likely to develop hypertension, heart disease, and diabetes and are less likely to die from these diseases; and tend to live longer than their inactive counterparts. In addition, exercisers feel better and younger throughout life and maintain their independence longer than sedentary women.

## RECENT RESEARCH

Both the Gittleman and Somer diets for women stress the importance of maintaining ideal body weight to minimize the risk of developing chronic diseases. A study published in the September 14, 1995, issue of the *New England Journal of Medicine* confirmed that the risk of death is far lower among women who are slimmest, while mortality from all causes rises rapidly as weight increases.

Researchers from Brigham and Women's Hospital in Boston analyzed data collected from 1976 to 1992 from 115,000 female nurses between the ages of 30 and 55. The researchers found that for women who added 40 pounds or more to their weight from age 18, the death risk was 60 percent higher than those who gained 10 pounds or less. The risk of death from heart disease for that group was seven times higher, and the risk of death from cancer was 50 percent higher. "Being overweight is second only to cigarette smoking as a cause of premature death," concluded Dr. JoAnn Manson, principal author of the study.

Given the differences in the two diets reviewed in this chapter, the best advice is for women to first clearly identify their dietary goals (Chapter 4). A nutritionist or dietitian can then help them select the most appropriate diet based on their goals, weight, health factors, and lifestyle. They can also provide detailed analyses of the unique risk each woman faces throughout her life cycles, especially during her child-bearing and pre- and postmenopausal years.

# 11

## Diets for Children

America's children are not as healthy as they were twenty years ago, and, according to several national studies, the main reason is that they are not eating adequate amounts of healthy, nutritious foods. Elizabeth Gong and Felix Heald, in "Diet, Nutrition, and Adolescence" in Shils et al., *Modern Nutrition in Health and Disease,* cite several national studies which show that American children consume substantially less than the recommended daily amounts of vitamin A, B12, folate, and C, and iron, zinc, and calcium. This problem is compounded by the fact that 60 to 80 percent of American schoolchildren are now estimated to exceed the RDAs for daily total fat, saturated fat, cholesterol, and sodium. Some studies also suggest that they overconsume daily amounts of protein. As a result, American children are now increasingly obese. A 1995 national nutrition survey published by the National Center for Health Statistics, for example, concluded that as many as 5 million American children aged 6 through 17 are severely overweight.

Three markedly different diets for children are analyzed in this chapter which directly address these problems. The first, developed by the Children's Nutrition Research Center (CNRC) at Baylor College, endorses the Food Guide Pyramid of the U.S. Department of Agriculture (USDA). The second, developed by Dr. Harold and Dr. Francine Prince, argues that the 1989 USDA-recommended four food groups do not provide sufficient amounts of vitamins B1, B6, and B12, zinc, iron, magnesium, and calcium. Therefore, the Princes' diet suggests optimal dietary amounts of these nutrients in excess of the RDAs. The third diet, the Shapedown Program, developed by Dr. Laura Mellin of the University of California at San Francisco, has drawn the attention of the Clinton administration for its effectiveness in treating childhood obesity.

## CHILDREN'S NUTRITION RESEARCH CENTER DIET

The Children's Nutrition Research Center (CNRC) was established as part of the Department of Agriculture in 1978 to study the nutritional needs of children, from infancy through adolescence, and pregnant and nursing women. It is operated by the Baylor College of Medicine in cooperation with Texas Children's Hospital in Houston. The CNRC conducts studies of the most important nutritional problems of American children, including the alarming increase in obesity in American children; high cholesterol levels in American school-age children; low calcium levels, especially in teenage American girls; and the lack of fruits and vegetables in the average daily diet of American children. The CNRC's dietary program for children appears in its quarterly publication *Nutrition and Your Child.*

### Required or Recommended Foods

The CNRC endorses the official USDA Food Guide Pyramid which was developed to help consumers and educators apply the USDA's dietary guidelines to adolescent food selection and preparation. The Pyramid recommends the following foods for children from bottom (most important) to least important:

- Bread, cereal, rice, and pasta group: 6 to 11 servings. Examples of one serving:
    1 slice of bread
    1 ounce of ready-to-eat cereal
    1/2 cup of cooked cereal, rice, or pasta
    3 or 4 small plain crackers
- Meat, poultry, fish, dry beans, egg, and nuts group: 2 to 3 servings. Examples of one serving:
    2 to 3 ounces of cooked lean meat, poultry, or fish
    1/2 cup of cooked dry beans, 1 egg, or 2 tablespoons of peanut butter
- Milk, yogurt, and cheese group: 2 to 3 servings. Examples of one serving:
    1 cup of milk or yogurt
    1 1/2 ounces of natural cheese
    2 ounces of processed cheese
- Fruits: 2–4 servings. Examples of one serving:
    1 medium apple, banana, or orange

## HOW TO ENCOURAGE CHILDREN
## TO EAT VEGETABLES

To make vegetables more appetizing, CNRC nutritionist Janice Struff suggests that you should:

- prepare vegetables in a new way by stir-frying them or sprinkling them with lowfat grated cheese;
- use vegetables as pizza toppings or add them to spaghetti sauce;
- offer carrot sticks, cherry tomatoes, cucumber slices, and other finger-food vegetables as snacks; serve raw vegetables with yogurt, salsa, and bean dips;
- cut vegetables in bite-size pieces;
- give children stalks of celery and let them scoop up their stew with an edible spoon;
- add extra crunch to tacos with a few slices of red or green bell pepper.

    1/2 cup of chopped, cooked, or canned fruit
    3/4 cup of fruit juice
- Vegetables: 3–5 servings. Examples of one serving:
    1 cup of raw leafy vegetables
    1/2 cup of other vegetables, cooked or chopped raw
    3/4 cup of vegetable juice

Obviously, the CNRC cautions, children aged 1 to 3 will need smaller portions. For example, 1/4 to 1/3 cup of cooked vegetables or 1/2 cup of salad is considered an appropriate serving of vegetables for children aged 4 to 8. Portions increase to 1/2 cup of cooked vegetables and 1 cup of salad for children aged 9 to 17.

*Green Leafy Vegetables.* According to the CNRC, one of the three recommended daily vegetable servings should be a green leafy vegetable such as spinach, romaine lettuce, or broccoli. These vegetables are rich sources of vitamins and minerals and help a child's body utilize carbohydrates, fat, and proteins. They also contribute to red blood cell formation, help strengthen muscles, and regulate growth. Vegetables also provide fiber which keeps the digestive system functioning properly and prevents constipation.

The winter 1995 issue of the CNRC's *Nutrition and Your Child* provides the following chart highlighting the importance of vegetables in children's diets:

**Vitamin A sources:** carrots, tomatoes, pumpkin, sweet potatoes, winter squash, and broccoli;

**Vitamin C sources:** Brussels sprouts, green pepper, cauliflower, snow peas, kale, potatoes, tomatoes, and kohlrabi;

**Vitamin B6** (Pyridoxine) **sources:** spinach, carrots, corn, lima beans, cabbage, and potatoes;

**Folic acid sources:** dried peas and beans, spinach, beets, asparagus, turnip greens, and broccoli;

**Vitamin E sources:** chard, peas, legumes, and turnip greens;

**Calcium sources:** bok choy, mustard greens, turnip greens, broccoli;

**Iron sources:** legumes, peas, potatoes with skins, asparagus, and artichokes.

*Fruit.* American children, according to the CNRC, also need to consume more fruits, vegetables, and whole grains and eliminate high-fat, high-sugar junk foods. Carbohydrates should constitute approximately 55 percent of the child's diet, and protein 10 to 15 percent. The CNRC stresses that children need to understand basic nutritional principles and should help parents plan menus for the week. It suggests making shopping lists and asking children to help parents select vegetables and main dishes.

One quarter of American children eat no fruits or vegetables on any given day, according to a national survey of 3,122 second to sixth graders cited in the June 1995 issue of *American Health.* The findings reaffirm the CNRC's diet recommendation that children should consume at least five servings of fruits and vegetables a day to reduce the risk of many cancers, including colon, breast, and prostate cancer.

*Fiber.* CNRC nutritionist Janice Stuff, R.D., states in the spring 1995 issue of *Nutrition and Your Child:* "The U.S. diet is highly refined and overprocessing removes much of the natural fiber that children and adults need. Fiber or roughage is an essential part of a healthy diet because, as noted, it aids in digestion, may reduce cholesterol and protects against colon cancer." It also prevents constipation, a common medical complaint in children.

Stuff argues that a 40-pound child needs 10 grams of fiber daily, compared to 15 to 20 grams for teens and 25 to 35 grams for adults. A child can consume 10 grams of fiber each day, she notes, by eating a sandwich using whole-wheat bread, a medium apple or pear, a 1/2 cup serving of vegetables, and a 1/2 cup serving of beans or lentils. She urges parents to slowly increase the amounts of dietary fiber to their children's diet and to encourage them to drink plenty of water.

Stuff suggests the following tips for adding fiber to a child's diet:

- Use whole-wheat bread for toast or sandwiches.
- Serve fresh fruit such as pears or apples with the skin.
- Offer nectarines and bananas.
- Make bean nachos using baked tortilla chips.
- Stir granola or berries into plain yogurt.
- Serve vegetables such as cooked corn, green beans, broccoli, or carrots.
- Add vegetables to pizza toppings and spaghetti sauce.
- Offer celery sticks or hot air–popped popcorn as a snack.
- Add raisins or berries to whole-grain cereal.

## Calcium-Rich Foods

The CNRC notes that more than half of American women over age 50 and three-fourths over age 75 have significant bone loss, which causes osteoporosis, causing more than 1.3 million fractures a year, most often in the hips, wrists, and spine. It adds that few American girls consume enough calcium to meet the RDA allowances of 1,200 milligrams daily for ages 11 to 24. Most girls in the United States, for example, consume only 800 to 900 milligrams daily, according to several nutritional surveys cited by the CNRC. According to CNRC, osteoporosis may have its origins in childhood. Bones are formed primarily in childhood, and without sufficient calcium intake, the body cannot build strong, dense bones. Several national studies have shown that more calcium intake during preteen and teen years results in stronger, healthier bones.

CNRC researcher Dr. Steven Abrams, who headed the study, suggests that the study's findings indicate that most American girls need to boost their calcium intake earlier than previously believed. "Bone-forming activity peaks earlier than might have been previously thought," he noted. He recommends that all children, especially girls, boost their calcium intake to at least 1,200 milligrams daily by the age of 8 instead of 11. The National Institutes of Health recently revised its guidelines for calcium intakes for ages 11 to 24 to a range of 1,200 to 1,500 milligrams per day. Studies suggest that a calcium intake up to 1,600 milligrams may be necessary for optimal bone growth. In one study of identical twins ages 6 to 14, the twins who consumed 1,612 milligrams of calcium developed denser bones than those who took 908 milligrams.

Other research studies by Dr. Abrams have shown that some children absorb calcium less efficiently than others, and that this tendency appears to be stress related. To adjust for possible hereditary factors, Dr. Abrams emphasizes that most children should consume extra daily servings of calcium. Approximately four servings of calcium-rich foods, such as milk or calcium-fortified orange juice, delivers approximately 1,200 milligrams, and a fifth serving is even better, according to Abrams.

### Soybean Substitutes for Cholesterol

The CNRC officially states that one excellent way to lower cholesterol levels in children is to serve soybean substitute dishes as main entrees. According to Dr. Wong, for example, people who consume substantial amounts of soybeans generally have lower total cholesterol levels. Soybean protein may slow the formation of cholesterol in the body, minimize the absorption of cholesterol, or somehow hasten the elimination of cholesterol. Preliminary data show that people with high cholesterol levels can lower their levels 10 to 15 percent by eating more soybean products.

### Eliminated or Restricted Foods

According to CNRC, most American children also consume too much fat. The CNRC diet endorses the guidelines issued by the American Academy of Pediatrics which recommend that children over age 2 should consume no more than 30 percent of calories from fat, with 10 percent or less from saturated fat. Children under 2 need more fat and should never be given lowfat products. On the average, American children currently consume approximately 35 percent of calories as fat, with 10 to 15 percent as saturated fat.

To reduce fat consumption, the CNRC advises broiling instead of frying, using smaller amounts of vegetable oil or a light coating of spray oil instead of butter or margarine, or using nonstick oils if possible. The skin should be removed from chicken and turkey, the visible fat trimmed, and fat drained off from cooled soups. In baking recipes, parents should substitute applesauce to reduce the amount of oil or fat and consider using egg

---

### OTHER RESTRICTED FOODS
### IN THE CNRC DIET

- **Salt:** Salt has been linked to high blood pressure in adults, and the CNRC strongly urges limiting high-salt foods such as pickles and meats such as bacon, hot dogs, and sausage. When baking, decrease the salt added by one-fourth or more.
- **Sugar-Rich Beverages:** Sodas are usually empty calories and may satiate children to the point where they do not have an appetite. Water is a critical nutrient for growing bodies, and the CNRC urges parents to serve water or lowfat milk with meals instead of sugar-rich sodas.

---

substitutes or egg whites rather than whole eggs. They also advise eliminating (or severely restricting) all high-fat foods such as cheese, cream sauces and creamed soups, fried food, mayonnaise and dressing, snacks, cakes, chips, and some microwave popcorns. They note that many lowfat lunch meats and cheeses, dressings, and yogurt are available. Sorbet, sherbet, frozen yogurts, and ice milk usually have less fat than ice cream.

### Vitamin and Mineral Supplements

According to the CNRC, a balanced diet normally provides all the essential vitamins and minerals. They do, however, consider most multivitamin/mineral supplements safe, although they are usually unnecessary. One exception may be iron supplements for children with iron deficiencies, which is common, especially in infants. Some teenagers may also be iron deficient, according to Dr. Kathleen Motil, a CNRC researcher. Children who do not take iron supplements should consume more beef, although nonmeat sources can be substituted, including whole grains, dried fruit, baked potatoes, pinto or kidney beans, and iron-fortified cereals. Parents can also add iron to their children's diets by cooking in cast-iron skillets.

### School Lunches

Children generally take the food habits they learn at home to school with them, which means that if they've been taught to eat and enjoy a balanced diet, they will continue to do so at school. One way to ensure this, according to the CNRC, is to visit your child's school to survey their menus and then discuss menu choices with the child. If choices at school include foods

## RECOMMENDED DAILY ALLOWANCES
## OF NUTRIENTS FOR NORMAL CHILDREN

| NUTRIENT | RECOMMENDED INTAKE PER DAY | | |
|---|---|---|---|
| | 1 to 3 years (Weight = 13 kg) | 4 to 6 years (Weight = 20 kg) | 7 to 10 years (Weight = 28 kg) |
| Energy (kcal) | 1,300 | 1,800 | 2,000 |
| Fat (g) | | | |
| Carbohydrate | | | |
| Protein (g) | 16 | 24 | 38 |
| Electrolytes and minerals | | | |
| Calcium (mg) | 800 | 800 | 800 |
| Phosphorus (mg) | 800 | 800 | 800 |
| Magnesium (mg) | 80 | 120 | 170 |
| Sodium (mEq)* | 13 | 20 | 28 |
| Chloride (mEq)* | 13 | 20 | 28 |
| Potassium (mEq)* | 26 | 36 | 40 |
| Iron (mg) | 10 | 10 | 10 |
| Zinc (mg) | 10 | 10 | 10 |
| Copper (mg)† | 0.7–1.0 | 1.0–1.5 | .1–2 |
| Iodine (μg) | 70 | 90 | 120 |
| Selenium (μg) | 20 | 20 | 30 |
| Manganese (μg)† | 1–1.5 | 1.5–2 | 2–3 |
| Fluoride (mg)† | 0.5–1.5 | 1–2.5 | 1–2.5 |
| Chromium (μg)† | 20–80 | 30–120 | 50–200 |
| Molybdenum (μg) | 25–50 | 30–75 | 50–150 |

that children do not eat or that are high in fat, help them pack their own lunches with nutrient-dense foods.

### Serve a Variety of Foods

The CNRC suggests that the best way to encourage nutritious eating habits in children is to serve a variety of nutrient-dense foods in attractive ways. Experiment with less familiar but more nutritious foods such as bulgur, lentils, split peas, and sweet potatoes. Children often have a tendency to eat the same foods over and over and to turn up their noses at new foods. The best strategy is to begin serving small portions of new foods and encouraging the child to sample them.

## RECOMMENDED DAILY ALLOWANCES OF NUTRIENTS FOR NORMAL CHILDREN (continued)

| NUTRIENT | RECOMMENDED INTAKE PER DAY | | |
| --- | --- | --- | --- |
| | 1 to 3 years (Weight = 13 kg) | 4 to 6 years (Weight = 20 kg) | 7 to 10 years (Weight = 28 kg) |
| **Vitamins** | | | |
| Vitamin A ($\mu$g RE) | 400 | 500 | 700 |
| Vitamin D ($\mu$g) | 0.10 | 10 | 10 |
| Vitamin E (mg $\alpha$-TE) | 6 | 8 | 7 |
| Vitamin K ($\mu$g) | 15 | 20 | 30 |
| Vitamin C (mg) | 40 | 45 | 45 |
| Thiamin (mg) | 0.7 | 0.9 | 1.0 |
| Riboflavin (mg) | 0.8 | 1.1 | 1.2 |
| Niacin (mg NE) | 9 | 12 | 13 |
| Vitamin $B_6$ (mg) | 1 | 1.1 | 1.4 |
| Folate ($\mu$g) | 50 | 75 | 100 |
| Vitamin $B_{12}$ | 0.7 | 1.0 | 1.4 |
| Biotin ($\mu$g)† | 20 | 25 | 30 |
| Pantothenic acid (mg)† | 3 | 3–4 | 4–5 |

*Minimal requirements rather than recommended.
†Estimated safe and adequate daily intake.
Data taken from Food and Nutrition Board, National Research Council, *Recommended Dietary Allowances, Tenth Edition.* Washington, D.C.: National Academy Press, 1989.
Source: Shils, Maurice, et al., *Modern Nutrition in Health and Disease* (Philadelphia, PA: Lea & Febiger, 1994): 784.

## THE FEED YOUR KIDS BRIGHT DIET

The Feed Your Kids Bright Diet was developed by Dr. Harold Prince and Dr. Francine Prince and is outlined in their book *Feed Your Kids Bright*. The Princes are both nutritionists and have authored or coauthored seven diet and recipe books.

### Basic Nutritional Approach

As parents, the Princes were concerned to provide the maximum amounts of essential vitamins and minerals for their young children for optimal health and brain development. They began by following the USDA diet, which is based on tables compiled by the USDA of nutrient contents of foods. However, the Princes found that several studies suggested that the USDA's 1989 well-balanced diet of four food groups did not appear to provide sufficient RDA amounts for vitamins B1, B6, and B12, zinc, iron, magnesium, and calcium because of food processing. The Princes concluded, "At best the well-balanced diet can only contribute to the RDA, not to the optimal dietary amounts necessary to ward off preclinical disorders that disrupt your kids' mental, emotional, and behavioral well-being."

## Recommended Foods

The Princes suggest that the basic idea of the USDA's well-balanced diet is sound, and that their diet for children provides added insurance because it contains eleven food groups. Their diet includes "265 best foods for your kids which are low in saturated fats and cholesterol, contain no added sugar and salt, and supply the right amounts of fiber — all factors in warding off nutrition-related disease." The Princes caution that their diet includes higher amounts of fats and cholesterol which they suggest children need until the ages of 3 to 5. They state that "by selecting servings from each food group, parents can ensure the best possible nutritional mix for the whole family." Their recommended eleven food groups are:

*Eggs.*

*Fish.* Fish and fish oil supplements contain polyunsaturated fats, the type of oil that has been found to prevent nutrition-related diseases such as coronary artery disease, diabetes, and cancer. Recommended fish include lowfat fish such as abalone, cod, flounder, gray snapper, haddock, hake, yellow perch, pike, pollock, white sea bass, scrod, skate, sole, and tilefish; and moderate-fat fish such as albacore, Pacific barracuda, all sea bass, bluefish, carp, catfish, halibut, herring, monkfish, porgy, redfish (ocean perch), swordfish, brook trout, tuna, and whiting.

*Meats.* The Prince diet recommends lean cuts of meat, and advises dieters to purchase "choice" rather than "prime" cuts. Lean meats contain saturated fats, which, the Princes suggest, may help prevent some diseases. But, they caution, dieters should not overconsume meats, because their saturated fats can only be metabolized in small quantities.

They also suggest that only chemical-free meats should be consumed, including: *Beef:* all cuts, as long as they are "choice"; lean cuts which are free of any chemicals; *Lamb:* only lean cuts including leg, loins, chops, and other loin cuts; shoulder chops; and rib chops; *Pork:* only the leanest cuts from "choice" grades including fresh ham and picnic pork; *Rabbit, venison, and veal:* only lean cuts in "choice" grades, including leg, loin cuts; round; rump; and shoulder chops; *Poultry:* chicken, Cornish hen, pheasant, quail, squab, and turkey (young, light, or dark meat).

*Dairy products.* The authors recommend whole milk for pregnant and nursing mothers and children up to age 5. For nonpregnant mothers, adults, and children aged 5 years and older, recommended dairy products include buttermilk, nonfat and skim milk, nonfat and whole dry milk; *Yogurt:* plain lowfat yogurt, plain whole-milk yogurt; *Cheese:* only unprocessed cheese including cottage cheese, farmer cheese, mozzarella, Parmesan, pot cheese, and ricotta cheese.

*Grains.* Barley, millet, rolled oats, Cream of Wheat, regular wheat germ, rice, wheat flakes, whole kasha (buckwheat oats), wild rice.

*Breads and crackers.* Arrowroot flour, baking soda, buckwheat flour, cornstarch, double-acting baking power without aluminum, dry yeast, pastas made from flour and water with no salt or other additives, rye flour, stone-ground whole-wheat flour, unbleached flour, whole-wheat pastry flour.

*Legumes, nuts, and seeds.* All nuts and nut butters (especially walnuts); almonds, peanuts, and Persian walnuts may be eaten if dieters take zinc supplements; dried beans, dried peas (including split peas and chickpeas, lentils, sesame seeds, sunflower seeds, tofu (soybean curd).

*Vegetables.* Asparagus, broccoli, Brussels sprouts, cabbage (cooked), chard, dark leafy lettuce, escarole, red leaf lettuce, romaine lettuce, scallions, chicory, Chinese cabbage, endive, cooked spinach and turnips, watercress, artichokes, bamboo shoots, cooked beets, carrots, celery, cucumber, eggplant, green beans, mushrooms, okra, onions, pumpkin, radishes, and yams.

*Fats.* Only cold-pressed vegetable oils. These include corn oil, cottonseed oil, peanut oil, safflower oil, sesame oil (except Oriental varieties), soybean oil, sunflower oil, virgin olive oil, and walnut oil.

*Sweets.* Carob powder and chips (unsweetened), date powder, dried un-processed fruits, fresh fruit juices (frozen juices are only permitted with supplements), uncooked, unfiltered honey (not for children under 1 year of age), raw nuts and nut pastes which contain no sugar or salt additives, sugar cane, sweet herbs (aniseed, marjoram, oregano, rosemary, sweet basil, tarragon), sweet spices (allspice, cinnamon, coriander, ginger, mace, sweet paprika).

*Herbs, spices, condiments, and flavorings.* The authors recommend only natural, unprocessed, or chemically treated herbs which, they state, are "replete with essential vitamins and minerals." They note that garlic is a nutritionally potent herb which has important medicinal properties.

*Condiments and flavorings.* Apple cider vinegar, balsamic vinegar, grain coffee (uncaffeinated), low-sodium vegetable seasoning, pure vanilla ex-tract, low-sodium soy sauce, smoked yeast, vanilla beans, and wine vin-egar.

## Protein-Rich Foods

The Princes suggest that the proteins most needed by growing children are best supplied by animal foods — meat, fish, poultry, cheese, milk, and plain yogurt. These are "complete proteins" because they contain all the essential amino acids in the right proportions which a growing body and brain require. "The only way to obtain complete proteins from plant foods," they add, "is to combine specific selections from the vegetable kingdom that together provide all the essential amino acids in the right proportion." They provide the following list of complementary proteins: rice and ses-ame seeds, rice and tofu, rice and beans, rice and lentils, beans and peas, beans and whole-wheat bread, beans and cracked wheat, beans and corn-meal, beans and cornbread, beans and tortillas, garbanzo beans and tahini (sesame seed paste), soybeans (roasted), sunflower seeds, and peanuts, lentils and barley, split peas and cornbread.

The authors cite national nutritionists who claim that vegetable pro-tein can meet the protein needs of pregnant and nursing women. They note, however, that a vegetarian diet may be low in folic acid and calcium, iron, and zinc, all of which are essential for young children.

## Restricted Foods

*Fiber-Rich Foods.* The authors note that diets that contain as much as 50 grams of dietary fiber daily block the absorption of brain-vital minerals: calcium, copper, iron, magnesium, phosphorus, and zinc. They state that deficiencies of these minerals may result in irritability, nervousness, insomnia, mood swings, anxiety, depression, memory loss, diminished attention span, impaired sense perception, fatigue, lack of motivation, and learning disabilities.

*Low-Protein Foods.* According to the Princes, children who do not consume the daily RDAs are liable to show symptoms of protein deprivation. The protein gap may be between 8 and 12 percent of daily proteins. On a high-carbohydrate diet, especially a pure vegetarian diet, children's protein consumption could drop into the gap. When children receive insufficient quantities of protein, they are vitamin and mineral deficient, particularly in vitamin A and folic acid, iron, zinc, manganese, magnesium, and copper. A high-carbohydrate diet may also create lowfat levels in a child's bloodstream, a condition which can deter a child's brain functioning. Sufficient fat levels are required to transport sufficient fat-soluble vitamins (A, D, E, and K) to sites in the brain where they are vitally needed.

*Carbohydrate-Rich Foods.* The authors state that the currently recommended high-carbohydrate diet (60 to 75 percent of total daily calories) is not the right diet for young children. A high-carbohydrate diet can create iron deficiencies. This, in turn, can decrease the body's ability to manufacture sufficient hemoglobin, the red blood cells that transport oxygen to the brain. Zinc deficiencies, they argue, can contribute to learning disabilities, memory loss, diminished attention spans, irritability, sluggishness, fatigue, lack of motivation, and anemia.

*Anti-Iron Foods.* Foods that contain phytates, phosphates, or polyphenols, according to the Princes, deplete heme iron stores in children (and, to a lesser degree, in adults) and should be restricted. Anti-iron foods include bran that contains phytates, cereals (phytates), cheese (phosphates), corn (phytates), (polyphenols), eggs (phosphates), finger millet (polyphenols), horse beans (polyphenols), legumes (polyphenols), cow's milk (phosphates), rice (phytates), sorghum (polyphenols), spinach (polyphenols), soybeans (phytates), tea (polyphenols), and red wine (polyphenols).

These anti-iron foods are harmless in a diet that supplies adequate amounts of meat, poultry, or fish, however. Meat, the primary source of heme iron, also increases the body's ability to use non-heme iron in potatoes and other vegetables when they are served with meat.

## Eliminated and Restricted Foods

According to the Princes, the "181 Worst Foods for Children" are:

- *Baked goods.* Bagels, baking powder, baking soda, brioches, brownies, cakes and crackers, cookies, cornbread, croissants, dietetic breads, doughnuts, gluten breads, pastries, pies, pumpernickel rolls, rye bread, salt sticks, Swedish flat breads, sweet rolls, white bread, Zwieback.
- *Beverages.* Alcohol, chocolate milk, cocoa, coffee, diet drinks, fruit-type drinks, instant drinks, soft drinks, including cola drinks, and tea (including most herb teas).
- *Breakfast foods.* Bacon, granola, ham, high-sugar cereals, sausages.
- *Canned, frozen, and instant foods.* Baking mixes, bouillon-type cubes, canned entrees, canned fruits, juices, soups, and vegetables, dessert mixes, frozen baked goods, prepared foods and meals and uncooked foods, instant breakfast mixes, powdered drink mixes, prepared stuffings, sauce mixes, seasoning mixes, and soup mixes.
- *Condiments, sauces, and salad dressings.* Chili sauce, chutney, horseradish, ketchup, mayonnaise, prepared mustards, salad dressings which are packaged or bottled, soy sauce, steak sauces, and Tabasco.
- *Cooked take-outs.* Barbecued poultry, French fries, fried chicken, fried fish, hamburgers, and rotisseried chicken.
- *Dairy products.* Coffee whiteners, dessert whips, egg whites, flavored yogurts, high-fat cheese (brie, Gruyère, Muenster, and gorgonzola), and all processed cheeses.
- *Delicatessen foods.* Bologna, coleslaw, fish salads, frankfurters, wursts (including liverwurst), cold cuts (including prosciutto), luncheon meats, meat salads, olives, pastrami, pickled vegetables (including pickles), salami, sauerkraut, and vegetable salads.
- *Desserts.* Candy, chocolate, custards, flavored gelatin, fruit toppings, ice cream and ice milk, all ices, jams and jellies, mousses, puddings, sherbets, and syrups.

- *Fats and oils.* All artificial foods and flavoring, including artificially colored butter, coconut oils, hardened white vegetable shortenings (hydrogenated vegetable fats), margarine (with additives), lard and other animal fats, and palm oil.
- *Fish.* Caviar and other roes, preserved or artificially colored fillets, raw fish, fish sticks, red snapper (which may be high in toxic mercury), and smoked fish, including Scotch salmon, Nova Scotia salmon, Norwegian salmon, and finnan haddie.
- *Meats and poultry.* Capon, duck, fatty cuts of meat, goose, kidneys, lungs, roaster chicken, self-basting poultry, and sweetbreads.
- *Produce.* Almonds, avocados, raw beets, cabbage, spinach, turnips and vegetable greens, cassava, coconut, corn and corn products (except corn oil), horseradish, kale, mustard greens, Pinon (female pine-seed) nuts, rape, rutabagas, soybeans and soybean products, and watercress.
- *Snacks.* Cheese puffs and similar snack items, cream-filled baked goods, dips, granola bars, peanuts, popcorn, potato chips, pretzels, salted nuts, seeds, snack-type fruit pies, and Persian walnuts.
- *Sugar and sugar substitutes.* Aspartame, beet sugar, blackstrap molasses, brown sugar, cane sugar, corn syrup, dextrins, dextrose fructose, glucose, high-fructose corn syrup (HFCS), processed honey, inert sugar, mannitol, maple syrup, NutraSweet, pancake syrups, raw sugar, saccharin, sorbitol, sucrose (table sugar), turbinado sugar, yellow-D, and xylitol.

## The Basic All-Family Menu Plan

The Princes provide a Basic All-Family Menu Plan that includes their 265 recommended foods. They are combined to supply the best possible quantities of nutrients in the most beneficial proportion by making selection from the author's eleven food groups. The menu plans are low in saturated fats and cholesterol and salt. They contain virtually no sugars, are moderate in fiber, have all the essential amino acids, and the right amount of calories. Thus, the menu is ideal for men and nonpregnant women, and it can be easily adapted with modifications for pregnant and breast-feeding women.

## Recipes

Having presented a basic Menu Plan, the authors also provide more than 100 pages of recipes, divided into three categories: Magic Mixers — recipes to make all recipes taste better; "junk food recipes" that are delicious and taste like junk food favorites but are entirely healthy; and Bright Cuisine recipes — healthy recipes for the whole family designed to provide essential nutrients for growing bodies and brains.

## Vitamins and Mineral Supplements

The authors note that processed foods, additives, fertilizers, and preservatives have diminished the supply of vitamins and minerals in foods, and even the best diet must be "supplemented to achieve optimal health levels for body and mind." They therefore recommend that children take daily supplements of all vitamins, as well as choline, calcium carbonate, magnesium oxide, zinc gluconate, iron (ferrous fumarate), manganese gluconate, copper gluconate, selenium, chromium acetate, iodine (potassium iodide), molybdenum (sodium molybdate), and magnesium trisilicat.

## THE SHAPEDOWN WEIGHT-LOSS DIET PROGRAM FOR CHILDREN

As noted, adolescent obesity is an increasing problem in the U.S. According to a recently published study, 75 percent of American teenagers have tried dieting, and 21 percent of adolescents and 27 percent of children suffer from obesity. According to *Weighing the Options,* an official report of the Food and Nutrition Board, obesity in the young has at least a 50 to 70 percent chance of persisting into adulthood.

The Shapedown Weight-Loss Program for Children, created by Dr. Laura M. Mellin, Director of the Center for Child and Adolescent Obesity at the School of Medicine, University of California, San Francisco, has proven clinically effective in helping obese children lose weight and implement lifestyles that reduce depression and improve their self-esteem. Mellin's Shapedown Weight-Loss Program for Children, which has received White House endorsement, is detailed in several articles that appeared in the *Journal of the American Dietetic Association.* More than 80,000 teenagers have graduated from the Shapedown program.

## Eligibility and Costs

Shapedown is for children (aged 6 to 12) and adolescents (13 to 19) who are obese, have an eating disorder, or are trying to improve their fitness and eating habits. Parents are required to concurrently join the Parent Program to ensure family involvement and support. Costs for the ten-week Shapedown program range from $150 to $325, which includes four workbooks. Costs for the Advanced Shapedown twenty-week continuing care program range from $100 to $200. There are no special foods or supplements required by the program.

The program is easily adaptable since it allows the individual and family to set their own limits, goals, and strategies for weight loss and maintenance. Children are taught how to identify and cope with emotional, sensory, social, and situational cues that trigger overeating patterns.

Children dieters begin the program by meeting with Mellin's staff to design a personalized program to break the cycle of overeating. They learn stress management, assertiveness skills, and relaxation techniques and are taught ways to develop a support system of friends and family members.

## Basic Nutritional Approach

The Shapedown Diet focuses on reducing a child's caloric density in the diet (for example, increasing consumption of nonfat milk products, fruits, vegetables, grains, and lowfat meats and decreasing high-fat foods and added fat), consuming regular meals, increasing exercise levels (for example, structured after-school sports, household chores, walking, and family physical activities), and decreasing sedentary activities such as watching television and playing video games.

Parents and children attend both separate counseling sessions and joint family sessions. Parents are encouraged to change the entire family's diet to include lighter and more nutritious foods, and to increase family activity time and exercise. Parents are also counseled in numerous methods of effective parenting, including listening techniques for improved family communication, use of verbal contracts or agreements for increased understanding and acceptability, setting limits, providing enhanced emotional support, and the general promotion of family closeness.

## Recommended Foods

Foods are divided by the Shapedown Program into four categories:

- Foods with less than 30 percent of their calories from fat, less than 10 percent from simple carbohydrates (sugar), and containing fewer than 30 calories per serving;
- Light foods with less than 30 percent of their calories from fat, 10 percent from sugars, but higher in overall calories than free foods;

- Heavy foods deriving more than 30 percent of their calories from fat or more than 10 percent of their calories from sugars;
- Junk foods that are mostly fat, high in calories, and offer little nutritional value.

Shapedown dieters are encouraged to eat foods primarily from the free and light categories, but not to the complete exclusion of the other two, so that they do not feel deprived. Recommended foods can be easily purchased at supermarkets or found in most restaurants, making dining out and traveling relatively easy. Weight-loss goals for children and adolescents are determined individually and can range from lack of new weight gain to a weekly weight loss of one-half to one pound. Rigid or very low calorie diets are discouraged so that weight loss is gradual and does not restrict growth, deplete lean muscle tissue, or create nutritional deficiencies.

Shapedown clients are enrolled in a group weight management program in which dietitians conduct fourteen weekly sessions for dieters and two parent sessions. Sessions use only Shapedown materials, and each session lasts 90 minutes, including a voluntary weigh-in. Registered dietitians serve as group leaders and conduct group interaction sessions, followed by an exercise session. Height and weight measurements are taken and questionnaires are presented at the beginning of fourteen weeks, at the end of the test group intervention, and one year after the completion of the program.

## Monitoring Weight Loss

The following measures are used in the Shapedown Program to monitor weight loss and maintenance: relative weight, weight-related behavior; caloric density of the diet; frequency of ingestion; quantity of food consumed; exercise and activity; internal/external cue responsivity; hyper-emotional-state eating; compulsive eating patterns; eating style; eating environment; and assertiveness. According to Mellin, these measurements have been demonstrated to reliably predict which children will become obese and which will not. The questionnaire also measures each child's knowledge of nutrition at the beginning and conclusion of the program. During the initial meeting, dieters complete a registration form that includes demographic and medical data.

With this information, the child and family can identify their healthful characteristics and those which might be the cause of the child's obesity. Some children learn, according to Mellin, that their obesity is due to the fact that their family is extremely tense, and, in fact, hypertensive. Mellin strongly believes that one of the reasons Shapedown has proven clinically effective is because it identifies the family problems underlying a child's obesity. By doing so, families do not focus unnecessarily on the symptom (obesity) and as a result scapegoat the child, but reframe the problem as related to family tension. Many families, according to Mellin, are surprisingly open to the computerized information provided by the Shapedown program and are more than willing to address the underlying disturbances.

Each Shapedown client is given an easy-to-follow workbook that is appropriate to the specific age group. Assignments, stories, and quizzes are designed to permit regular monitoring of the client's diet and exercise activities. Record keeping by dieters is considered vital to success, and their workbooks are reviewed weekly as a precondition to attending weekly group sessions where they discuss family issues that contribute to their weight problems.

## Behavioral Modification

The overall goals of the program are to create positive lifestyle changes in the child and to address self-esteem, depression, communication, and parental difficulties, not just for the sake of appearance and general well-being but also to reduce the future risk of major diseases associated with obesity, such as diabetes, heart disease, and certain forms of cancer.

Since childhood obesity has been linked with child-parent conflicts, parent and family counseling is an important factor in Shapedown's success. Leonard Epstein and colleagues at the University of Pittsburgh School of Medicine have conducted similar programs that prove the effectiveness of family-based obesity treatment programs. Epstein reported in the November 1990 issue of the *Journal of the American Medical Association,* for example, that after ten years in one of his studies, children in a parent-child treatment group reduced their weight by 15 percent.

## Physical Activity

Shapedown encourages its dieters to gradually and consistently increase their level of physical activity, to cultivate their peer relationships, and to communicate their feelings and attitudes to their parents. Parents are, in turn, taught how to support their child's weight-loss efforts, and this includes altering their (parents') dietary and exercise patterns and improving their communication with their children.

Clients learn to calculate their target heart rates and develop individual exercise programs that increase their physical endurance, flexibility, and strength. Dieters are encouraged to engage in any form of safe exercise that interests them, from walking to karate to modern jazz dance. Shapedown provides an "exercise summary" booklet with specific recommendations, and the weekly meetings include a physical activity session.

One other weight-loss program for children should be noted here. The Jenny Craig weight-loss program (Chapter 6) also offers its Adolescent Program for children aged 13 to 17. This twelve-month program is based on the same nutritional, psychological, and exercise principles as the adult program, but includes a special menu plan and supporting educational materials designed specifically for the young client (for example, a parental-managed reward system and strategies for managing peer pressure and handling popular snacks and fast foods).

## RECENT RESEARCH

As role models and food providers, parents are the most important influence on a child's eating behavior. *Weighing the Options* cites a number of studies, summarized below, that detail how parents can encourage healthy dietary and exercise habits:

1. If parents themselves adopt prudent and nutritious diets, the children are more likely to follow their example.

2. Education and parental support are critical in helping children lose weight, improve their social lives, self-esteem, and academic performance.

3. Parents can effectively instill healthy eating habits in their children by encouraging them to spontaneously make their own informed food choices. The more control parents exert over their child's diet, the less self-regulation the child will display.

4. Parents must limit their children's television viewing to prevent harmful eating habits, including obesity. A 1985 study by Dietz and Gortmaker found a direct, positive relationship between television viewing and childhood obesity in a national sample of children and adolescents from diverse socioeconomic backgrounds. One way that television contributes to obesity is by displacing more vigorous activities, thereby reducing physical activity (or promoting inactivity) and increasing food and snack consumption, particularly of the nonnutritious foods frequently advertised. Television viewing has been shown to be associated with significant reductions in

resting metabolic rate among obese and nonobese girls, although these results were not replicated in a 1994 study by Dietz.

5. Parents should encourage schools to provide lowfat, nutrient-dense foods in school lunch programs. The USDA subsidizes school lunches by providing cash reimbursements and entitlement commodity foods. Most school lunch menus, however, offer high-fat meat meals and few vegetarian alternatives. Nevertheless, several studies have shown that children will readily adapt to lowfat plant-based diets. A 1994 pilot research project conducted by nutritionist Colin Campbell in Trumansburg, New York, demonstrated that if parents and school officials educate their children about diverse foods options, both the parents and children adopt healthier dietary habits.

6. Parents must also protect their families from exposure to pesticides, herbicides, fungicides, and other biocides, including the multiple residues that commonly occur on single servings of fruits and vegetables and drinking water (U.S. Department of Agriculture National Food Consumption Surveys). More than 80 percent of peach, apple, and celery samples contained residues of more than one pesticide; 10 percent of the servings, even after washing and preparation, had four or more pesticides. A 1990 EPA survey found that 10.4 percent of community water system wells and 4.2 percent of rural domestic wells contained one or more pesticides, which are not removed by the standard water treatment technologies.

Some experts suggest that widespread, low-level exposures to pesticides in the environment may be contributing to rising rates of some cancers in children and adults. A study reported in the January 1995 issue of *American Journal of Public Health* of children under age 15 found a strong association between home use of pesticides in the yard and soft-tissue sarcoma and between use of pest strips and leukemia. Consuming a wide variety of organic fruits and vegetables grown without agrochemicals reduces the risk of repeated exposure to the same pesticides, and varying the source of produce can also lower the risk of toxic reactions.

Raising a healthy child is a demanding and time-consuming job, and because in many families both parents work, it is often difficult for them to monitor their child's eating habits. The diets reviewed in this chapter, along with the studies cited above, document how important it is for parents to adapt self-regulating nutrition and exercise lifestyles in their children at the earliest age possible.

# 12

## Diets for the Elderly

M ichelangelo was carving his *Pietà* shortly before he died at age 89. Verdi finished his opera *Falstaff* at age 80. Titian created his greatest masterpieces in his late 80s. "I am still learning," the 80-year-old Goya scrawled on a drawing.

Most of us know elderly persons who refuse to give in to the infirmities of old age. These people stay young the old-fashioned way — they exercise, keep their minds agile with hobbies, and eat nutritious foods.

As a result, the elderly are at a higher risk of developing essential nutrient deficiencies. Surveys cited in *The Mayo Clinic Diet Manual,* for example, report that elderly Americans often have decreased intakes of vitamins A, B2, B6, and C. Other studies have reported similar low intakes of vitamins B1, D, folate, niacin, zinc, and calcium.

In response to a growing concern for improving the diets of elderly Americans, several national health agencies sponsored the 1991 Nutrition Screening Initiative, which created level I and II screening tools to help dietitians and physicians assess the risk of poor nutritional status.

The three diets reviewed in this chapter assist in the national effort to improve the nutritional status of elderly Americans. The first diet, Dr. Ray Walford's Anti-Aging Plan, is the most extreme. Walford believes that poor nutrition is a primary cause of the aging process. He argues that most of the elderly who develop chronic diseases such as heart disease, stroke, and cancer consume *more* calories than they need, and recommends a calorie-restrictive diet. The second, developed by Dr. Elizabeth Somer, adapts her healthy woman's diet (see Chapter 10) to suit the specific needs of elderly women. Her diet recommends increasing the consumption of foods containing vitamins B6, B12, and D as well as calcium beyond the current RDAs, and decreasing vitamin A intake. The third diet, developed by Dr. Marie Feltin, and published by the American Association of Retired Persons, focuses on the unique dietary problems of elderly women.

## THE WALFORD ANTI-AGING PLAN DIET

Dr. Ray Walford received his medical degree from the University of Chicago in 1948 and has been a professor of pathology at the UCLA School of Medicine since 1966. His anti-aging diet is presented in his book, *The Anti-Aging Plan.* Dr. Walford has authored more than 250 scientific articles and was a delegate to the 1994 White House Conference on Aging.

### Basic Nutritional Approach

In the Introduction to *The Anti-Aging Plan,* Walford relates that he was an adviser to Biosphere 2, the one-year experiment in which he and seven other scientists lived in a massive closed ecological space on the Arizona desert near Tucson which housed more than 3,800 carefully selected species of plants and animals. Walford states that "we could only grow food enough to provide each member of the experiment with approximately 1,800 calories per day for the first six months." Nevertheless, he believes their 1,800-calorie diet of nutrient-dense vegetables, grains, complex carbohydrates, legumes, and fiber was ideal. He observes that the Biospherians on this calorie-limited diet decreased their average weight by 26 (men) and 15 pounds (women); cholesterol levels dropped by 68 points from average levels of 191 to 125; and blood pressure levels decreased from an average of 110/75 to 90/58 after only three months.

The diet Walford presents in *The Anti-Aging Plan* is a gourmet version of the Biosphere diet, which "is low in calories and fat, high in nutrient-rich calories, satisfying, tasty, and easy to prepare." The overall intake, Walford states, is 1) generally moderate in protein, with emphasis on vegetable as opposed to animal protein sources; 2) low in fat with an emphasis of "quality" fats; 3) high in fiber; and 4) low in simple sugars but rich in complex carbohydrates.

The diet provides approximately 75 to 80 percent of calories as complex carbohydrates, 10 percent as saturated fat, and 10 to 20 percent as protein. According to Walford, the amount of "complete protein a person requires daily is approximately 0.015 ounces per pound of body weight — which equals about two ounces per day, depending on the person's size." This amount is required to replace the protein the body loses daily in the form of discarded cells and proteins broken down, or "turned over," through metabolism. Walford argues that his essentially vegetarian diet should provide adequate protein intake for most people. He advises dieters who feel they might need more protein to consume more nonfat milk or buttermilk, which both provide "complete" proteins.

## Required Foods

Walford's diet focuses on combining the most nutrient-dense lowfat foods: vegetables, which are low in fat (especially saturated fats) and cholesterol, and high in fiber; and legumes (various types of beans), which are low in fat and high in complex carbohydrates.

*Vegetables.* Walford notes that vegetarians tend to have lower incidences of many chronic diseases. For this reason, his is a vegetarian diet which requires the Brassica class of vegetables: kale, broccoli, collards, cauliflower, Brussels sprouts, mustard greens, and turnip greens. Besides containing beta-carotene, vitamin C, and high amounts of fiber, these vegetables are also excellent sources of calcium — important for dieters who restrict their intake of dairy products. Several studies, he adds, have linked a reduction in cancer risk with consumption of large amounts of Brassica vegetables, which, Walford suggests, should be eaten raw.

*Legumes and Grains.* Legumes and grains are required on Walford's anti-aging diet, because they are low in fat, and high in complex carbohydrates and fiber. He specifically recommends beans, oats, and brown rice. These foods are required because they help stabilize blood glucose levels. He notes that by consuming 75 to 80 percent of daily calories as complex carbohydrates, the Biospherians were able to lower their blood glucose levels by an average of 20 percent within a six-month period.

*Fiber.* According to Walford, fiber lowers blood cholesterol levels, adds fecal bulk, aids in colonic function, and helps metabolize sugar. In addition, fiber helps regulate appetite because it is filling but adds no calories. The average daily fiber intake in most Western diets, he observes, is approximately 20 grams. He states, however, that an average-sized person should consume at least 40 grams of total fiber daily. It may be necessary to gradually work up to this level to avoid temporary flatulence and bloating. He recommends starting by consuming 1/2 cup cooked black beans, 2 slices whole-wheat bread, 1/4 cup rolled oats, or 1/4 cup oat bran daily.

Most vegetarians will consume considerably more than 40 grams daily. The Biospherians consumed between an average of 45 and 60 grams daily. "This," states Walford, "played a role in their weight loss and contributed to marked improvement in both aging and biomarker health indices."

## Recommended Foods

In Chapter 9, "Tips, Tricks, Technique and Shortcuts," Walford lists foods he highly recommends along with the required vegetables and legumes: bran flakes, oat and wheat bran, kombu (a seaweed), nori (sea lettuce), nonfat dry milk, brewer's yeast, shiitake mushrooms, soybeans, and wheat germ.

## Eliminated Foods

Low-nutrient, high-calorie foods that are high in simple carbohydrates such as sugar are eliminated on Walford's diet. He specifically mentions all processed and refined foods, ice cream, lemon meringue pie, pecan pie, hamburger, doughnuts, and whipped cream.

## Restricted Foods: Alcohol

While Walford notes that alcohol is not a nutrient-rich food, dieters who consume only 1,800 calories daily may consume 100 to 200 calories of alcoholic beverages (one to two drinks daily) on his diet. He does not recommend this, although he notes that consuming alcohol is much healthier than consuming sugar. Some domestic beers and wines, he cautions, contain as many as fifty-two chemical additives and should be avoided. German beer and French wines are the best because they contain no additives.

## Vitamin and Mineral Supplements

According to Walford, scientific research suggests that elderly dieters should consume at least or exceed the RDAs of all essential nutrients. He specifically recommends taking the following vitamin and mineral supplements:

> **Vitamin A:** 25,000 IUs (international units)
> **Vitamin E:** 300 IUs (preferably vitamin E succinate or vitamin E acetate)

In Chapter 8, "Your Nutrient-Rich Kitchen," Walford provides the following list of required or recommended foods which dieters should always have on hand:

**Grains and cereals.** Brown rice, wild rice, barley, buckwheat, bulgur, couscous, millet; rolled oats; and wheat bran.

**Flour and pasta.** Whole-wheat flour; oat flour; whole-wheat pastry flour; cornmeal; whole-wheat pasta (spaghetti, macaroni, lasagna, shells); brown rice pasta; and soya noodles.

**Legumes.** Black beans; black-eyed peas; garbanzo beans; kidney beans; lentils; lima beans; white beans; pinto beans; and soybeans.

**Nuts and seeds.** Almonds; filberts (hazelnuts); walnuts; pumpkin seeds; sesame seeds; sunflower seeds; peanut butter and sesame butter (tahini).

**Seaweeds.** Kombu; nori; arame.

**Oils.** Canola oil spray; olive oil spray; olive oil; sesame oil; and walnut oil.

**Dried fruits.** White figs; papaya; raisins; and currants.

**Dry staples.** Nonfat dry milk; tapioca; dried vegetable or chicken broth; brewer's yeast; arrowroot and cornstarch thickeners; baking powder; baking soda; shiitake mushrooms; Chinese dried mushrooms; and cream of tartar.

**Canned staples.** Evaporated skim milk; tomato products; green chilies and salsa; water-packed sardines and tuna; chestnuts; legumes; water chestnuts; and artichoke hearts.

**Condiments and flavorings.** Balsamic and raspberry vinegars; rice wine, cider, tarragon; Dijon mustard; capers; hot sauce; low-sodium soy sauce; lemon and lime juice; sake; cooking wine; and vanilla.

**Frozen foods.** Corn; peas; orange, pineapple, and apple juices; chopped spinach and broccoli.

**Herbs.** Balsamic; bay leaves; chives; cilantro; dill; dried horseradish; garlic powder; marjoram; dried mustard; onion powder; oregano; rosemary; sage; tarragon; and thyme.

**Spices.** Allspice; black mustard seed; cardamom; cloves; chili powder; cinnamon; coriander; cumin; fennel seed; ginger; nutmeg; paprika; black, white, and cayenne pepper; red pepper flakes; saffron; and turmeric.

**Vitamin C:** 0.5 grams (500 milligrams)
**Selenium:** 100 micrograms (preferably products labeled "organically bound")
**Magnesium:** 0.5 to 1 gram
**Chromium picolinate:** 200 micrograms
**Coenzyme Q10:** 20 milligrams

## Physical Activity

Physical activity is not a required part of Walford's diet, although he notes its many medical benefits, including:

1. Exercise increases cardiovascular fitness, decreases susceptibility to heart attacks and strokes, improves carbohydrate metabolism, improves brain function, and delays some of the age-related deterioration of skeletal muscles.
2. Exercise increases beneficial high-density lipoprotein (HDL) levels in the blood and lowers the level of low-density lipoproteins (LDL). Exercise also benefits the cholesterol/HDL ratio (a better predictor of heart disease than the cholesterol level alone).

Walford cautions, however, that animal experiments have clearly shown that while exercise may increase a person's general health, it will not increase their maximum life span. Walford believes his anti-aging plan, which combines diet with exercise, does both, however, and "to a much greater degree than exercise alone." With a doctor's approval, he recommends beginning a program of moderate exercise, "more or less equivalent to fifteen miles of jogging per week." An alternative for nonrunners, he adds, is to take a brisk 30-minute walk three times a week.

## Anti-Aging Benefits of the Walford/Biosphere Diet

In summarizing the benefits for both elderly persons and people who hope to delay the onset of aging, Walford states that his diet:

1. Reduces risk of (and may reverse) coronary heart disease and arteriosclerosis.
2. Reduces high blood pressure.
3. Reduces risk of various cancers.
4. Reduces risk of osteoporosis and diverticulitis.

5. Improves appearance by helping dieters to lose weight, maintain weight loss, and decrease their percentage of body fat.
6. Retards mental dysfunctioning.
7. Maintains longer sexual functioning.
8. Keeps the immune system "younger": a stronger immune system helps elderly persons fight off bacterial or viral infection, strengthens the liver which detoxifies poisons, helps the kidneys purify the blood, strengthens connective tissue, maintains the body's hormonal systems, and helps repair DNA.
9. Helps increase average life span (along with exercise).

## ELIZABETH SOMER'S DIET FOR THE ELDERLY

Elizabeth Somer suggests that her lowfat, nutrient-dense Healthy Woman's Diet can be easily adapted for elderly persons. She states that there is a "wealth of information" showing a strong link between a lowfat nutrient-dense diet and improved health, reduced risk of disease and slowed progression of age-related processes. Most specialists agree, she adds, "that good food choices can have profound effects on the quality of life and longevity."

### Basic Nutritional Approach

Somer's diet for the elderly limits fat to less that 30 percent and saturated fats to no more than 7 percent of total calories. She contends that excessive fat consumption has been linked with numerous diseases, including heart disease and diabetes. High-fat diets also cause considerable excess weight and body fat problems in elderly persons. While some fat is necessary for the proper absorption of the fat-soluble vitamins, Somer argues that diets limited to even 20 percent fat calories or less still supply ample fat for normal digestion.

Elderly dieters, she cautions, must ensure that they consume all the essential vitamins and minerals which have been proven to reduce the risk of disease, improve immune function, and slow the aging process. Because of the possible reduction in the absorption utilization of some nutrients, Somer states that even healthy seniors "should aim for intakes about 25 percent higher than present RDAs." These additional RDAs, she adds, can be usually obtained in adequate amounts from foods in her diet as long as enough of these foods (at least 2,000 calories) are consumed daily. When dietary habits fall short, or if calorie intake is lower than this, Somer recommends that elderly persons take moderate-dose vitamin and mineral supplements.

### Required or Recommended Foods

Somer does not identify specific required foods in her diet for the elderly. She does, however, highly recommend:

- *Breads.* 100 percent whole-wheat bread, whole-wheat bagels, pita bread and rolls, English muffins, French bread, cornbread, pumpernickel, and corn tortillas.
- *Crackers and snacks.* RyKrisp, Akmak, or other lowfat, whole-wheat crackers, low-salt corn chips, rice cakes, graham crackers, tortilla chips, pretzels, and air-popped popcorn.
- *Cereals.* Nutri-Grain cereal, Grape-Nuts, shredded wheat, puffed wheat and puffed rice, whole-grain hot cereal such as oatmeal, wheat germ, and kasha.
- *Noodles, rice, and other grains.* Whole-wheat, spinach, and "enriched" noodles, long-grain or short-grain brown rice, wild rice, millet, cracked wheat or bulgur, barley, tabouli mix, Spanish rice, rice and wheat pilaf (packets can be omitted for the latter four if sodium is a concern).
- *Flour.* Whole-wheat, rye, oat, and unbleached white flours (although less nutritious than the whole-grain varieties).
- *Fruits.* All fresh fruits; canned fruits in their own juices; all 100 percent fruit juices; canned, bottled, or frozen concentrate.
- *Vegetables.* All fresh or plain frozen vegetables except avocados and olives, all 100 percent vegetable juices, tomato sauce and paste, marinara sauce, salsa, and artichoke hearts canned in water.
- *Beans and peas.* All dried beans and peas, canned cooked dried beans and peas, packaged bean mixes, and peanut butter in small quantities.
- *Meat, chicken, and fish.* Chicken (with skin removed before cooking), extra-lean beef (less than 9 percent fat by weight), extra-lean pork, turkey (with skin removed before cooking), canned tuna packed in water, and all fresh and frozen unprocessed fish.
- *Milk and eggs.* No-fat cheeses, lowfat mozzarella cheese, nonfat or one percent fat plain yogurt, milk or buttermilk, nonfat, lowfat, or dry curd cottage cheese, lowfat Parmesan cheese, partially skimmed swiss and

ricotta, and one to two eggs weekly (preferably using only the egg white).

- *Beverages.* Mineral water, diet soda, tea, and decaffeinated coffee and tea.
- *Spices and flavorings.* Garlic powder, selected spices and herbs (including dill), mustard, sugar substitute, clam juice, and pimiento.
- *Oils and fats.* Low-calorie margarine and mayonnaise, nonfat salad dressing, safflower oil, dry roasted nuts such as almonds, and sunflower seeds.
- *Sweets and desserts.* Jams (preferably all-fruit, no-sugar variety), angel food cake, sherbet, vanilla wafers, Dole frozen fruit bar and Fruit Ice, and Healthy Choice ice cream.

*Protein.* According to Somer, the elderly need as many essential amino acids as younger adults, although older people need to get these from less food. Thus, they should ensure that they consume "high-quality protein foods" daily, balanced with complex carbohydrates. She notes that many elderly people living at home do not consume enough milk or its equivalent in cheese because of difficulties with purchasing and storage. Meat is also often omitted because it is difficult to chew. As a result, the elderly tend to have low hemoglobin levels, and many complain of feeling fatigued or apathetic. Somer advises elderly dieters to consume 12 percent of total daily calories as protein.

*Fiber.* Somer states that adequate daily fiber intake is especially important for elderly dieters because it helps alleviate constipation. Fiber helps offset the effects of diminished muscle tone and peristalsis. In order to avoid abdominal discomforts, dietary fiber should be increased gradually while adequate amounts of liquid are consumed. She advises that fruits, vegetables, and whole-grain cereals must be consumed each day to maintain the health of the intestinal tract. In addition, some fibers, with the exception of wheat bran, help bind and eliminate cholesterol from the body.

*Carbohydrate.* As noted in Chapter 10, Somer's basic Healthy Woman's Diet recommends consuming daily amounts of a wide variety of complex carbohydrate foods, which provide essential vitamins and minerals.

*Water.* Somer cautions that elderly persons often need to be reminded to drink fluids because they are likely to be somewhat insensitive to their own thirst signals. They should drink six to eight glasses a day, enough to bring their urine output to about 1,500 milliliters (6 cups) per day.

## Eliminated or Restricted Foods

Somer does not eliminate any foods from her diet for the elderly because it is not practical. "Any realistic lifelong nutrition plan," she writes, "must include a person's favorite foods, or it is likely to fail. Remember that nothing is forbidden but everything counts." She does, however, restrict foods high in fat, salt, and sugar.

*Fat.* Somer advises elderly dieters to restrict fat in order to reduce caloric intake, and also to retard the development of atherosclerosis. She argues that high-fat intakes also interfere with calcium absorption and help promote osteoporosis. An appropriate daily fat level is 20 percent of calories, of which about half should be from polyunsaturated fat to contribute the essential fatty acids and to displace the saturated fat thought to contribute to high levels of cholesterol in the blood.

*Salt.* Somer advises all elderly persons to restrict daily salt intake. She notes that excessive salt consumption has been directly linked with hypertension, congestive heart failure, and cirrhosis of the liver. Her diet restricts all high-sodium convenience and processed foods. Since reducing excessive salt intake "has no harmful side effects," she advises elderly dieters to limit salt intake to no more than 6 grams daily, adding that 4 grams or less is even healthier.

*Sugar.* Somer states that "a little sugar in the diet is safe," but cautions that most Americans consume an average of 20 percent of daily calories with sugar. She recommends restricting sugar intake to no more than 10 percent.

## Vitamin and Mineral Supplements

Somer believes that the current RDAs for many vitamins and minerals are too low for the over-65 group. She suggests that if elderly people conscientiously follow her dietary guidelines, they will not need to take a vitamin-mineral supplement. It is often difficult for elderly dieters, however, to follow her diet because they do not plan, purchase, or prepare their own foods. In that event, they should consider a supplement(s) that provides approxi-

## TIPS FOR THE ELDERLY

Dr. Elizabeth Somer provides the following helpful tips for elderly persons who wish to ensure they are consuming nutrient-dense foods:

- *Storing foods.* Casseroles, soups, and other dishes can be prepared in bulk and then divided into individual portions for easy reheating at a later time. Since standing and cooking can be tiring, it is helpful to have a chair or stool at a suitable height for the counter or stove.

- Seniors often have trouble chewing and thus should consciously choose foods that are softer, such as ground meat, mashed potatoes, cottage cheese, peanut butter, oatmeal, applesauce, and soft-cooked vegetables. Meats, vegetables, and grains prepared in stews and soups are also easier to chew.

- Seniors with diminished taste buds can season sweet potatoes, squash, and fruits with allspice, cinnamon, and ginger. Sauce, meat dishes, and other vegetables can be seasoned with nutmeg; ham or pickled dishes can be seasoned with cloves. Seasonings that replace salt include basil in tomato-based soups, meat stews, and Italian sauces; dill in seafood or chicken dishes, cream sauces, and spinach; garlic for meats, seafood, chicken, mushrooms, potatoes, and tomatoes; and oregano in tomato sauces, asparagus, zucchini, and beets.

- Seniors trying to avoid weight gain should reduce their fat intake, eat smaller portions, broil or bake foods rather than fry them, purchase only extra-lean meats (labeled 9 percent or less fat) and trim off excess fat, use fresh or unsweetened canned fruits for dessert, and limit the use of desserts, fats, oils, and alcohol.

mately 100 to 200 percent of the U.S. RDAs or 125 percent of the RDAs for vitamin D, the B vitamins, calcium, chromium, copper, iron, magnesium, manganese, selenium, and zinc. Beta-carotene, vitamin C, and vitamin E can be consumed in slightly higher amounts, according to Somer, with no known harmful effects, and, in fact, large doses of these nutrients might be beneficial. The chart below shows the RDA's and Somer's optimal dietary allowances for the elderly:

| Nutrient | RDA | ODA |
|----------|-----|-----|
| Protein | 50 grams | 62 grams |
| Vitamin A | 4,000 IU | 5,000 IU |
| Vitamin D | 200 IU | 400 IU |

| Nutrient | RDA | ODA |
|---|---|---|
| Vitamin E | 12 IU | 15 IU |
| Vitamin K | 65 mcg | 80 mcg |
| Vitamin C | 60 mg | 75 mg |
| Vitamin B1 | 1 mg | 1.25 mg |
| Vitamin B2 | 1 mg | 1.5 mg |
| Niacin | 13 mg | 16 mg |
| Vitamin B6 | 1.6 mg | 2 mg |
| Folic acid | 180 mcg | 400 mcg |
| Vitamin B12 | 2 mcg | 2.5 mcg |
| Calcium | 800 mg | 1,000–1,500 mg |
| Phosphorous | 800 mg | 1,000 mg |
| Magnesium | 280 mg | 350 mg |
| Iron | 10 mg | 12.5 mg |
| Selenium | 55 mcg | 60 mcg |
| Copper | 1.5–3 mg | 3 mg |
| Manganese | 2–5 mg | 5 mg |
| Fluoride | 1.5–4 mg | 4 mg |
| Chromium | 50–200 mcg | 200 mcg |
| Molybdenum | 75–250 mcg | 250 mcg |

## Physical Activity

Somer stresses the importance of exercise in her diet program for the elderly, noting that many of the symptoms of old age, including increased body fat, weak and stiff muscles, brittle or porous bones, low energy, and increased risk of disease are related to a sedentary lifestyle. She recommends aerobic activity such as walking, bicycling, swimming and water aerobics, and strength-training or weightlifting, which increase muscle strength and flexibility and reduce the risk of disease and premature aging.

## THE DIET FOR WOMEN OVER 50

The Diet for Women Over 50 was developed by Dr. Marie Feltin, a physician with the Urban Medical Group in Boston and medical director of the Independent Living Primary Care Program. Her diet is detailed in *A Woman's Guide to Good Health After 50*, published by the American Association of Retired Persons (AARP).

## Basic Nutritional Approach

After reviewing an impressive amount of clinical studies, Feltin suggests that an elderly woman's nutritional needs will depend on her body size, metabolic rate, state of health, and level of physical activity. She recommends that elderly persons follow the caloric guidelines recommended by the National Academy of Science, adding that persons who are very physically active will need to more closely adopt the nutritional guidelines for younger people:

1. Adults between the ages of 50 and 75 should eat only 90 percent of the calories that those under 50 consume, or approximately 1,800 calories daily, depending on their level of activity.
2. Adults above 75 years of age should eat only 75 to 80 percent of calories that those under 50 eat, or about 1,600 calories daily.
3. Older adults should divide their daily caloric intake so that it contains approximately 12 percent protein, 30 percent fat, and the remainder (more than 50 percent) complex carbohydrates.

## Required and Recommended Foods

Feltin describes separately the importance of protein, carbohydrate, fat, and fiber, but she does not discuss individually recommended or required foods. Instead, she advises elderly women to follow the Four Basic Food Groups and Recommended Daily Servings:

| Recommended Food Group | Daily Servings | Sample Servings (measurements are for 1 serving) |
|---|---|---|
| Milk | 4 | 1 cup milk |
| | | 1 cup yogurt |
| Meat and Dairy | 2 | 2 eggs |
| | | 2 oz. cheddar cheese |
| | | 2 oz. lean cooked meat |
| | | 1/2 cup creamed cottage cheese |
| Fruits and Vegetables | 4 | 1 medium-sized apple |
| | | 1 cup raw broccoli |
| | | 1/2 cup orange juice |
| | | 1/2 cup cooked spinach |

| Recommended Food Group | Daily Servings | Sample Servings (measurements are for 1 serving) |
|---|---|---|
| Grains | 4 | 1 slice bread |
| | | 1/2 cup cooked cereal |
| | | 1/2 cup cooked pasta |
| | | 1/2 cup cooked rice |

*Protein.* Feltin suggests that meats, egg, and soybeans contain all the essential amino acids. Other foods, such as beans and peas, have some but not all the essential amino acids. However, when consumed with rice or wheat, the combination provides all the essential amino acids. Nevertheless, she does not list (other than in her daily sample menu) specific foods or amounts that elderly women should consume daily. She does suggest that women eat more chicken, veal, fish, and tofu rather than beef, and that they serve three-ounce servings per meal rather than the eight-ounce servings (which butchers and fish sellers recommend and which restaurants serve regularly). She also notes that the body uses more protein during sickness, and that women should increase their protein intake when they are sick.

## Eliminated or Restricted Foods

Feltin's book does not list categories of eliminated or restricted foods. Instead, she provides the following guidelines outlining restricted foods:

- Restrict fats to 30 percent of the diet; reduce the consumption of foods that contain hidden fats, such as doughnuts and luncheon meats.
- Restrict fats from meat by substituting fish at least three times a week.
- Restrict saturated fat oils by substituting plant-based oils, including corn and corn oil margarine, safflower oil, and vegetable oil.

## Daily Meal Plans

Feltin provides two sample daily menus based on her food recommendations:

**Day 1** (approximately 1,800 calories)
**Breakfast**
1/2 cup grapefruit juice
1/2 cup oatmeal
1/3 cup lowfat milk

1 tablespoon brown sugar
1 slice whole-wheat bread
1 teaspoon margarine
coffee

**Lunch**
Grilled mozzarella cheese (1 ounce) and tomato (1/8 tomato)
sandwich
Baked apple
1 cup lowfat milk

**Snack**
tea
2 oatmeal-raisin cookies

**Dinner**
3 1/2 oz. broiled chicken, white meat
1/2 cup mixed rice, green peas, and mushrooms
1/3 cup cucumbers, sliced
1 tablespoon oil
1 slice rye bread
1 teaspoon margarine
1/2 cup pineapple chunks
tea

**Snack**
2 cups popcorn
1 tablespoon margarine

**Day 2** (approximately 1,800 calories)
**Breakfast**
1 orange, sliced
1/2 cup unenriched grits
2 slices bacon
tea

**Lunch**
1 cup cream of tomato soup
1/3 cup tuna salad in a half-slice of whole-wheat pita bread
1/5 of a head lettuce
1 cup apple juice

**Snack**
(same as day 1)

**Dinner**
1 cup beef stew
1 cup enriched rice
1/2 cup coleslaw
1 slice whole-wheat bread
1 teaspoon margarine
1/2 cup raspberry sherbet
**Snack**
1 6-oz. cup of cocoa
1 bran muffin (small)

## Lactose Intolerance

Feltin also suggests that many elderly persons find it especially difficult to digest lactose, the main sugar found in milk. One result is that they often notice gas, cramps, and diarrhea after drinking milk. This, she suggests, is due to the fact that lactase levels decrease with age, and to remedy this, she advises elderly women to drink smaller amounts of milk, or to drink soybean milk, which is available at many health food stores. Women can also try LactAid, a product that provides the deficient enzyme from yeast and helps them digest milk. Fermented dairy products such as live-culture yogurt, buttermilk, and some cheese may also be easier to digest, because they contain less lactose than milk.

## Vitamins and Mineral Supplements

According to Feltin, most elderly women who eat a balanced daily diet from the four food groups will not need to take vitamin or mineral supplements. For example, she advises elderly women to consume the following nutrients daily in natural foods:

**Vitamins**

| | |
|---|---|
| Vitamin A | 800 mcg |
| Vitamin D | 5 mcg |
| Vitamin E | 8 mg |
| Vitamin C | 60 mg |
| Vitamin B1 | 1 mg |
| Vitamin B2 | 1.2 mg |
| Vitamin B6 | 2 mg |
| Vitamin B12 | 3 mcg |

| Niacin | 13 mg |
|---|---|
| Folic acid | 400 mcg |
| **Minerals** | |
| Calcium | 1,200–1,500 mg |
| Phosphorus | 800 mg |
| Magnesium | 300 mg |
| Iron | 10 mg |
| Zinc | 15 mg |
| Iodine | 150 mcg |
| Sodium | 1,100–3,300 mg |
| Potassium | 1,875–5,625 mg |
| Chloride | 1,700–5,100 mg |

Foods are safer and more natural sources of most essential nutrients than pills, she observes, and "'wise women will be pill-free whenever possible." She adds, however, that women with increased risk for specific chronic diseases may need to take calcium (for osteoporosis), iron (for iron deficiency anemia), or potassium supplements (women with high blood pressure or who take diuretics).

## Alcohol

According to Feltin, alcohol consumed in moderate doses is more beneficial than harmful to the health of elderly persons. She cites several studies that have concluded that people who have one to two drinks of alcohol live longer than those who abstain. Moderate drinkers, she adds, tend to have higher levels of high-density (good) lipoproteins in their blood which reduces their risk of arteriosclerosis and may help the heart by relieving stress and lessening tension in arterial wall muscles. She defines one drink as:

1/2 ounce of 80-proof distilled spirits
one 12-ounce glass of lager beer
one 5-ounce glass of French wine
one 4-ounce glass of American wine
one 3-ounce glass of sherry

## Physical Activity

In Chapter 2, "Your Musculoskeletal System," Feltin cites many medical benefits of exercise for elderly women. She suggests that the easiest way to grow physically fit is exercise daily, and she specifically recommends walking. She cautions that walking steps should be brisk to build up endurance, as well as to limber and strengthen joints and muscles. She also recommends weight-bearing exercises (especially for women with osteoporosis), yoga, exercise classes, ballroom dancing (swing, jazz, tap, modern dance, and ballet), swimming, aerobics, and Nautilus machines.

### Behavioral Modification

In her chapter entitled "Eating Problems of Older Women," Feltin identifies a number of lifestyle changes that commonly occur in elderly women which can jeopardize their nutritional status:

- Loneliness can lead to unbalanced diets, especially overeating or undereating.
- Women may find it more difficult to cook for themselves or their husbands.
- Once children leave or a husband or partner passes away, many women tend to lose interest in regular eating and let their good eating habits deteriorate.
- Poor health can interfere with eating.
- It often is more difficult to keep perishables such as milk, fruits, and vegetables on hand.
- The diminished sense of taste and smell that accompanies age can decrease a woman's interest in eating.
- Drugs taken for medical or psychological conditions often interfere with the body's ability to absorb vitamins and minerals.
- Several research teams have found that women over 55 often have diets low in calcium, protein, vitamin A, thiamine (B1), and iron, and that women over the age of 65 often eat too little food to meet their energy needs.

## RECENT RESEARCH

Although the role of vitamins and minerals in delaying the aging process is still debated by scientists, one public health organization, the Alliance for Aging Research, officially advises elderly persons to consume daily vitamin C, E, and beta-carotene supplements to reduce the risk of life-threatening medical disorders such as heart disease and cancer. According to an article in the May 1994 issue of the *Tufts University Diet and Nutrition Letter,* the

**ANTIOXIDANT RECOMMENDATIONS OF
THE ALLIANCE FOR AGING RESEARCH**

- **Vitamin C:** 250 to 1,000 milligrams, or 4 to 16 times the U.S. RDA of 60 milligrams
- **Vitamin E:** 100 to 400 International Units (IUs), the equivalent of 3 to 13 times the U.S. RDA of 30 IUs
- **Beta-carotene** (a relative of vitamin A found only in plant foods): 17,000 to 50,000 IUs, or 3 to 10 times the recommended vitamin A allowance of 5,000 IUs

Alliance's recommendations were developed after convening a panel of respected scientific experts from research and academic institutions around the country. The panel reviewed more than two hundred studies of antioxidants conducted over the last twenty years, which collectively suggest that elderly persons should consume larger amounts than the U.S. RDAs of vitamins C, E, and beta-carotene to combat free radicals — the highly toxic molecules which are produced as a natural byproduct during the chemical process of oxidation.

If free radicals are left unchecked, they can, according to the Alliance, damage the cells inside various tissues, potentially leading to the development of clogged arteries, various cancers, and other debilitating conditions. The Alliance's official report concluded that illness and poor health due to antioxidants can be minimized if elderly dieters maintain optimum nutrition, including taking its recommended supplements.

# 13

## Vegetarian Diet Programs

A vegetarian diet was good enough for Buddha, Plato, Socrate, Hippocrates, Ovid, Aristotle, Shelley, Tolstoi, George Bernard Shaw, and Mahatma Gandhi, and the authors of diets reviewed in this chapter argue it should be good for all of us as well.

More than 14 million Americans currently consider themselves vegetarians. The increasing popularity of vegetarian diets reflects an increasing awareness of many Americans that vegetarian lifestyles have been linked with reduced risks of chronic diseases. Dr. C. Everett Koop, former Surgeon General of the Public Health Service, in his 1988 *Report on Nutrition and Health*, expressed "major concern" about the average American diet's disproportionate consumption of animal foods high in fats "at the expense of foods high in complex carbohydrates and fiber — such as vegetables, fruits, and whole-grain products — that may be more conducive to health." And while guidelines from the U.S. Departments of Agriculture and Health and Human Services advise 2 to 3 daily servings of milk and the same of foods such as dried peas and beans, eggs, meat, poultry, and fish, they recommend 3 to 5 servings of vegetables, 2 to 4 servings of fruits, and 6 to 11 servings of bread, cereal, rice, and pasta — in other words, 11 to 20 plant foods but only 4 to 6 animal foods.

The three diets reviewed in this chapter reflect the evolution of recent American scientific thinking on vegetarian diets. When Michio Kushi first introduced his macrobiotic diet to Americans in the late 1940s, he argued that it could reduce the risk of heart disease and cancer. His claim was hotly contested by American nutritionists who contended that vegetarian diets could be dangerous because they did not provide enough high-quality protein. Vegetable proteins, they suggested, did not supply all the essential amino acids.

---

**TYPES OF VEGETARIANS**

In its pamphlet *Eating Well — The Vegetarian Way,* the American Dietetic Association defines vegetarians as people who do not eat meat, poultry, or fish, but rather consume primarily plant foods: vegetables, legumes, grains, seeds, and nuts. The three main classifications include:

- Strict vegetarians exclude all animal products, such as meat, poultry, fish, eggs, milk, cheese, and other dairy products. Many vegans also do not eat honey.

- Lactovegetarians exclude meat, poultry, fish, and eggs but include dairy products.

- Ovolactovegetarians exclude meat, poultry, and fish but include eggs and dairy products. Most vegetarians in the United States follow this type of diet.

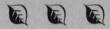

---

The American health researcher Gary Null, author of the second diet in this chapter, conducted several studies which found that when different vegetarian foods were combined in appropriate ways, they provided better amino acid profiles with more fiber and less fat and excess protein than meat-based diets.

Kushi and Null's arguments that vegetarian diets are nutritionally more sound and medically more beneficial have been endorsed by several national health organizations including the American Dietetic Association (ADA) and the Mayo Clinic. The *Mayo Clinic Diet Manual,* the third diet reviewed, enthusiastically endorses vegetarian diets for children, adults, and, in some cases, hospitalized patients.

## KUSHI MACROBIOTIC DIET

Michio Kushi came to the United States shortly after World War II upon completing studies at Tokyo University. He helped introduce the dietary approach of his former professor, Dr. George Oshawa (the founder of macrobiotics), to the West. Kushi founded the East West Foundation, Kushi Institute, Kushi Foundation, and Macrobiotics International. His diet is detailed in *The Book of Macrobiotics: The Universal Way of Health, Happiness and Peace,* coauthored by Alex Jack.

## Basic Nutritional Approach

Kushi defines macrobiotics as a philosophy of "living consciously." The goal is to realize health and happiness by living in harmony with the natural order of the universe, which includes eating a simple, traditional diet based on natural whole foods. His macrobiotic diet consists of 50 to 60 percent whole cereal grains daily, 20 to 25 percent fresh vegetables, 5 to 10 percent beans and bean products, and 5 to 10 percent soups. "Occasional supplemental foods" include fish and seafood (less fatty varieties), seasonal fruits (cooked, dried, and rarely fresh), nuts and seeds, natural nonaromatic and nonstimulant beverages, and natural, unprocessed seasonings and condiments.

## Required and Recommended Foods

Kushi does not specifically state that particular foods are required on his diet. His diet does require, however, that cereal grains, vegetables, beans and bean products, and soup be consumed daily.

*Whole Cereal Grains.* Kushi's diet allows dieters to choose whole grain cereals for each meal, and must include either brown rice, whole-wheat berries, millet, barley, corn, buckwheat, rye, or oats. Whole-grain products (such as cracked wheat, rolled oats, noodles, pasta, bread, baked goods, and other flour products) may occasionally be substituted, although Kushi warns that the nutrients they contained are substantially less than grain consumed in whole form.

*Vegetables.* Vegetables represent 25 to 30 percent of daily food in the Kushi macrobiotic diet, prepared in such ways as steaming, boiling, baking, salads, marinades, and pickles. Vegetables should include root vegetables (carrots, cabbage, and radishes), leafy green vegetables (kale, collard greens, broccoli, turnip and mustard greens, and watercress), and ground vegetables such as onions, squash, and cucumbers. Kushi suggests avoiding vegetables that historically originated in the tropics (such as tomato and potato).

*Beans and Bean Products.* Cooked beans or bean products such as tofu and tempeh comprise 5 to 10 percent of Kushi's macrobiotic diet. He suggests preparing these foods individually, cooking them together with grains, vegetables, or sea vegetables, or serving them in the form of soup. Although all dried and fresh beans are suitable for consumption, Kushi points out that the smaller varieties such as adzuki beans, lentils, and chickpeas contain less fat and oil and are preferable for regular use.

*Sea Vegetables.* Sea vegetables are excellent sources of vitamins and minerals, according to Kushi, and should comprise about 5 percent of total food volume. He specifically recommends nori which is used as wrapper for sushi rolls; wakama (added to soups); arame and hiziki, which can be added to grains, vegetable dishes, and salads; powdered kelp (a soft salt substitute); and agar (a substitute for gelatin in aspics and jelled desserts). Kushi recommends that these sea vegetables be seasoned with a moderate amount of tamari soy sauce, sea salt, or brown rice vinegar.

*Seafood.* Kushi's macrobiotic diet allows a small amount of fish or seafood a few times per week for people in good health. White-meat fish, he notes, generally contains less fat than red-meat or blue-skin varieties. Kushi recommends consuming grated daikon, horseradish, fresh ginger, or mustard as a condiment to "help detoxify the body."

*Soup.* According to Kushi, one or two small bowls of soup, comprising 5 to 10 percent of daily food intake, should be consumed daily. He recommends that soup broths be made with miso or tamari soy sauce to which varieties of land and sea vegetables (including wakame, kombu, carrots, onions, cabbage, and Chinese cabbage) should be added during cooking. Soups made with grains, beans, land vegetables, and seafood may also be prepared as part of this category.

*Seeds and Nuts.* Kushi states that seeds and nuts, lightly roasted and seasoned with sea salt or tamari soy sauce, may be enjoyed as occasional snacks. However, he recommends not overconsuming nuts and nut butters as they are high in fats and difficult to digest.

*Fruit.* Kushi's macrobiotic diet permits only fruits grown in the dieter's local climate zone. They can be consumed as snacks or desserts several times a week, preferably cooked or naturally dried. Raw fruits can be eaten "in moderate volumes," but only during their growing season. Temperate-climate fruits are suitable for occasional use, especially apples, pears, peaches, apricots, grapes, berries, and melons. Tropical fruits such as grapefruit, pineapple, and mangoes are permitted, but only if the dieter lives in the tropics. He does not recommend natural fruit juices because they are usually too concentrated for regular use, although occasional consumption is permitted in very hot weather.

*Desserts.* People in good health may eat desserts in moderate volume two or three times a week, including cookies, pudding, cake, pie, or other sweets. Kushi prefers naturally sweet foods such as apples or dried fruit that can often be used in dessert recipes without additional sweetening. He recommends avoiding sugar, honey, molasses, chocolate, carob, or other sweeteners that are refined, extremely strong, or of tropical origin.

*Cooking Oil.* For daily cooking, Kushi recommends only naturally processed, unrefined vegetable oil. Dark sesame oil is preferable, although light sesame oil, corn oil, and mustard seed oil are also suitable. For special occasions, other unrefined vegetable oils such as safflower oil, olive oil, and walnut oil may be used.

*Beverages.* Kushi recommends that only spring or well water be used for drinking, preparing tea and other beverages, and for general cooking. Commonly consumed macrobiotic beverages include bancha twig tea (also known as kukicha), and grain-based teas or traditional, nonstimulant herbal teas. Green tea, fruit juice, soymilk, beer, wine, and sake are permitted on his diet, but should be served less frequently.

## Eliminated or Restricted Foods

Kushi eliminates all meat from his diet because he believes it has been directly associated with many chronic diseases. He argues that meat is harder to digest than plant foods, produces toxins that accumulate in the liver, kidneys, and large intestine, destroys bacterial culture (especially those that synthesize the B vitamins), and causes degeneration of the villi of the small intestine, where metabolized foodstuffs are absorbed into the blood.

Kushi further notes that saturated fatty acids from meat and other animal products accumulate in and around vital organs and blood vessels, often leading to cysts, tumors, and hardening of the arteries. Saturated fat also raises the amount of cholesterol in the blood, further contributing to the buildup of atherosclerotic plaque.

*Dairy Products.* Kushi contends that casein — the protein in cheese, milk, cream, butter, and other dairy foods — cannot be assimilated easily and accumulates in an undigested state in the upper intestine, where it produces toxins, and leads to a weakening of the gastric, intestinal, pancreatic, and biliary (bile-producing) systems. He further asserts that modern medical studies have begun to link dairy food consumption with a wide variety of disorders, including cramps and diarrhea, multiple forms of allergy, iron-deficiency anemia (in infants and children), atherosclerosis, heart attacks, arthritis, and several forms of cancer.

*Sugar.* Kushi eliminates all processed sugars from his diet and strongly recommends restricting foods such as fruit juices, which contain excess natural sugars. Simple sugars, he contends, help release fatty acids into the bloodstream. They are stored in the more inactive places of the body such as the buttocks, thighs, and midsection, and in the heart, liver, and kidneys. This buildup of excess fat can lead to various forms of cancer, including tumors of the breast, colon, and reproductive organs.

### Recipes

Kushi admits that initially many Americans will find his macrobiotic diet somewhat bland. He urges dieters to be creative in adding the natural seasonings and spices he recommends, and provides a number of excellent macrobiotic recipes.

### Vitamin and Mineral Supplements

Kushi does not endorse taking vitamin and mineral supplements because his diet supplies all essential nutrients, and some supplements can be toxic. Some vitamin C capsules, he contends, originate from potatoes, tomatoes, and other solanaceous (nightshade) plants that have been associated with arthritis and other disorders. The best sources of vitamin C, he notes, are leafy green vegetables that contain no sugar — collard greens, kale, parsley, turnip greens, and broccoli.

Vitamin B12 supplements are not necessary because tempeh, spirulina, kombu, and wakame are excellent sources. He adds that his diet contains sufficient amounts of all minerals in "proper proportions," and cautions that taking megadose mineral supplements can either block the absorption of other essential nutrients or increase the body's normal requirements.

Excessive amounts of zinc, for example, can cause anemia by inhibiting copper absorption and interfering with proper calcium absorption. Similarly, excess iron or selenium can cause a zinc deficiency.

Kushi notes that Western dietitians commonly make the mistake of suggesting that milk and other dairy foods supply the most calcium of any foods and that the best source of iron is liver or other animal-quality foods. He presents several charts that show that many lesser-known foods supply these nutrients, sometimes in proportionately greater amounts than meat or dairy foods.

**Calcium Content (milligrams per average serving)**

| | |
|---|---|
| Cheese, various (1 slice) | 100–350 |
| Cow's milk (1 cup) | 288 |
| Sesame seeds | 331 |
| Sardines with bones | 372 |
| Broccoli (large stalk) | 246 |

**Iron Content (per 100 grams)**

| | |
|---|---|
| Calf liver | 8.7 |
| Millet | 6.8 |
| Chickpeas | 6.9 |
| Soybeans | 7.0 |
| Parsley | 6.2 |

### Behavioral Modification

Kushi stresses that macrobiotics is a complete lifestyle, not just a diet, and that meditation, prayer, and self-reflection enhance the harmony which his diet produces within the body. He concludes, "By mentally changing ourselves, our body changes, just as by changing our physical condition, our mental condition also improves. Through meditation and similar mental and spiritual exercises, we can return to our infinite source, empty our minds of our troubles, and come back to the everyday world refreshed and inspired to begin anew."

## GARY NULL'S VEGETARIAN DIET

Gary Null, well-known holistic health and nutrition author, was a competitive runner who discovered that he was allergic to many of the high protein staples on his vegetarian regimen, including eggs, milk, wheat germ, and brewer's yeast. He often experienced fatigue as a runner and could not improve his pace. Nevertheless, after five years of research and hundreds of interviews with leading experts, Null claims that he discovered new high-protein vegetarian food combinations that provided more high quality protein than most meat foods. His vegetarian diet is detailed in *Vegetarian Handbook: Eating Right for Total Health.*

## Basic Nutritional Approach

Null states that his Protein Combination Project used computers to compare the protein pattern of more than one hundred commonly eaten foods. He argues that he was able to design vegetarian food combinations that provided more complete protein than meat sources such as beef, chicken, veal, pork, or milk. "The protein in these combinations, in fact," he states, "exceeded that of beef, chicken, veal, pork, and milk in quality."

Null cautions that because the human body is unable to store substantial amounts of protein, his vegetarian food combinations must be consumed in the same meal. It should be noted that the American Dietetic Association's (ADA) position on vegetarian diets modifies Null's argument. The ADA suggests that adequate amounts of amino acids can be supplied by a variety of vegetarian foods on a daily basis — and that they do not need to be consumed together in one meal. According to the ADA, the mixture of proteins from grains, legumes, seeds, and vegetables provides a complement of amino acids so that deficits in one food are made up by the others. Not all types of plant foods need to be eaten at the same meal, since the amino acids are combined in the body's protein pool.

## Required or Recommended Foods

Null's diet, closely following Kushi's macrobiotic diet, recommends that vegetarians consume

- 50 to 60 percent of food as grains
- approximately 30 percent as fresh vegetables
- 10 percent as soups
- 10 percent as beans and bean products
- 5 percent as sea vegetables

Null includes in his appendix a protein combination list that outlines hundreds of high-quality vegetarian food combinations. They are listed in general order of quality, starting with those whose protein is closest in quality to that of the egg. Unfortunately, he does not provide a list of the essential and nonessential amino acids — or, equally important, vitamins and minerals — that each of his food combinations provides. He does, however, present more than one hundred vegetarian recipes.

Null explicitly states that most of his plant protein combinations need to be cooked, because it helps break down the cell wall structure of vegetables, which makes them easier to digest and allows for the complete release of their protein content. He specifically recommends steam cooking which he suggests lessens the risk of toxicity (beans, for example, must always be cooked) and preserves protein, vitamin, and mineral content. Certain classic meat-cooking techniques, such as charcoal broiling and pan frying, on the other hand, he adds, can render animal foods carcinogenic.

*Legumes and Grains.* Grains and legumes are required foods in Null's macrobiotic diet, providing as much or more high-quality protein as animal products. Vegetarian combinations of rice and beans — for example, chickpeas and sesame seeds or peanut butter and wheat — he contends, not only provide as much protein as animal food but are more easily metabolized by the body.

*Soy Protein Foods.* Null's recipes are high in soybeans and soybean products, which, he notes, have been used as a primary source of protein in Japan for more than three thousand years. Soybean products he recommends include tofu, tempeh, and miso. Tofu, or bean curd, is an easily digestible protein source made from coagulated soy milk. It absorbs the flavor of other foods or spices added to it, and is an ideal base for many dishes. Burgers made from tofu, for example, boast lower saturated fat and as much or more protein, depending on the recipe used. Tofu is low in the amino acid methionine, although it forms a complete protein when it is complemented by whole grains such as brown rice or wheat.

Many of Null's recipes also incorporate tempeh or fermented soybeans, which are usually sold in sheets or patties and have a meatlike texture. Three ounces of tempeh contain 19.5 grams of protein and supply eight essential amino acids.

Miso is a fermented paste made from a mixture of soybeans, salt, and water. Some variations contain barley, rice, chickpeas, or barley malt. Miso is usually added as flavoring to soups, sandwich spreads, gravies, dressing, and dips. It is easily digested and contains live lactobacillus culture and other digestive enzymes that can be well utilized by the body. Null suggests that starting a meal with a cup of miso soup helps prepare the stomach for proper digestion of the meal to follow.

*Spirulina and Chlorella (Algae).* Spirulina and chlorella, both single-celled algae, are very high in protein. According to the *Alternative Health and Medicine Encyclopedia,* spirulina is the only food that contains all essential and nonessential amino acids. Thus, it makes an ideal breakfast food — usually prepared as a green energy drink for breakfast, mixed in a blender with pineapple juice and a banana. Null suggests that a spirulina algae drink is the ideal breakfast for vegetarians because of its high concentration of protein (60 percent), amino acids, beta-carotene, vitamin B12, gamma-linoleic acid, and essential minerals and natural pigments. Spirulina also supplies an easily absorbable source of calcium, potassium, manganese, copper, silicon, and zinc.

*Calcium-Rich Foods.* Like Kushi, Null suggests that many vegetable sources of calcium are better than cow's milk. He specifically lists leafy vegetables such as cauliflower, sesame seed, soy beans, carob flour, fresh and dried fruits, and sea vegetables. He advises women at risk for osteoporosis who cannot consume adequate amounts of calcium on his vegetarian diet to take calcium lactate, calcium citrate, or calcium gluconate supplements.

## Eliminated and Restricted Foods

Null's diet totally eliminates meat and meat products because they create "biochemical imbalance, mental distraction, and spiritual lethargy." He also eliminates refined oils, simple carbohydrates, refined sugar products, stimulants such as coffee and colas, and processed, chemically treated foods.

*Meat.* Although meat is an excellent source of protein, Null states that it often provides too much protein and fat for health. Excess protein can lead to cell damage and acceleration of the aging process. Most meat is also high in fat calories, and the overconsumption of meat is one reason that an increasing number of Americans are obese.

Store-bought meats are also increasingly toxic, according to Null, because they contain chemicals administered to livestock, including antibiotics, hormones, pesticides, and fungicides, some of which may be carcinogens. In addition, meat foods, because they are difficult and time-consuming to digest, may spread toxins throughout the body, further weakening the immune system. Finally, Null contends excess meat protein metabolism produces a byproduct called urea, which stresses the kidneys.

## Restricted Foods: Eggs and Dairy Products

Eggs, milk, and dairy products such as cheese, yogurt, and butter can cause allergic reactions in some people, and for this reason, Null argues that these foods should either be eliminated or severely restricted. To reduce cholesterol, he recommends eliminating cream and substituting skim or lowfat milk for regular milk. Even though butter is a saturated fat, Null recommends it instead of margarine, unless dieters are allergic to dairy products. Milk products often combine with certain grains and legumes to increase their protein content, and he specifically recommends using plain yogurt as a sour-cream-like garnish on rice and beans.

## Vitamin and Mineral Supplements

Vitamin B12 is manufactured by microorganisms, and many Western nutritionists used to argue that, as a result, it was not produced in fruits and vegetables. Null notes, however, that B12 is present in fermented vegetarian foods such as miso, soy sauce, tempeh, and yogurt. He suggests that vegetarians can meet their RDA for vitamin B12 by consuming large amounts of tempeh and miso, which are both high in this vitamin, since it is produced by bacteria during fermentation. Miso contains about .17 micrograms of B12 per 100 grams (.03 micrograms per tablespoon). Tempeh contains 3.9 micrograms per 100 grams. Depending on the type of miso, protein quantity can range from 12 to 20 percent, a more usable protein than beef, because its net protein utilization is 72 percent compared to 67 percent for a hamburger. According to Null, miso accounts for nearly 10 percent of the protein intake in modern Japan, and is relied upon as a primary food staple.

For macrobiotic dieters who still find it difficult to consume their daily RDAs of vitamin B12 in natural foods, Null suggests that they take vitamin B12 supplements.

## Iron

Like Kushi, Null points out that plant foods provide only non-heme iron whose absorbability is influenced by other foods in the diet, especially vitamin C or ascorbic acid. As a result, he advises lactovegetarians and strict vegetarians to include substantial amounts of vitamin C–rich foods in their diets to increase iron absorption — specifically leafy green vegetables, dried fruits such as apricots, figs, and raisins, and blackstrap molasses and yeast, to guarantee proper iron absorption.

## Vegetarian Rotational Diet Plan

There is increasing evidence, Null states, "that frequent consumption of the same food can lead to a food allergy which may affect the way we feel and think." Foods such as wheat, corn, dairy products, and beef, for example, have been so overconsumed by many Americans that they have developed food allergies or food intolerances.

In order to prevent the development of new allergies, Null outlines a four-day rotational vegetarian diet in which dieters consume different foods for each. Certain foods such as leafy green vegetables, he states, do not need to be rotated as conscientiously, because they are not as apt to cause allergies. Rice is also safe for most people, although Null advises against eating it every day.

## Menu Planner

Null cautions that many macrobiotic diets contain too much tamari, miso, and other high-sodium foods, which draw water out of the blood cells and dehydrate the tissues. Excessive sodium can also increase heart rate and blood pressure levels. Many macrobiotic recipes also overutilize sea vegetables which, although high in calcium, are too high in sodium. Null states that his macrobiotic diet is safe, contains normal sodium levels, and features dark leafy greens, which are important sources of beta-carotene, vitamins E and B12, and calcium.

# THE MAYO CLINIC VEGETARIAN DIET

The Mayo Clinic Vegetarian Diet is presented in *Mayo Clinic Diet Manual: A Handbook of Nutritional Practices,* edited by Jennifer Nelson, R.D.

### Basic Nutritional Approach

According to Nelson, the nutritional goal of vegetarian diets is to 1) supply an adequate caloric intake to meet energy needs; and 2) supply a balanced intake of all essential amino acids, vitamins, and minerals. She states that a well-planned vegetarian diet that consists of a variety of unrefined fresh foods supplemented with milk and eggs (ovolactovegetarian diet) meets all known nutrient needs. She cautions, however, that some vitamins and minerals are in lower concentrations or absent in plant foods — and that vegetarian dieters must make sure that they take supplements and that their caloric intake is sufficient to meet energy needs.

Like Null and Kushi, Nelson contends that vegetarian foods can easily supply recommended protein levels as long as foods are carefully combined. Meat, chicken, fish, eggs, and milk products contain all the essential amino acids, and are called "complete" or high-quality protein foods. Grains, dried beans and peas, nuts, seeds, and vegetables contain varying amounts of the essential amino acids and therefore are called "incomplete" proteins.

Unlike Null, Nelson cites more recent research which indicates that not all the essential amino acids must be consumed at each meal. She explains that the body maintains an "amino acid" pool, and normal protein metabolism is maintained as long as complementary proteins are consumed sometime during the day. For example, an English muffin at breakfast and a bowl of lentil soup at lunch will provide ample amounts of all essential amino acids for normal body functions. Even vegetarian exercisers and athletes can consume enough protein to meet the extra demands of sports as long as three servings of a milk product, two or more servings of cooked dried beans and peas, and at least 2,000 calories of nutrient-dense foods are consumed daily.

### Recommended Foods

In "Planning and Evaluating Vegetarian Diets," the authors present a scheme for planning a nutritionally adequate vegetarian diet. It divides foods into four essential groups, two of which must always be combined in any meal. The scheme can also be used to evaluate the adequacy of vegetarian dietary practices, the *Manual* suggests.

> **Group A:** Whole grains and cereals: wheat, rye, barley, corn, millet, oats, rice, buckwheat, triticale, and bulgur.

**Group B:** Legumes: peanuts, peas, mung beans, broad beans, black-eyed peas, lentils, lima beans, soybeans, black beans, kidney beans, garbanzos, chickpeas, and navy beans.

**Group C:** Nuts and seeds: cashews, pistachios, walnuts, brazil nuts, almonds, pecans, pumpkin seeds, squash seeds, sunflower seeds, sesame seeds, filberts, and pine nuts.

**Group D:** Vegetables: potatoes, dark green vegetables, other vegetables.

According to the *Manual,* food group A, whole grains and whole-grain products should be used in generous amounts each day because they are important sources of protein, iron, and riboflavin in addition to acting with group C (nuts and seeds) and group D (vegetables) to form complete proteins. The authors suggest that in order to yield a balance of amino acids, a vegetarian's daily meal plan should include foods from groups A, B, C, and D. Different types of foods whose proteins complement one another should be eaten over the course of the day.

### Sample Meal Plan

The *Mayo Clinic Diet Manual* also provides a sample meal plan which they call a "modified food guide for vegetarian diets."

- Legumes, nuts, and seeds (including nut butters): 2 tablespoons or 1/2 cup cooked;
- Milk, milk products, fortified soybean milk, or meat analogs: 1 cup or 1 item;

- Vegetables (especially dark green): 1 cup raw or 1/2 cup cooked;
- Fruits (rich in vitamin C): 1 item or 1/2 cup canned.

Nelson notes that this adult meal plan may fall short of calcium and energy requirements for women and calcium, protein, and energy requirements for men. Thus, she recommends that larger serving sizes be used in this meal to fulfill all requirements for both men and women.

## Eliminated and Restricted Foods

Nelson's diet does not eliminate any foods. It does, however, endorse the 1990 *Dietary Guidelines for Americans,* published by the Human Nutrition Information Service of the United States Department of Agriculture, which advises dieters to restrict high-fat and cholesterol foods, salt, sugar, and alcohol.

*High-Fat and High-Cholesterol Foods.* Fat intake should be limited to less than 30 percent of calories, with less than 10 percent of calories from saturated fat. Most people can keep their blood cholesterol at a desirable level by consuming the recommended amounts of vegetables, fruits, and grain products, choosing lean fish and poultry instead of meat, and consuming only lowfat dairy products. High fats and oils are restricted. Sugars should also be used sparingly, especially if calorie needs are low. Because sugars can contribute to tooth decay, excessive snacking should be avoided.

*Salt.* Nelson notes that most Americans consume much more salt and sodium than they need. All high-sodium foods are restricted on her diet because they have been linked with several diseases, including high blood pressure.

*Alcohol.* Drinking alcoholic beverages has no net health benefits, according to Nelson, and is linked to many health problems and accidents. Therefore, she advises dieters who drink alcoholic beverages to use moderation. Moderate drinking she defines as no more than one drink per day for women and two drinks per day for men. One drink may be 12 ounces of beer, 5 ounces of wine, or 1 1/2 ounces of 80-proof distilled spirits.

## Vitamin and Mineral Requirements

Nutrients that may be lacking in vegetarian diets include high-quality protein, vitamin B12, vitamin D, riboflavin, calcium, zinc, and iron. An

## VITAMIN AND MINERAL SUPPLEMENTS FOR CHILDREN

Nutritionists do not recommend vitamin supplements for vegetarian children across the board. According to Dr. Michael Kapler, a vegan and the author of *Pregnancy, Children and the Vegan Diet,* there is no need for a vitamin supplement unless there is good reason to suspect a child is not getting enough of a particular nutrient. Kapler believes vitamin supplementing is largely unnecessary for children who eat a balanced diet, though he does agree that the practice provides a measure of "vitamin insurance." For toddlers, he recommends one dropperful a day of a commercial vitamin and a standard child's multivitamin once a day for adolescents.

individual's intake should be assessed for nutritional adequacy and supplemented accordingly. Additionally, there may be times when certain individuals may be at nutritional risk if their vegetarian diet is not carefully planned. Such periods include pregnancy and lactation, growth stages, and when health problems or disease limits the intake or increases nutrient requirements beyond normal. Except for the vegan diet, most vegetarian menus contain ample protein from dairy products and/or eggs, grains, beans, and nuts.

*Vitamin B12 Foods.* According to Nelson, ovovegetarian and lactovegetarian diets normally provide an intake of vitamin B12. Strict vegetarians, however, may need to take vitamin B12 supplements or consume more fortified breakfast cereals, soybean milk (fortified with vitamin B12), or commercial meat analogs fortified with vitamin B12. Sea plants, such as seaweed and algae, may contain some B12, although Nelson believes they are too variable to be considered a reliable source.

*Riboflavin, Calcium, Vitamin D, Iron, and Zinc.* Nelson asserts that ovolactovegetarians will be able to meet their needs for calcium and riboflavin from dairy products. Pure vegetarians, however, will need to consume more vegetables in order to satisfy their daily requirements. Excellent sources of calcium for strict vegetarians include dark green leafy vegetables (foods high in oxalic acids, such as spinach, chard, and beet greens may lessen calcium availability), some nuts and seeds, and fortified soybean milk. Those

### RECOMMENDATIONS OF THE AMERICAN DIETETIC ASSOCIATION FOR VEGETARIANS

1. Minimize intake of less nutritious foods such as sweets and fatty foods.

2. Choose whole or unrefined grain products instead of refined products.

3. Select a variety of nuts, seeds, legumes, fruits, and vegetables, including good sources of vitamin C to improve iron absorption.

4. Choose lowfat varieties of milk products, if they are included in the diet.

5. Avoid excessive cholesterol intake by limiting eggs to two or three yolks a week.

6. Vegans should make sure they consume properly fortified food sources of vitamin B12, such as fortified soy milks or cereals, or taking a supplement.

7. Infants, children, and teenagers should have adequate intakes of calories, iron, and vitamin D, taking supplements if needed.

8. Consult a registered dietitian or other qualified nutrition professional, especially during periods of growth, breast-feeding, pregnancy, or recovery from illness.

9. If breast-feeding premature infants or babies beyond 4 to 6 months of age, give vitamin D and iron supplements to the child from birth or at least by 4 to 6 months, as your doctor suggests.

10. During pregnancy, take iron and folate (folic acid) supplements.

individuals who do not consume milk or soybean milk in adequate quantities may need supplemental calcium. Vitamin D supplements or consumption of vitamin D–fortified foods is imperative for pregnant women, infants, and children who do not consume animal foods.

She notes that the absorption availability of iron and of zinc can be increased by consuming fortified grains and cereals, although some brans contain phytates which tend to reduce iron and zinc absorption. The proportion of iron available for absorption can also be increased by consuming foods rich in ascorbic acid in the same meal. Excellent sources of iron include enriched cereals and grains, legumes, dates, prunes, raisins, and greens. Good sources of zinc include leavened breads, legumes, nuts, and spinach.

## RECENT RESEARCH

The National Cancer Institute (NCI) states in its 1995 booklet *Diet, Nutrition, and Cancer Prevention: The Good News* that vegetarian diets may reduce the risk of some cancers. According to the NCI, vegetables from the cabbage family (cruciferous vegetables) may reduce cancer risk; diets low in fat and high in fiber-rich foods may reduce the risk of cancers of the colon and rectum; and diets rich in foods containing vitamin A, vitamin C, and beta-carotene may reduce the risk of certain cancers.

However, the available evidence does not demonstrate that it is total fiber, or a specific fiber component, that is related to the reduction of risk of cancer. Although the NCI acknowledged that high intakes of fruits and vegetables rich in beta-carotene or in vitamin C have been associated with reduced cancer risk, it believes the data are not sufficiently convincing that either nutrient by itself is responsible for this association.

The National Cholesterol Education Program (NCEP) also officially states that there is "strong" evidence showing that vegetarians have decreased risks for obesity, constipation, lung cancer, and alcoholism. It adds that there is "good" evidence that they have decreased risks for hypertension, coronary artery disease, type II diabetes, and gallstones. According to NCEP, the evidence is "poor" that vegetarian diets lower the risks of breast cancer, diverticular disease of the colon, colonic cancer, calcium kidney stones, and osteoporosis. It also suggests that death rates for vegetarians are similar or lower than for nonvegetarians, although these are influenced by vegetarians' adoption of many healthy lifestyle habits in addition to diet, such as abstinence or moderation in the use of alcohol and cigarettes, being physically active, resting adequately, seeking ongoing health surveillance, and seeking guidance when health problems arise.

# 14

## High-Performance Sports Diets

**M**ilo of Crotona, a legendary wrestler of the ancient Greeks who was never once brought to his knees during five Olympiads (532 to 516 B.C.), reputedly ate gargantuan amounts of meat to increase his stamina prior to competing. More recently, Don Kardong, an Olympic marathon runner, boasted of his huge intake of ice cream, soda pop, cookies, pastries, and beer.

While the authors of the three high-endurance sports diets reviewed in this chapter do not advocate either of these nutritional regimens, they unanimously agree that a high-carbohydrate diet is the best choice for competitive athletes. Sports always involve muscle exertion, and carbohydrate foods play a vital role in exercise performance because they are the most important source of glycogen and blood glucose. The authors disagree, however, as to what percentage of an athlete's training diet and event diet should consist of carbohydrates, and they also make different recommendations as to what vitamin and mineral supplements (if any) are beneficial.

### DR. LOUISE BURKE'S SPORTS PERFORMANCE DIET

Dr. Louise Burke presents her high-performance sports diet in *The Complete Guide to Food for Sports Performance.* Burke initially trained as a triathlete and competed in seven international Ironman events. She holds a Ph.D. in sports nutrition and currently serves as dietitian at the Australian Institute of Sport.

## Basic Nutritional Approach

While Burke acknowledges that no single eating plan will meet the nutritional needs of every athlete, she feels certain goals are common to all sports. The basic principles of her everyday training diet (which holds the most potential to influence sports performance) are as follows:

1. Consume a wide variety of foods. Doing so prevents athletes from overconsuming any one food or overexposing themselves to particular food chemicals. A varied diet, she contends, also offers greater opportunities for flexibility, enjoyment, and adventure with food.

2. Reduce fats and oils. While fats and oils in foods can provide essential fatty acids and fat-soluble vitamins, they do not supply the fuel needs of exercising muscles during strenuous activity (unlike carbohydrates). They can also add body fat. Burke warns, however, that dietary fat should not be eliminated from the diet, and recommends restricting fats and oils to less than 30 percent of total caloric intake.

3. Increase intake of nutritious carbohydrates to at least 50 to 60 percent of total calories. Higher levels should be set for endurance athletes and those undertaking lengthy daily training sessions.

4. Regularly restore both fluid and electrolyte levels with a sports drink after strenuous exercise or a little salt at the next meal. Avoid salt tablets.

5. Maintain day-to-day fluid balance during training, and weigh yourself both before and after exercise sessions so any fluid losses can be replaced.

6. Use alcohol sensibly. Do not consume alcohol in the twenty-four hours prior to competition, and if any soft tissue injuries or bruising occurs during an event, avoid alcohol for the next twenty-four hours. Limit social consumption to several drinks per occasion, and use nonalcoholic alternatives whenever possible.

## Recommended Foods

Like the authors of the other two diets in this chapter, Burke essentially advocates a high-carbohydrate diet. She notes that the critical source of fuel for exercising muscles comes from the body's carbohydrate stores. The stores are depleted after 90 minutes of continuous intense exercise and must be continually replenished. The more people exercise, the greater their dietary carbohydrate needs will be.

*Carbohydrates.* Nutritious, unrefined carbohydrate-rich foods that Burke recommends in order to attain a minimum target of 50 to 60 percent of total calories include bread, breakfast cereals, pasta and noodles, rice and other grains, starchy vegetables, legumes, dry biscuits, and rice cakes (all of which are complex carbohydrates), as well as fruit, fruit juice, canned and dried fruit, milk and yogurt, and liquid meals such as Sports Nutrition Supplement (all of which are simple carbohydrates). Also recommended are lowfat cakes, biscuits, and desserts, which contain significant amounts of both simple carbohydrate (sugar) and complex carbohydrate (flour).

*Protein.* According to Burke, recent research has shown that protein requirements are also increased by exercise. She suggests that athletes consume approximately 12 to 15 percent of their total calories as protein and advises them to choose lowfat protein foods that supply other essential nutrients such as calcium and iron.

Recommended protein-rich foods include:

| Animal Foods | Vegetable Foods |
|---|---|
| Grilled fish | Whole-grain bread |
| Tuna or salmon | Wheat flakes (cereal) |
| Lean beef or lamb | Untoasted muesli |
| Veal | Cooked pasta or noodles |
| Turkey or chicken | Cooked brown rice |
| Rabbit or venison | Cooked lentils |
| Eggs | Cooked kidney beans |
| Cottage cheese | Baked beans |
| Nonfat yogurt | Cooked soybeans or tofu |
| Skim milk | Nuts |
| Liquid meal supplements | Seeds (such as sesame) |

*Fiber.* Fiber, Burke explains, affects metabolism of food in the body in such ways as aiding digestion, and regulating blood glucose and blood cholesterol levels. Fiber also adds bulkiness and volume to foods, making meals more filling, which is disadvantageous for athletes with heavier energy needs. Burke advises athletes to consume only fiber found naturally in foods, such as fruits and vegetables, as this ensures they get a mixture of fiber types.

## Restricted Foods

Burke assumes that athletes already consume a healthy diet, and does not specifically eliminate or restrict any foods. As noted, however, she recommends reducing fats and oils to less than 30 percent of total caloric intake. For small eaters and those trying to lose weight, it may be necessary to cut back fat intake to 12 to 20 percent to allow for other nutrient needs.

*Sugar.* Although sugar itself is not the direct cause of any disease, apart from its contribution to tooth decay, Burke urges athletes to restrict sugar to approximately 10 percent of total daily calories. There are, she notes, occasions when moderate amounts of sugar are appropriate, for example, in a sports drink consumed during and after prolonged training sessions.

## Preparing for General Sports Competition

Burke presents the following guidelines for athletes preparing for general sports competition — that is, events consisting of up to 80 minutes of continuous exercise:

- In the absence of muscle damage, rest 24 to 36 hours before the event, and eat a high-carbohydrate diet to allow the storage of adequate muscle glycogen.
- Schedule training so sessions that could potentially damage muscles (such as hard running or working with heavy weights) take place early in the week, allowing time for muscles to recover.
- Consume a diet that provides 9 to 10 grams of carbohydrates for every kilogram (2.2 pounds) of body weight. Thus, a 110-pound athlete should eat 450 to 500 grams of carbohydrate during the day preceding competition, while a 176-pound athlete should consume 700 to 800 grams of carbohydrate.
- If extra carbohydrate is needed, increase consumption of complex carbohydrate foods and reduce the protein component of meals.
- Drink plenty of fluids, especially if competing in a hot environment.
- Consume a good pre-event meal (see "the pre-event meal" below).

## Carbohydrate Loading for Endurance Events

Burke describes carbohydrate loading as "probably the most talked about yet least understood nutrition topic in sport." She recommends it only for

Burke's carbo-loading diet, like Dr. David Nieman's, is a moderate regimen. Dr. Stephen Van Pelt, a sports physician at St. Francis Hospital in San Francisco and a member of this book's medical advisory board, notes that high-endurance competitive athletes typically use a much more extreme carbo-loading regimen. Because such programs substantially stress the body of even the most conditioned athlete, they can be used only two or three times a year. On an extreme carbo-loading program, Van Pelt suggests that on the first day (usually six days before the competition) an exhausting exercise is usually performed, followed by two days of a low-carbohydrate diet with further bouts of exhausting exercise. Thereafter, a carbohydrate-rich diet (75 to 80 percent) is consumed for three days, during which no hard exercise is performed. To avoid excessive depletion of muscle glycogen stores, Van Pelt recommends a normal mixed diet for the first three days (50 percent carbohydrate) after which the carbohydrate-rich diet can be consumed. At the same time, shorter periods of exercise are performed also on days four and five, and rest is normally taken only on the day preceding the competition.

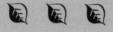

those competing in endurance sports that involve more than ninety minutes of continuous high-intensity exercise using the same muscle groups, because these will challenge the capacity of the athlete's normal fuel stores.

And, because endurance athletes undergo a daily cycle of depletion and loading of muscle glycogen stores in their training, the simplified technique she recommends involves seventy-two hours of pre-event tapering off of exercise and a high-carbohydrate intake of 10 grams/2.2 pounds of body weight per day. This will cause an overloading of glycogen in the trained muscles, enabling competition performance to continue for a longer period of time at an optimal pace.

Burke also counsels athletes to carefully monitor fat intake during this period and to drink plenty of fluids so their bodies are well hydrated for a long event. During the final twenty-four hours, if athletes wish to race feeling light, she suggests switching to low-fiber foods, making extra use of compact sugar foods, and possibly even using a combination of liquid meal or high-carbohydrate supplements to supply some or all of their carbohydrate needs.

## Carbohydrate-Loading Menu Plan

Burke presents a sample carbohydrate-loading menu plan that provides approximately 600 grams of carbohydrate per day, which is suitable for a 132-pound athlete to meet the 10-gram-per-day recommendation. This menu is appropriate for carbohydrate-loading days only, as it does not meet all nutritional goals for everyday eating.

**Breakfast:**
2 cups of Wheaties with 1 cup skim milk
1 cup sweetened canned peaches
1 cup of sweetened fruit juice
**Snack:**
2 slices of thick toast with a scrape of margarine and 1 tablespoon of honey
1 cup of a sports drink
**Lunch:**
2 large bread rolls with light salad
1 can of soft drink
**Snack:**
1 large piece of unbuttered coffee cake
1 cup of fruit juice
**Dinner:**
3 cups of boiled rice (made into a light stir-fry with small amounts of lean ham, peas, corn, and onion)
1 cup of fruit juice
**Snack:**
2 crumpets with a scrape of margarine and 1 tablespoon jam
Tea or coffee

## The Pre-Event Meal

The major goals of the pre-event meal, according to Burke, are to increase liver glycogen and fluid levels; fill the stomach to a point of comfort so that athletes do not feel hungry or suffer gastrointestinal upsets; and leave them feeling confident and ready. Toward this end, she offers the following suggestions:

- Plan the day so the final larger meal is eaten four hours before the event, and any snacks one to two hours in advance.

## BURKE'S PRE-EVENT MEAL IDEAS

- Breakfast cereal, skim milk, and fresh or canned fruit
- Muffins or crumpets with jam or honey
- Pancakes with syrup
- Toast and baked beans
- Baked potatoes with lowfat filling
- Creamed rice (made with skim milk)
- Spaghetti with tomato or lowfat sauce
- Rolls or sandwiches with banana filling
- Fruit salad with lowfat yogurt
- Liquid meal supplement

- Choose high-carbohydrate, lowfat foods that ensure easy digestion and increase carbohydrate fuel supplies.
- Avoid foods that cause discomfort or upsets.
- Drink plenty of fluids leading up to the event.
- People who suffer precompetition nerves may find that drinking liquid meal supplements is helpful because they are high in carbohydrates and low in fat and bulk, as well as being easy to digest.
- Avoid consuming large amounts of sugar 30 to 60 minutes before exercise.

### Vitamin and Mineral Supplements

Burke suggests that athletes who consume the RDA for essential vitamins and minerals by eating a balanced diet will not need to take any supplements. Athletes on very restricted diets (including strict vegetarian diets), however, or those with low-energy intakes (such as athletes who are on weight-loss diets), may need to take supplements and should consult a sports dietitian.

*Iron.* According to Burke, iron is an important nutrient in sports performance because it is a component of oxygen carriers in the blood (hemoglobin) and in the muscles (myoglobin). Iron also interacts with enzymes that promote exercise metabolism, and iron deficiencies will reduce the oxygen supply to muscles as well as slow down some metabolic reactions. She recommends that athletes with very low iron stores (who may complain of fatigue and poor recovery from training) add iron-rich foods to their daily diet.

Burke discusses the two different forms of dietary iron: heme iron that is found in some animal foods (and which generally has more iron overall and is well absorbed) and non-heme iron (which is poorly absorbed). Good sources of heme and non-heme iron include:

| Heme Iron Foods | Non-Heme Iron Foods |
|---|---|
| Liver | Spinach |
| Liver pâté | Fortified breakfast cereals |
| Oysters | Lentils/kidney beans (cooked) |
| Lean steak | Almonds |
| Chicken (dark meat) | Dried apricots |
| Salmon | Whole-wheat bread |
| Fish | Eggs |

Burke warns that athletes (such as vegetarians or those who eat only carbohydrates) whose diets are based heavily or solely on plant iron foods may find that their iron intake is inadequate or poorly absorbed. She also counsels that combining non-heme iron meals with a vitamin C food enhances iron absorption — for example, orange juice with breakfast cereal or tomatoes with a spinach omelet.

*Calcium.* Calcium is an essential mineral for athletes because it forms 99 percent of the body's bone content. Burke recommends meeting the RDA for calcium from food sources, including milk (skim, 1%, 2%, or fortified soy), reduced-fat cheese, cottage cheese, nonfat yogurt, sardines (oil drained), oysters, almonds, salmon (with bones), tahini, spinach (cooked), tofu, and lowfat ice cream.

## ELIZABETH SOMER'S HEALTHY WOMAN'S DIET

Elizabeth Somer, author of *The Essential Guide to Vitamins and Minerals* and *The Nutrition Desk Reference,* presents her dietary recommendations in *Nutrition for Women.*

### Basic Nutritional Approach

Somer claims that her Healthy Woman's Diet, with its emphasis on lowfat, nutrient-dense, minimally processed foods, will both maximize athletic performance and ensure optimal health throughout life. She recommends that women engaged in moderate to vigorous physical activity consume at least 60 percent of total calories as carbohydrates in fruits, vegetables, whole-grain breads and cereals, and cooked dried beans and peas.

Athletes (who exercise five or more hours a week or who compete in athletic events) and recreational exercisers alike should divide food intake into several small meals and snacks throughout the day, eating every three to four hours. Somer further suggests never skipping breakfast, and combining protein and carbohydrate during the midday meal to avoid fatigue in the afternoon.

## Recommended Foods

Somer's Healthy Woman's Diet consists mainly of pasta, fruits, vegetables, cooked dried beans and peas, and small amounts of lean meat, chicken, and fish (no more than six ounces per day). Her diet recommends consuming twelve or more daily servings of grains, four or more servings of fruit, one to two servings of cooked dried beans and peas, and five or more servings of vegetables.

*Carbohydrates.* According to Somer, carbohydrates are the primary fuel used by athletes engaged in anaerobic sports (such as tennis, volleyball, and sprinting, which involve short, intense bursts of energy) and by endurance-sports athletes, such as race walkers, runners, swimmers, cross-country skiers, and cyclists. The amount of carbohydrates in the diet, she asserts, is directly related to athletic performance.

Consumption of a high-carbohydrate diet such as the Healthy Woman's Diet results in a greater buildup of muscle glycogen and power output during training than the moderate-carbohydrate diet (45 to 55 percent of total calories as carbohydrates) typically consumed by athletes, adds Somer. And for those who consume less than 45 percent of total calories as carbohydrates, the results can also include increased tension, depression, fatigue, anger, mental confusion, and reduced vigor.

Somer believes that the way the body uses carbohydrates before, during, and after exercise is directly influenced by the amount of carbohydrate consumed on the days prior to, and the hours after, the event. A high-carbohydrate diet consumed during the week prior to an endurance event will have a greater impact on stocking the body's glycogen stores than will a big pre-event meal the night before.

## GUIDELINES FOR REPLENISHING CARBOHYDRATES

According to the National Center for Nutrition and Dietetics, muscles replenish stored carbohydrates most efficiently within the first two hours following exercise. Therefore, athletes should eat or drink 200 to 400 carbohydrate calories as soon as possible after exercise, and then again two hours later. Some 200 to 400 calorie suggestions include:

- two pieces of fruit such as a banana and orange or apple
- 12 ounces of fruit juice cocktail such as cranberry, or fruit juice such as grapefruit or orange
- one cup of nonfat frozen or regular yogurt topped with one cup of blueberries or raspberries
- one cup of grapes and one bagel
- one ounce of cereal with 1/2 cup skim milk and 1/2 sliced banana
- one cup of lowfat vegetable soup with one pita pocket
- one bran, blueberry, or cranberry lowfat muffin with one cup of skim milk

Source: *Nutrition Fact Sheet: Athletes Fuel Up for Fitness.*

*Sports Drinks.* Somer recommends that athletes drink easily digested forms of carbohydrates such as fruit juices or carbohydrate-rich sports drinks during lengthy aerobic exercise (i.e., one hour or more of running, brisk walking, cycling, swimming, or aerobic dance sessions) because they help slow the rate of muscle glycogen depletion, maintain blood sugar concentrations, and prevent subsequent fatigue. She notes that the ideal proportion of glucose to water in sports drinks remains controversial and may vary for each individual athlete.

Somer cautions that drinks containing too much carbohydrate slow the rate of emptying from the stomach and limit the delivery of fluids to the body during exercise. Beverages containing glucose polymers, such as maltodextrin, help maintain a high blood sugar level when consumed during endurance events and do not affect fluid replacement any more than water ingestion does. She adds that isotonic beverages are preferable because they can provide as much as 40 percent of carbohydrate calories expended during the latter stages of moderately intense, long-term exercise.

*Protein.* Somer points out that because the typical American diet supplies two to three times the recommended amount of protein, it should be more than adequate to meet all protein needs of athletes and exercisers. The only exception may be women bodybuilders, who might need as much as 1.5 to 2 grams of protein for every 2.2 pounds of body weight (compared to the "typical" reference person who needs 0.8 grams of protein for every 2.2 pounds of body weight). Therefore, a 138-pound female bodybuilder might need as much as 126 grams of protein, or more than double the recommended protein intake of 50 grams for the average woman, depending on the frequency, intensity, and duration of her workouts.

On the other hand, Somer notes, excessive protein intake can interfere with strength-training and health. Any protein consumed in excess of the body's needs is broken down for energy or stored as fat. The waste products of this process are toxic to the liver and can damage the kidneys. In the kidneys' attempt to eliminate protein fragments from the body, extra water is lost, which can result in dehydration and potential mineral deficiencies.

To avoid excessive intake while ensuring adequate protein consumption, Somer recommends that bodybuilders and weight lifters follow the dietary guidelines outlined in her Healthy Woman's Diet and consume an additional one or two ounces of protein-rich meat, chicken, or fish. Foods should be eaten in small doses throughout the day, especially prior to and following a workout session.

*Fluids.* Dehydration resulting from inadequate fluid replacement is the most common contributor to reduced athletic performance, according to Somer. Dancers, for example, typically lose two to three pounds of water during a performance, while runners can lose five pounds or more of water during a race. Gradual dehydration develops unless the entire fluid loss is replaced.

Since thirst is a poor indicator of fluids needs, a general rule is to drink twice as much water as is needed to quench it. Somer advises that athletes and exercisers drink water prior to, during, and following all training and sports events as well as regularly throughout the day.

*Potassium-Containing Beverages.* Somer argues that the consumption of beverages that contain potassium rather than water during intense exercise probably has no additional effect on minimizing exercise-induced disturbances in blood electrolytes or blood volume. Athletes who consume electrolyte-replacement drinks, for example, show no differences in body temperature, blood volume, or blood levels of potassium, chloride, calcium, or sodium compared with athletes who consume non-electrolyte-containing drinks. In addition, she notes, any potassium lost during exercise can be replaced by eating a few high-potassium fruits and vegetables such as bananas and potatoes.

## Preparing for Endurance Events

Somer believes that athletes preparing for a marathon, triathlon, or other strenuous endurance event should consume a higher-carbohydrate diet (70 to 75 percent) than normal the week before their event, and drink extra water to ensure optimal hydration.

She recommends that they also consume a moderate-size, high-carbohydrate meal that is easily digested the night before their event. A pre-event meal or snack (within one to three hours beforehand) should consist of easily digested carbohydrates such as cereal, toast, and fruit. This snack should be light — less than 500 calories of lowfat foods.

During the event, Somer counsels athletes to consume ample water and/or diluted sports drinks containing glucose polyesters or a combination of glucose polyesters and fructose that help maintain blood sugar levels and prevent glycogen depletion. For exercise sessions lasting more than 90 minutes, consuming approximately 100 calories of carbohydrate every 30 minutes helps maintain blood sugar levels and allows athletes to continue exercising longer without "hitting the wall" or tiring. After the event or training session, athletes should begin replenishing their glycogen stores by consuming a high-carbohydrate snack such as a bagel with fruit or a bowl of Cheerios.

## Sample 3,000-Calorie Meal Plan for Endurance Athletes

The following meal plan, according to Somer, meets or exceeds the RDA for all vitamins and minerals. It consists of 125 grams of protein (16% of total calories), 508 grams of carbohydrate (65%), and 19% fat.

**Breakfast:**
Two cups of Cheerios
1 slice of whole-wheat toast with 1 teaspoon of margarine
1 medium peach

1 cup of nonfat milk
**Snack:**
Whole-wheat bagel with 2 tablespoons of peanut butter
1/2 cup of raisins
**Lunch:**
Cheese sandwich consisting of 2 ounces of cheese, 2 slices of whole-wheat bread, lettuce, mustard, and 1 teaspoon of mayonnaise
1 cup of tossed green salad with 2 tablespoons dressing
1 medium orange
**Snack:**
1 cup of apple juice
3 ounces of mixed dried fruit
**Dinner:**
Linguini with clam sauce consisting of 3 ounces of clams, 1/2 cup low-fat milk, onions, celery, garlic, 1 tablespoon cornstarch, and 3 cups of pasta
3 spears of broccoli
2/3 cup of three-bean salad
**Snack:**
1/2 cup of nonfat milk

## Sample 3,500-Calorie Meal Plan for Bodybuilders

By way of comparison, Somer recommends the following meal plan for bodybuilders, which consists of 161 grams of protein (18 percent of total calories), 581 grams of carbohydrate (63 percent), and 19 percent fat. It also meets or exceeds the RDA for all vitamins and minerals.

**Breakfast:**
2 slices of whole-wheat toast with 1 tablespoon of peanut butter
1 cup of whole-wheat cereal with 1 cup of lowfat milk
1 cup of orange juice
**Snack:**
1 cup of mixed fruit salad
1 cup of lowfat cottage cheese
6 graham crackers
1 cup of apple juice
**Lunch:**

Tuna sandwich consisting of 2 ounces of tuna, 2 slices of bread, and lettuce

Pasta salad consisting of 1/2 cup macaroni, 1/2 cup of peas and carrots, and 2 teaspoons mayonnaise

1 cup tomato juice

2 cups of raw broccoli with 1 cup of nonfat yogurt dip

**Snack:**

1 1/4 cups of blueberries

3 ounces of mixed dried fruit

**Dinner:**

Beef stroganoff that consists of 3 ounces lean beef, 1 cup noodles, 2 tablespoons peppers, 2/3 cup tomato sauce, and 1/4 cup sour cream

1 ear of corn on the cob

**Snack:**

1/3 cup sherbet

2 cups of raw carrots

## Vitamin and Mineral Supplements

Somer states that her Healthy Woman's Diet provides RDA levels of most of the antioxidant nutrients such as vitamin C and beta-carotene, as well as ample amounts of all other nutrients, including magnesium, zinc, chromium, the B vitamins, and copper. However, because it is difficult to obtain the 200 IU or more of vitamin E recommended to combat free radical exposure from dietary sources alone, moderate-dose supplementation might be considered.

Somer advises that athletes engaged in frequent strenuous training and competition may benefit from taking a moderate-dose vitamin-mineral supplement to ensure adequate intake of all nutrients. There is no reason, however, to take megadose levels (more than ten times the RDA) of any nutrient at any time, nor is there any need for protein powders or other fabricated nutritional products.

*Magnesium.* According to Somer, intense physical training increases the need for magnesium, which serves numerous roles in the development and maintenance of muscle tissue. For example, magnesium helps convert glycogen to energy, regulates muscle building and relaxation, helps muscles and nerves communicate, and regulates heartbeat and blood pressure.

Strenuous exercise lowers magnesium concentrations in muscles and blood, which can affect performance and general health. In addition, hormone levels, such as norepinephrine and epinephrine (adrenaline), rise in response to strenuous exercise, and these hormones also increase urinary loss of magnesium.

Although RDA levels of magnesium might be adequate for the recreational exerciser, Somer suggests that higher amounts may be necessary for women engaging in strenuous activity.

*Calcium.* Female athletes who do not consume adequate amounts of calcium are at increased risk for stress fractures, shin splints, weakened or porous bones, strains, poor ability of bone fractures to heal, and ultimately osteoporosis. Increased loss of calcium is also caused by stress, low vitamin D intake or insufficient exposure to sunshine, high protein or fiber intakes, abuse of antacids or diuretics, and in periods of inactivity, such as when recovering from an injury.

Calcium is especially important for female athletes such as competitive runners who are amenorrheic — that is, they have stopped menstruating. Once considered a harmless side effect of intense athletic training, this condition is now recognized as very harmful to long-term health and athletic performance because of resultant loss of bone mass. Somer claims that a primary treatment is reduction in exercise training and increased weight gain and/or calorie consumption, as well as increasing calcium intake to 1,000 to 2,500 milligrams per day.

*Iron.* Distance runners are most likely to develop iron-deficiency anemia, although any athlete is at risk. Symptoms include reduction in the ability to maintain the same speed over a long period of time (race performance time), increased heart rate, decreased oxygen consumption, increased blood lactic acid concentrations, decreased exercise tolerance, and compromised exercise performance. Other symptoms of iron deficiency include lethargy, irritability, poor concentration, and headache. Iron deficiency in athletes can result from poor dietary intake, increased metabolic requirements, increased breakdown of red blood cells caused by training (called footstrike hemolysis), and/or increased iron losses in sweat.

Somer notes that as many as 80 percent of exercising women consume inadequate amounts of iron; she does urge anyone exhibiting symptoms of a deficiency to undergo blood tests to ensure iron status is optimal.

## IDEAS FOR THE TRAINING TABLE

Good sources of iron, according to the American Dietetic Association, include lean red meat, dark turkey meat, clams and oysters, iron-fortified cereals, legumes, dried apricots, and lima beans.

The American Dietetic Association suggests the following combination foods or meal ideas that are high in carbohydrates, rich in protein, and low in fat:

- Chili made with kidney beans and lean beef.
- Vegetable stir-fry with lean pork cubes, chicken, shrimp, or tofu served over rice.
- Soft-shell corn tortillas filled with vegetarian refried beans and topped with tomato sauce or salsa and lowfat cheese.
- Grilled fish kabobs (chunks of fresh fish alternating with cherry tomatoes, green pepper, and pineapple on a skewer) served on brown rice.
- Lentils (alone or mixed with lean ground beef) in spaghetti sauce on whole-wheat pasta.
- Green peppers stuffed with a mixture of lean ground turkey and brown rice. Add a mixed green salad, and finish the meal with angel food cake topped with strawberries.
- Strips of lean roast sirloin served with a baked potato, steamed carrots and cauliflower, and whole-wheat rolls.
- Chicken salad (made with reduced-calorie mayonnaise, lemon zest, and tarragon) on rye bread with tomato slices and sprouts. Serve with vegetable soup, whole-wheat crackers, and cantaloupe slices.

Source: Cooper, Linda Howt, et al., *Winning Sports Nutrition* (Tucson: University of Arizona, 1994).

## DR. DAVID C. NIEMAN'S SPORTS MEDICINE DIET

Dr. David C. Nieman, who outlines his recommended dietary principles in *Fitness and Your Health,* is one of the leading U.S. researchers on sports nutrition and a fellow of the American College of Sports Medicine. A specialist in exercise and the immune system, Nieman is in charge of the health promotion degree program at Appalachian State University. He wrote *Fitness and Sports Medicine: An Introduction.*

## Basic Nutritional Approach

Nieman asserts that the two most important nutritional principles associated with improved endurance performance are high intake of dietary carbohydrates and water. The following are his seven major dietary guidelines, as also summarized by the National Research Council, the American Heart Association, the National Cancer Institute, and the U.S. Department of Agriculture.

1. Eat a variety of foods. The more than forty nutrients needed for good health should come from a variety of foods, not from only a few highly fortified foods or supplements.
2. Maintain a healthy weight by being physically active and consuming a variety of foods low in calories and fat, such as fruits, vegetables, whole grains, nonfat dairy products, and fish or poultry.
3. Choose a diet low in total fat, saturated fat, and cholesterol. Total dietary fat intake should represent less than 30 percent of total calories, with saturated fat contributing less than 10 percent. Cholesterol intake should be below 300 milligrams a day.
4. Choose a diet with plenty of vegetables, fruits, and grain products so as to increase consumption of carbohydrates and fiber while reducing fat and cholesterol intake. According to Nieman, most authorities recommend consuming at least 55 percent of calories from carbohydrates.
5. Use sugars in moderation.
6. Use salt and sodium in moderation.
7. Limit alcoholic beverages to no more than two drinks a day (men), or no more than one drink a day (women). One drink is defined as 12 ounces of regular beer, 5 ounces of wine, and 1.5 ounces of distilled spirits.

Nieman explains that a diet following the above principles, which he defines as a "prudent diet," is one that enhances health and is advocated for fitness enthusiasts (those exercising three to five days a week, 15 to 30 minutes per session). Several adaptations beyond this diet (as detailed below) are beneficial for the competitive or endurance athlete who trains more than one hour a day.

## Recommended Foods

Nieman suggests choosing at least the lower number of daily servings from each of the following food groups: vegetables (3 to 5), fruits (2 to 4), bread, cereals, rice, and pasta (6 to 11), lowfat milk, yogurt, and cheese (2 to 3), lowfat meats, poultry, fish, dry beans and peas, eggs, and nuts (2 to 3).

The most important dietary principle for both fitness enthusiasts and athletes to adhere to is a diet that is 55 to 70 percent carbohydrate, emphasizes Nieman, as body carbohydrate stores (glycogen) are the primary fuel source for working muscles. When muscle glycogen levels drop too low, the ability to exercise decreases, and people feel more fatigued and are more prone to injury.

As time spent in endurance activity increases, Nieman urges reducing the quantity of fat in the diet and replacing it with carbohydrate. Recommended sources include grain products (pasta, bagels, breads, brown rice, cereals), tubers (potatoes, yams), legumes (kidney beans, pinto beans), dried fruits (raisins, dates), and fresh fruits and vegetables. He notes that approximately 2,500 calories of dietary carbohydrate lead to near maximal replenishment of muscle glycogen following a strenuous training bout.

*High-Carbohydrate Foods.* Nieman provides a list of high-carbohydrate foods (one-cup portions) in descending order of carbohydrate content (shown as grams of carbohydrate). He notes that the foods high in sugar should be consumed in moderation because excess simple sugars in the diet can result in vitamin and mineral deficiencies:

| | |
|---|---|
| Honey (272) | Pancake syrup (238) |
| Jams/Preserves (224) | Molasses (176) |
| Chopped dates (131) | Raisins (115) |
| Prunes (101) | Grape-Nuts (94) |
| Whole-wheat flour (85) | Uncooked dried apricots (80) |
| Boiled sweet potato (80) | Sweetened applesauce (51) |
| Brown rice (50) | Prune juice (45) |
| Kidney beans (42) | Cooked rolled wheat (41) |
| Cooked macaroni (39) | Cooked lentils (39) |

*Water.* Nieman considers drinking water to be the second most important dietary principle for those who exercise, and notes that as little as a two percent decrease in body weight caused by water loss (primarily from sweat) can compromise performance. Fluid replacement immediately prior

---

### FOOD HINTS

To decrease the amount of fat in the diet, the American Dietetic Association provides the following suggestions:

- Trim the fat from meats and remove the skin from chicken.
- Try reduced-calorie mayonnaise and salad dressings.
- Substitute tomato-based sauces for pasta for cream or cheese-based sauces.
- Use sauces and salad dressings sparingly.
- Eat baked, broiled, roasted, or steamed foods instead of fried foods.
- Substitute bagels, English muffins, or toast for croissants, Danish, and doughnuts.
- Use nonstick sprays for cooking.
- Choose water-packed tuna and leaner meats such as round or loin cuts.

Source: Cooper, Linda Howt, et al., *Winning Sports Nutrition* (Tucson: University of Arizona, 1994).

---

to, during, and after exercise can dramatically reduce the adverse effects of dehydration: fluid replacement helps slow down the increase in core body temperature, maintain plasma volume and cardiac output, improve endurance, and lessen the risk of heat injury.

According to Nieman, most sports nutrition experts recommend that people drink 200 to 400 milliliters (7 to 14 ounces) of water for every 20 minutes of exercise, or 500 milliliters (2 cups) for every 30 minutes. The water should be 40 to 50 degrees Fahrenheit (refrigerator-cold), when consumed during exercise. This coldness does not interfere with gastric emptying (or cause cramps), says Nieman, and helps stabilize the core temperature of the body.

*Fluids Containing Electrolytes.* According to Nieman, athletes competing in events lasting less than four hours do not risk depleting stores of electrolytes (sodium, potassium, and chloride), because the electrolyte content of sweat is very low. However, those engaging in events exceeding four hours in duration are urged to drink fluids containing electrolytes. He recommends consuming a sports drink that contains 4 to 10 percent carbohydrate of any type (glucose polymer, glucose, or sucrose) in volumes of 7 to 14 ounces every 15 to 20 minutes. The importance of carbohydrate in an

## HOW MUCH FLUID DO ATHLETES NEED?

Most athletes must make a conscious effort to drink fluids at all times during the day. In addition, they need plenty of fluids before, during, and after a session. The American Dietetic Association offers the following guidelines:

- 2 to 2 1/2 hours before a competition or workout: drink at least 2 cups of fluid.
- 15 minutes before a competition or workout: drink another 2 cups of fluid.
- Every 15 to 20 minutes during a competition or workout: drink 1/2 to 1 cup of fluid.
- After a competition or workout: drink 2 cups of fluid for every pound lost during the session; continue to take in fluid throughout the day.

Source: Cooper, Linda Howt, et al., *Winning Sports Nutrition* (Tucson: University of Arizona, 1994).

electrolyte fluid is that it helps prevent the exercise-induced drop in blood glucose levels, even when muscle glycogen levels are low.

*Protein.* Recent studies, according to Nieman, have concluded that the contribution of protein as an energy source during endurance training is between 5 and 15 percent, instead of virtually nothing, as was previously thought. The actual amount of protein utilized during such exercise depends on intensity, duration, and fitness status.

The American Dietetic Association advises that endurance athletes consume one gram of protein daily per kilogram (2.2 pounds) of body weight. For athletes involved in unusually heavy training, more than 1.5 grams per kilogram may be required. A good rule for endurance athletes, Nieman adds, is to keep caloric intake of protein at 12 to 15 percent of their diet. Regardless of exercise level, this should provide sufficient protein, because caloric intake generally rises with energy expenditure. Most endurance athletes, he notes, currently keep their caloric intake at 12 to 15 percent of their diet and have no need to supplement their diet with protein powders.

## Caffeine

Nieman notes that the American College of Sports Medicine does not recommend the use of caffeine for performance enhancement. In addition, the International Olympic Committee has banned caffeine at levels greater than 15 micrograms per milliliter of urine. Nieman notes that if an athlete is not carbohydrate-loaded and not accustomed to the use of caffeinated beverages, drinking two to four cups of coffee one hour before exercise may prolong time to exhaustion by 7 to 19 percent. However, caffeine increases urine output (thereby contributing to dehydration), and may increase the incidence of premature ventricular contractions in susceptible individuals. In addition, regular and heavy consumption may increase blood cholesterol and increase the risk of heart attacks.

## Sample One-Day Menu

Nieman presents a sample one-day menu consisting of 3,500 calories, 79 percent of which is carbohydrate. This, he suggests, is the type of diet recommended for the average male runner training for long endurance events. It is also recommended for carbohydrate loading during the three-day period before a long endurance race. This sample diet meets the RDA for all nutrients and follows the guidelines of Nieman's diet. Most of the calories are consumed during breakfast and lunch, with a lighter supper to allow for a better night's rest. Portions, foods, and calories are listed below:

**Breakfast:**
1 cup Grape-Nuts (404)
2 cups of 2% lowfat milk (242)
1 whole banana (105)
1/2 cup seedless raisins (247)
2 cups orange juice (224)
1 piece whole-wheat bread (84)
2 teaspoons honey (43)
**Lunch:**
2 pieces whole-wheat bread (168)
1 tablespoon peanut butter (96)
2 whole apples (162)
2 cups cooked brown rice (464)
2 cups mixed vegetables (105)
1 teaspoon seasonings (5)

1 cup lowfat yogurt (231)
2 whole bagels (330)
**Supper:**
1/2 fresh tomato (12)
1/2 cup loose-leaf lettuce (5)
2 ounces cooked chicken (108)
2 pieces whole-wheat bread (168)
1 tablespoon low-calorie dressing (35)
2 cups canned pineapple juice (278)

## Vitamin and Mineral Supplements

According to Nieman, most studies have found that athletes (because they tend to eat more than sedentary people) exceed 67 percent of the RDA for all vitamins and minerals measured, except iron for females. He adds that no convincing research evidence shows that supplementation enhances performance, hastens recovery, or reduces the rate of injury for healthy, well-nourished adults in athletic training.

And, while Nieman admits that heavy endurance exercise increases the need for many nutrients — including iron, zinc, copper, magnesium, chromium, vitamin B6, riboflavin, and ascorbic acid — he argues that these demands are generally met by the athlete's increased consumption of conventional foods.

In addition, Nieman notes that problems are associated with high intakes of vitamins and minerals; namely, that the dietary excess of one nutrient may have a detrimental effect on another. High intakes of fat-soluble vitamins A, D, E, and K, for example, can be toxic in themselves, and also block the action of other nutrients. He concludes that the best nutritional resource for optimum athletic performance is proper eating habits.

## RECENT RESEARCH

In *Modern Nutrition in Health and Disease,* Hultman, Harris, and Spriet present the most current and comprehensive survey of recent findings concerning the role nutrition plays in athletic performance. The guidelines below summarize their findings. It is a summary of nutritional guidelines for high-endurance physical activity (80 minutes of continuous exercise):

1. Follow the national dietary guidelines developed by the USDA, the National Research Council, and other organizations: a) follow a varied diet that supplies all essential nutrients from a variety of foods; b) the diet

should be low in fat, saturated fat, and cholesterol, and high in vegetables, fruits, and grain products; c) maintain a healthy weight; d) use sugar and salt in moderation; e) drink alcoholic beverages in moderation, if at all.

2. Increase daily caloric intake. Athletes with normal body weights who exercise regularly will need to consume higher amounts of calories than average sedentary Americans because of their high working capacities, high intensity training levels, elevated basal metabolic rates, and greater-than-normal lean body masses.

3. Consume 55 to 70 percent of daily calories as complex carbohydrate. Most nutritionists agree that body carbohydrate stores (glycogen) are extremely important because they are the primary fuel source for the working muscles. When muscle glycogen levels decrease drastically, the ability to exercise is compromised; athletes experience more fatigue and are more prone to injury. Carbohydrate is essential both for the maintenance of the liver glycogen stores and for the rapid resynthesis of muscle glycogen. A loss of liver glycogen during exercise results in a decrease in blood glucose content, and a lack of muscle glycogen decreases the work capacity.

4. According to Hultman, Harris, and Spriet, the optimal carbohydrate diet should include complex saccharides, such as starch in bread, pasta, potatoes, rice, and cereals, and not simple sugars such as glucose and sucrose. Starch and other complex carbohydrates are digested more slowly in the intestine and are absorbed over a longer period of time. The result is that a larger fraction is deposited in the glycogen stores; less is deposited as fat.

5. Consume large amounts of water during training and the event. Studies have shown that as little as a 2 percent drop in body weight caused by water loss (primarily from sweat) compromises the ability to exercise. Severe depletion of water (dehydration) can cause death. Sports medicine experts advise drinking two cups of water immediately before the exercise event, one cup during the exercise session, and two additional cups after the session.

6. If performing a sports event exceeding four hours in duration, athletes should consume more electrolytes (sodium, potassium, and chloride) in fluids. Most athletes competing in sporting events lasting less than four continuous hours will normally consume all the electrolytes they need in a balanced diet. During prolonged exercise, it is recommended that athletes consume carbohydrate in concentrations of 4 to 10 percent in fluids to prevent exercise-induced declines in blood glucose levels.

7. It is not necessary for athletes to take vitamin and mineral supple-

ments if they consume a balanced diet: studies have not shown that supplements improve performance in high-endurance events, hasten recovery, or reduce the rate of injury for healthy, well-nourished adults.

8. The consumption of extra protein does not increase athletic performance in high-endurance sporting events. Contrary to popular opinion, weight lifters need less protein (on a gram per kilogram basis) than endurance athletes. Muscle mass can be increased only by heavy-resistance exercise training. The consumption of large quantities of protein has no effect on muscle mass.

9. Rest and consume carbohydrates before endurance events. The best scheme for endurance athletes preparing for exercise events that will last longer than 60 to 90 minutes is to taper off the exercise gradually during the week preceding the event, while consuming more than 70 percent carbohydrate the three days immediately prior to the competition. If the exercise event lasts less than 90 minutes, carbohydrate loading is unnecessary.

10. The use of ergogenic aids such as steroids is unethical, and in some cases dangerous. The use of these aids may expose athletes to the risk of injury to ligaments and tendons. There is also some evidence that steroid use is linked with cancer, fetal damage, heart disease, prostate enlargement, sterility, and severe psychiatric problems.

# Part Four

# 15

## Diets for Osteoporosis

According to the June 1994 issue of the *Tufts University Diet and Nutrition Letter*, 24 million Americans — 80 percent of them women — suffer from osteoporosis, a progressive condition in which bones lose mass and become extremely brittle and prone to injury under the slightest amount of stress.

Osteoporosis begins when the rate of bone loss exceeds the ability of the body to make new bone. Both men and women lose some bone mass as they age, but the rate of loss is much slower in men (who have denser bones to begin with) than in women, and osteoporosis is rarely a problem. Conversely, according to Butler and Rayner in *The Best Medicine: The Complete Health and Preventive Medicine Handbook,* women who live to the age of eighty usually lose a third to two-thirds of their entire skeleton and up to six inches of their height.

The process of bone loss typically begins in a woman's mid-thirties, approximately ten to fifteen years before the onset of menopause, at a rate of 0.5 to 1 percent a year. This loss increases to 2 to 5 percent in the first ten years following menopause, and then tapers off to about 1 percent per year. In the decade after menopause, women typically lose 5 to 10 percent of the bone-sustaining minerals in their spines alone. As a result, according to the National Osteoporosis Foundation, one-third of American women over sixty-five suffer spinal fractures and 15 percent break their hips because of osteoporosis.

Although estrogen deficiency is considered the leading cause of osteoporosis, the body's ability to absorb sufficient amounts of calcium also plays an important role. This is because bone formation is strongly dependent on adequate dietary calcium, and if the body's stores of this nutrient are depleted, bone replacement and repair are impaired. Other factors that favor development of this debilitating condition include smoking, excessive use of alcohol, taking certain prescription drugs, and exposure to the toxic chemical cadmium.

Many health professionals argue that osteoporosis can be prevented by improved nutrition and by implementation of healthy lifestyles, which include regular exercise and minimal use of tobacco and alcohol. The osteoporosis diets discussed in this chapter typically advise increasing the consumption of foods rich in calcium such as hard cheese, milk, and yogurt. Diet supplementation with calcium carbonate, calcium citrate, or calcium phosphate is also helpful in improving calcium absorption. Other important vitamins and minerals include vitamin D and phosphorus (which aid calcium absorption), magnesium (60 percent of the body's supply is in bones), and zinc (which aids bone calcification and is known to speed healing).

## KEYS TO UNDERSTANDING OSTEOPOROSIS

Jan Rozek is a registered nurse who also writes a syndicated column for senior citizens. Her diet, presented in *Keys to Understanding Osteoporosis*, was written with resources provided by the National Osteoporosis Foundation and the National Institutes of Health.

### Basic Nutritional Approach

Rozek, who strongly contends that osteoporosis is preventable and treatable, advocates following the best possible diet. She specifically recommends that women consume 50 to 65 percent of total daily calories as carbohydrates; 12 to 20 percent as protein; no more than 30 percent as fats (preferably 25 percent), and no more than 10 percent of total fat intake as saturated fat; and 30 (but not more than 35) grams of fiber.

### Recommended Foods

Rozek advises people to consume balanced daily amounts of nutrients from the four basic food groups: dairy products, proteins, grains, fruits, and vegetables.

*Dairy Products.* Foods from the dairy group supply proteins, vitamins, and minerals and are the best source of dietary calcium. Rozek recommends consuming two to four servings daily, especially lowfat and nonfat milk and milk products such as cheese, ice milk, and yogurt.

*Proteins.* Two servings daily are recommended from this group, which provides protein, vitamins, iron, and other minerals. Fish canned with bones (such as sardines and salmon) and tofu processed with calcium sulfate are excellent calcium sources, as are canned shrimp and cooked soybeans and navy beans. Rozek advises dieters to bake or broil (rather than fry) all foods to minimize saturated fat, to serve only lean meat, and to substitute fish and poultry for meat whenever possible.

*Grains.* This group, abundant in fiber, iron, B vitamins, and other vitamins and minerals, supplies complex carbohydrates, boosts energy, and is an inexpensive source of protein. Rozek recommends four or more servings daily of breads, cereals, and other whole-grain or enriched products.

Good sources of calcium from the grain group include English muffins, fortified oatmeal, and pancakes and waffles (with egg/milk added).

*Fruits and Vegetables.* Four or more daily servings are recommended from this group, which provides vitamins, minerals, and fiber. A citrus or other fruit or vegetable high in vitamin C should be consumed daily, as well as a dark green or yellow vegetable high in vitamin A at least every other day. Dark green vegetables such as spinach, broccoli, chard, kale, collards, beet and turnip greens, and Chinese cabbage are the richest sources of calcium.

*Vitamins and Minerals.* The following foods are also recommended as good sources of important vitamins and minerals.

- Vitamin D: fish liver oils, fortified cereals, and dairy products
- Magnesium: green leafy vegetables, whole grains, seafood, dried beans, milk, and nuts
- Zinc: oysters, herring, liver, fish, milk, and whole grains

## Restricted Foods

Certain foods add sugar, fat, alcohol, salt, and calories and provide little nutritional value. Rozek suggests including small amounts only after people have balanced their diet with nutritious choices from the four food groups. These restricted foods include candy, desserts, jams, and other sweets, soft drinks and alcoholic beverages, salad dressings, sauces, gravies, condiments, potato chips, and other such snack foods.

## Meal Planning

Rozek advises people to choose recommended servings from each food group and combine them in creative ways to suit individual tastes, traditions, and income. Not all food groups need to be included at each meal, although the consumption of a variety of foods from each group on a daily basis will provide a nutritionally balanced diet and help maintain healthy weight levels.

She further suggests that people record daily servings from each food group as well as daily calcium intake to assess their diet until they have learned the components of a balanced diet and can include adequate amounts without close record keeping.

## Sample Daily Menu

Rozek recommends the following one-day sample menu, which provides 1,423 milligrams of calcium, compared to the RDA of 1,200 to 1,500 milligrams:

> **Breakfast:**
> Whole-grain cereal, 1 ounce
> Soft-boiled egg
> Grapefruit half
> Bran muffin
> Skim milk, 4 ounces
> **Lunch:**
> Roasted chicken, 3 ounces (1/2 breast, boneless/skinless)
> Potato, boiled, 1 medium
> Chicken gravy, canned, 2 tablespoons
> Creamed broccoli, 1/2 cup
> Salad: pear (1/2 canned, juice pack) and cottage cheese (1/4 cup low-fat)
> Whole-wheat dinner roll with 1 teaspoon diet margarine
> Skim milk, 4 ounces
> **Snack:**
> Baking-powder biscuit with strawberry jam
> Hot almond herbal tea

**Dinner:**
Bean soup, homemade, 1 cup
4 saltines
Tossed salad: 1 cup (lettuce, tomato, mushrooms, broccoli, spinach)
with ranch-type, lowfat dressing
Angel food cake (1/12 of cake)
Ice milk, 1/2 cup
**Evening Snack:**
Cocoa, 1 cup
2 graham crackers

## Vitamin and Mineral Supplements

Rozek advises that while it is best to consume vitamins and minerals from natural foods, this is not always possible. For example, 42 percent of all Americans take in less than 70 percent of the RDA for calcium. If making up the difference with a calcium supplement, people should read labels carefully to determine the amount of elemental calcium (the actual calcium received) that is contained.

---

### WAYS OF ADDING CALCIUM
### TO THE DAILY DIET

- Use tofu (soybean protein) which, like dry milk, can be added to many dishes to increase calcium and protein intake.
- Serve the calcium-laden trio of broccoli, collards, and kale as often as possible.
- Substitute skim or lowfat milk or part milk whenever possible in recipes that call for water.
- Top salads, casseroles, soups, eggs, vegetables, corn chips, baked goods, and other dishes with lowfat grated cheese, heating to melt when appropriate.
- Add cottage cheese to crepes, gelatin desserts, vegetables, and casseroles.
- Blend 1 to 2 tablespoons of cornstarch with yogurt as a substitute for cream cheese and sour cream for more calcium and less saturated fat.
- Use buttermilk made from skim milk instead of milk in pancakes, biscuits, and baked goods. It contains the same amount of calcium but is much lower in fat.

---

Calcium is best absorbed if taken in divided doses several times a day with meals, or within one and a half hours afterward. This is because the presence of food in the stomach stimulates acid secretion needed to dissolve the calcium. Absorption is further aided when people drink eight ounces of fluid with their supplement. Most preparations dissolve within fifteen to thirty minutes.

Other important vitamins and minerals include vitamin D and phosphorus (which aid calcium absorption), magnesium (60 percent of the body's supply is in bones), and zinc (which aids bone calcification and is known to speed healing). Conversely, Rozek warns that an excess of sodium increases excretion of calcium.

## Physical Activity

Rozek emphasizes that bone mass is built primarily in response to the pressure of weight bearing and the tension of muscles. Exercise is an important part of her osteoporosis diet, because it works in concert with important nutrients such as calcium to increase bone density. Regular

---

### CALCIUM SUPPLEMENT TIPS

- Calcium is best absorbed if taken in small amounts throughout the day.
- Avoid taking more than 500 to 600 milligrams at one time.
- Avoid taking calcium with high-fiber meals or with bulk-forming laxatives. Fiber can interfere with absorption.
- Drink six to eight glasses of fluid a day.
- Do not take an iron supplement at the same time as a calcium tablet because calcium can block iron absorption.
- Calcium-carbonate tablets should be taken with food.
- Calcium-fortified foods — certain brands of cereal, fruit juice, and bread that have added calcium — are now being marketed.
- Calcium intake should not exceed 2,000 milligrams a day (experts recommend 1,000) because a high dose can increase the likelihood of developing kidney stones. People with a history of kidney problems should consult their doctor before starting high-calcium supplementation.

weight-bearing exercise can prevent and somewhat restore bone loss, she claims, and she urges dieters to design a personal program that includes exercises for flexibility, strength, and cardiorespiratory endurance.

## Behavioral Modification

Rozek believes that physical, psychological, and social problems often attend osteoporosis and psychological therapies are often overlooked. She therefore provides guidelines to nurture self-esteem, stay in control, cultivate a positive attitude, and build a support system of people who foster a sense of belonging, closeness, and security.

# THE BRITISH NATIONAL OSTEOPOROSIS SOCIETY DIET

Clare Dover is a highly respected English medical writer who suffers from osteoporosis. She developed the British National Osteoporosis Society Diet, found in her book *Osteoporosis*, which was written in association with the National Osteoporosis Society.

## Basic Nutritional Approach

Dover contends that osteoporosis, rather than being an inevitable part of aging, is largely preventable and treatable by taking preventive measures such as eating a diet high in calcium and exercising regularly to build strong bones. She notes that calcium consumption in the U.S. and England has declined. In England, for example, calcium intake has decreased from an average of 1,040 milligrams a day for men, women, and children to 817 milligrams. Dover attributes this decline to decreased consumption of milk and, to a lesser extent, white bread.

## Recommended Foods

Dover emphasizes that the best sources of calcium are milk, cheese, and yogurt, which are easily absorbed by the body. Adults who are concerned about clogging their arteries or weight gain can reduce intake of dairy fat by selecting lowfat milks, cheeses, and yogurts, which contain equal or even higher levels of calcium than full-fat varieties.

Alternatives for those who cannot or do not wish to drink ordinary milk include commercial calcium-fortified soy milk and soybean curd.

## DIETARY CALCIUM TIPS

- Drink a glass of milk with meals.
- Stir some milk or yogurt into soups.
- Choose calcium-rich vegetables such as broccoli and green beans.
- Make yogurt-based salad dressings.
- Serve a white sauce with fish or vegetables.
- Sprinkle grated cheese over soups and pasta.
- Eat dried apricots or lowfat cheeses as snacks.
- Use fruit-flavored fromage frais (a cheeselike topping) on fruit and desserts.
- Add grated cheese to pastry crusts.
- Make yogurt dips to serve with raw vegetables.
- Top baked potatoes with yogurt and chives or grated cheese.
- Make milkshakes by blending milk with fruit yogurt.

*Calcium-Rich Foods.* Dover's diet recommends the following calcium-rich foods:

- Dairy foods such as lowfat yogurt, skim milk, cottage cheese, and cheddar cheese.
- Canned fish with fish bones in an edible form, such as sardines and salmon.
- Nuts and seeds, especially Brazil nuts, almonds, and sesame seeds.
- Mineral water and tap water from hard-water areas, both of which can provide about 220 milligrams of calcium a day. (Tap water from soft-water areas, however, provides virtually no calcium.)
- Vegetables, especially green varieties such as spinach, broccoli, winter cabbage, and watercress.
- Dried fruit such as figs, prunes, and apricots.
- Legumes such as baked beans and red kidney beans.

Dover cautions that the calcium in spinach, broccoli, and nuts is not as well absorbed by the body as calcium from dairy food sources. Substances such as oxalates in vegetables and fiber in cereals may impair the absorption of calcium from the small intestine, thereby reducing the amount that is actually available to the body.

## Physical Activity

Dover stresses the importance of exercise in keeping bones healthy and strong. She specifically recommends weight-bearing exercises, including walking, weight training, jogging, tennis, dancing, and step aerobics. Dover believes that they must be performed at least three times a week, and preferably on a daily basis.

## PREVENTING AND REVERSING OSTEOPOROSIS DIET

In his book *Preventing and Reversing Osteoporosis,* Dr. Alan Gaby argues that osteoporosis — which causes at least 1.2 million fractures in women each year — is not only preventable but can most likely be reversed as well. Dr. Gaby is the past president of the American Holistic Medical Association, writes a regular column for the *Townsend Letter for Doctors,* and is a member of the Ad-Hoc Advisory Panel of the National Institutes of Health, Office of Alternative Medicine. He authored *Vitamin B6: The*

---

### THE FIFTEEN BEST CALCIUM SOURCES

The May 1995 issue of the *Mayo Clinic Health Letter* recommends consuming three cups of milk per day and one or two servings of any of the following foods to obtain more than 1,000 milligrams of calcium:

| Food | Calcium (milligrams) |
| --- | --- |
| Milk (skim and lowfat), 1 cup | 300 |
| Tofu set with calcium, 1/2 cup | 258 |
| Yogurt, 1 cup (a lowfat brand) | 250 |
| Orange juice (calcium-fortified), 8 ounces | 240 |
| Ready-to-eat cereal (calcium-fortified), 1 cup | 200 |
| Mozzarella cheese (part skim), 1 ounce | 183 |
| Canned salmon with bones, 3 ounces | 181 |
| Collards, 1/2 cup cooked | 179 |
| Ricotta cheese (part skim), 1/4 cup | 169 |
| Bread (calcium-fortified), 2 slices | 160 |
| Cottage cheese (1 percent fat), 1 cup | 138 |
| Parmesan cheese, 2 tablespoons | 138 |
| Navy beans, 1 cup cooked | 128 |
| Turnips, 1/2 cup cooked | 125 |
| Broccoli, 1 cup cooked | 94 |

*Natural Healer* and coauthored the reference manual *Nutritional Therapy for the 1990s.*

### Basic Nutritional Approach

Gaby argues that more than twice as many osteoporotic fractures occur today, compared with thirty years ago, and suggests that osteoporosis is partly due to the typical Western diet, with its high proportion of refined sugar, white flour, fat, salt, caffeine, and canned and processed foods. His nutritional approach recommends that refined sugar, caffeine, and alcohol be restricted and that protein and sodium intake be moderate. Whole grains should be consumed rather than refined grains because the refining process depletes many of the vitamins and minerals needed to maintain healthy bones. Heavily processed foods should be avoided, since processing may destroy important nutrients. Avoid cola beverages, which contain excessive amounts of phosphorus that may adversely affect calcium metabolism.

### Recommended Foods

Gaby does not specifically discuss any foods or nutrients that have been proven to prevent osteoporosis. He does stipulate, however, that calcium-rich foods are important, with the proviso that calcium alone is not effective. He advises dieters to reduce their consumption of junk foods and increase their intake of whole grains, fruits, vegetables, nuts and seeds, beans, and other unprocessed foods.

Gaby also contends that proper attention to food allergies may reduce the likelihood of people developing osteoporosis. This is because bones are living tissue — like the brain, heart, respiratory system, joints, and skin — and therefore are similarly affected by allergies. Continual ingestion of allergenic foods can cause damage to the gastrointestinal tract, resulting in malabsorption and deficiencies of nutrients that increase the risk of osteoporosis.

His allergy-elimination diet, which should be practiced under medical supervision to avoid the possibility of nutrient deficiencies, recommends:

- Cereals including oatmeal, oat bran, cream of rye, puffed rice, and puffed millet.
- Grains and flour products such as rice cakes and crackers, rye bread with no wheat, Oriental noodles, flour made from buckwheat, rice,

potatoes and beans, rice or millet bread, cooked whole grains including oats, millet, barley, buckwheat groats (kasha), rice, macaroni, spelt (flour and pasta), brown rice, amaranth, and quinoa. Most of these grains are available at health food stores.

- Legumes (beans) including soybeans, tofu, lentils, peas, chickpeas, navy beans, kidney beans, black beans, and string beans. Dried beans should be soaked overnight. Canned soups such as split pea and lentil that do not contain additives are also permitted, as are bean dips without sugar, lemon, or additives.
- All vegetables except corn.
- Proteins from meat, chicken, fish, tuna packed in spring water, turkey, grain, or bean casseroles. Shellfish is not restricted from an allergy standpoint, but is not considered particularly healthful. Beef and pork may be eaten unless otherwise specified. Lamb rarely causes allergic reactions, and may be used even when other meats are restricted.
- Nuts and seeds, either raw or roasted (without salt or sugar), as well as nut butters from peanuts, almonds, cashews, walnuts, sesame seeds, and sesame tahini.
- Oil and fats, including sunflower, safflower, olive, sesame, peanut, flaxseed, and soy oils (either cold-pressed or expeller-pressed). Once people have completed food testing, they are encouraged to use butter instead of margarine.
- Snacks including celery, carrot sticks, or other vegetables, fruit in moderation (not citrus), unsalted fresh nuts and seeds, and wheat-free cookies.
- Beverages including herb teas (no lemon or orange), distilled or spring water in glass bottles, seltzer (salt-free), Perrier, pure fruit juices without sugar or additives (which should be diluted with 50 percent water), almond nut milk, and soy milk without corn oil. Cafix, Inka, and Roma may be used as coffee substitutes.
- Sweeteners such as honey and real maple syrup, up to three teaspoons a day, as well as barley malt and fruit juice (not citrus).
- Thickeners such as rice, oat, millet, barley, soy, or amaranth flours, as well as arrowroot and agar.
- Spices and condiments including salt in moderation, pepper, herbal spices without preservatives or sugar, garlic, ginger, onions, ketchup and mustard from the health food store (without sugar), wheat-free tamari sauce, and vitamin C crystals in water as a substitute for lemon juice.

- Miscellaneous may include sugar-free spaghetti sauce and fruit-only jellies without sugar, honey, or lemon juice.

## Eliminated Foods

A typical elimination diet, Gaby explains, prohibits all foods containing sugar (which may deplete the body of calcium), wheat, dairy products, corn products, eggs, citrus fruits, coffee, and tea (because caffeine ingestion may contribute to bone loss), alcohol (a known risk factor for osteoporosis when consumed in excess amounts), and all food additives. If chronic symptoms disappear or improve considerably while on the diet, people are probably allergic to one or more of the foods eliminated.

Specifically, Gaby recommends that people on an elimination diet avoid the following foods:

- Dairy products, including milk, cheese, butter, yogurt, sour cream, cottage cheese, whey, casein, sodium caseinate, calcium caseinate, and any food containing these.
- Wheat found in most breads, spaghetti, noodles, pasta, most flour, baked goods, durum semolina, and many gravies.
- Corn, including any product with corn oil, vegetable oil from an unspecified source, corn syrup, corn sweetener, dextrose, glucose, corn chips, tortillas, and popcorn.
- Egg whites and yolks, and any product containing eggs.
- Citrus fruits, including oranges, grapefruits, lemons, limes, and tangerines.
- Coffee, tea, and alcohol, except herbal teas (both caffeinated and decaffeinated coffee and tea should be avoided).
- Refined sugars, including table sugar and any foods that contain it, such as candy, soda, pies, cake, and cookies.
- Honey and maple syrup may be allowed for some people, one to three teaspoons daily, as determined on an individual basis.
- Food additives, including artificial colorings, flavors, preservatives, texturing agents, and artificial sweeteners. Most diet sodas and other dietetic foods contain artificial ingredients and must therefore be avoided.
- Chicken and iceberg lettuce should be avoided completely; turkey or other varieties of lettuce may be substituted.
- Any other food eaten more than three times per week should be consumed no more than every fourth day while on the elimination diet.

## Vitamin and Mineral Supplements

Deficiencies of one or more vitamins and minerals can promote osteoporosis. Gaby believes that even if a person's diet emphasizes wholesome, nutrient-rich foods, vitamin and mineral supplementation may be worthwhile.

For individuals who wish to take supplements to reduce their risk of osteoporosis, he recommends the following range of suggested daily doses to correct nearly all deficiencies and to meet most requirements that are higher than normal:

*Minerals:*
- Calcium (400 to 1,200 milligrams)
- Magnesium (200 to 600 milligrams)
- Zinc (10 to 30 milligrams)
- Copper (1 to 2 milligrams)
- Manganese (5 to 20 milligrams)
- Boron (1 to 3 milligrams)
- Silicon (1 to 2 milligrams)
- Strontium (0.5 to 3 milligrams)

*Vitamins:*
- Vitamin B6 (5 to 50 milligrams)
- Folic acid (0.4 to 5 milligrams)
- Vitamin C (100 to 1,000 milligrams)
- Vitamin D (100 to 400 units)
- Vitamin K (100 to 500 micrograms)

## Physical Activity

Gaby believes that physical activity plays a crucial role in maintaining bone mass, due primarily to the repetitive physical stress applied to bones. He agrees with most specialists that only weight-bearing exercises are capable of increasing bone density, and recommends that people with osteoporosis — after first consulting with their physician — engage in some type of regular exercise (three or four times a week for 30 minutes) to promote optimal health.

## Estrogen and Progesterone Therapy

Past studies have consistently shown that estrogen and progesterone hormone replacement therapy sharply reduces the risk of developing osteoporosis. According to Gaby, a "growing body of evidence indicates that natural progesterone may be more important than estrogen in treating postmenopausal osteoporosis." As evidence, Gaby cites new research by Dr. Jerilynn C. Prior, of the Division of Endocrinology and Metabolism, University of British Columbia in Vancouver, which shows that progesterone stimulates bone formation by binding to osteoblasts, the cells that build new bone.

Gaby also discusses the research of Dr. John Lee of Sebastopol, California, who studied the effects of natural progesterone on one hundred postmenopausal women, aged 38 to 83 (the average age was 65.2 years). Lee found that the progesterone cream therapy increased bone mineral density in 63 women by an average 10 percent after the first six to twelve months of therapy. Some patients showed a 20 to 25 percent increase in bone mineral density. Many of the women receiving progesterone therapy commented that their mobility and energy level improved and that their lower sex drive returned to normal. Side effects, according to Lee, were virtually nonexistent. Gaby concludes that natural progesterone appears to be extremely effective for preventing and treating osteoporosis, and that the use of progesterone may eliminate the need for estrogen replacement therapy in many cases, although he cautions that more clinical research is needed.

## Skim Milk

In the August 1992 issue of *Prevention*, Dr. George Blackburn writes that women of all ages (especially those at risk of osteoporosis), should consume high daily levels of vitamin D and calcium. The most beneficial source, he adds, is fortified skim milk, because it contains the most readily absorbable type of calcium along with all the essential amino acids and special protein substances that promote bone and muscle growth.

According to Blackburn, everyone (except infants) should consume at least two 8-ounce servings of dairy products daily. (Americans typically consume less than half this amount). Skim milk contains virtually no fat and a minimum of calories, and people who drink it tend to consume fewer caffeine-containing beverages such as coffee and tea, fewer sugary soft drinks, fewer sugary calorie-laden foods and juices, and less fat-heavy whole milk and other whole-milk dairy products. By switching to skim milk exclusively, Blackburn suggests that people can reduce their risk of osteoporosis and decrease their total fat intake to 25 percent of calories (most Americans currently consume 37 percent of daily calories from fat).

### Soybean Milk

In the April 1994 issue of the *Journal of Nutritional Science and Vitaminology* N. Omi reports that soybean milk is an excellent source for increasing bone mineral density (BMD) and mechanical bone strength. Based on a study he conducted at the Department of Food and Nutrition at Japan Women's University in Tokyo, he concludes that peptides in soybean milk accelerate intestinal calcium absorption.

## VEGETARIAN DIETS

In his book *Dr. Dean Ornish's Program for Reversing Heart Disease,* Ornish maintains that the real cause of osteoporosis in this country is not insufficient calcium intake, but rather excessive excretion of calcium in the urine. Even calcium supplementation is often not enough to make up for the increased calcium excretion. Vegetarians, however, excrete much less calcium, says Ornish, which is why they have very low rates of osteoporosis, even though their dietary intake of calcium is lower than those who eat meat.

Ornish cites a study conducted at University of Texas Medical School at Dallas that compared urinary excretion of normal subjects who were given two different diets: one diet contained only vegetable protein, the other contained only animal protein. Both diets had the same amount of protein, sodium, potassium, calcium, phosphate, and magnesium. Patients on the animal protein diet excreted 50 percent more calcium in their urine than those on the vegetable protein diet. The researchers concluded that the inability of the subjects to compensate for the animal protein–induced loss of calcium in their urine might predispose them to develop osteoporosis as well as kidney stones.

# 16

## Diets for Arthritis

Approximately 37 million Americans — or one out of every seven (including 285,000 children) — have arthritis, a general term for more than one hundred diseases affecting many different parts of the body, most often joints. The word "arthritis" literally means joint inflammation ("arth" = joint; "itis" = inflammation). The most common types include rheumatoid arthritis, osteoarthritis, systemic lupus erythematosus, scleroderma, gout, ankylosing spondylitis, psoriatic arthritis, infectious arthritis, fibrositis, bursitis, and tendinitis. Each has its own characteristics and affects each sufferer differently.

People of all ages can develop arthritis, which is usually chronic and may last a lifetime. Dr. Jean-Pierre Pelletier of the University of Montreal estimates in the May 1995 issue of *Healthy Way* that the average American now has a 50 percent chance of suffering from arthritis by the age of 50.

The most common type of arthritis is osteoarthritis, a degenerative disease that has apparently always been part of the human condition. It has been found in the 40,000-year-old skeletons of Neanderthal men, 7,000-year-old mummies from Egypt and Peru, and 3,000-year-old skeletons from the Indian subcontinent. Approximately 97 percent of people older than 65 will exhibit some X-ray evidence of osteoarthritis, which is chronic and involves the breakdown of cartilage and other joint tissues, and 50 percent will have evidence that is significant.

Unlike rheumatoid arthritis and gout, osteoarthritis is not a metabolic or systemic disease; that is, if it occurs in one joint (any place in the body where two bones meet), it does not necessarily spread to others. With osteoarthritis, cartilage (a tough, elastic tissue that covers the ends of bones and lubricates them, while also acting as a shock absorber) gradually wears away. As a result, a person's bones grind against each other, eventually causing considerable pain and swelling.

Symptoms usually begin slowly and may seem minor. One or two joints, for example, may ache or feel mildly sore, especially with movement. A few sufferers, however, feel constant nagging pain. The symptoms are usually most extreme after the joints have been under- or overexercised for a long period. The muscles around affected joints may also become weak and affect coordination and posture. Osteoarthritis most commonly occurs in the joints that bear the most weight — the hips, knees, spine, fingers, thumbs, and big toes.

In contrast, rheumatoid arthritis is an autoimmune disease affecting the entire body that inflames many different tissues, but especially the membranes that line the joints. Eventually, outgrowths of the inflamed tissue begin to invade and damage the cartilage in the joints, causing them to become deformed.

The effects of rheumatoid arthritis differ from person to person. They are often mild (causing only minor discomfort at times and no joint deformity), but usually keep coming back and eventually become chronic. Early in the disease, most people feel tired, sore, and achy. The joints stiffen, then swell and become tender, eventually making full motion difficult and painful. The symptoms are often worse in the morning and after long periods of sitting or lying still. Often the joints on both sides of the body are affected, that is, both hands, both feet, or both hips.

Because it is a systemic disease, rheumatoid arthritis may also cause fatigue, weight loss, anemia, fever, and often crippling pain. Other possible changes include inflammation of the eyes, pleurisy (fluid in the lungs), and lumps under the skin (especially on the backs of the elbows) that come and go and usually don't cause problems.

The formulators of the diets reviewed in this chapter believe that nutritional therapies can help treat osteoarthritis and rheumatoid arthritis and relieve their accompanying symptoms.

## THE ARTHRITIS RELIEF DIET

The Arthritis Relief Diet, developed by Dr. James Scala, is detailed in his book *The Arthritis Relief Diet*. Dr. Scala received his Ph.D. in biochemistry from Cornell University and has taught nutrition at various universities and medical schools in the United States and abroad. A frequent guest on radio and television talk shows to discuss nutrition-related health issues, he has authored two other books, *Eating Right for a Bad Gut* and *The High Blood Pressure Relief Diet.*

Scala contends that the common denominator underlying most of the one hundred forms of arthritis is inflammation, which is moderated by diet. He believes that his Arthritis Relief Diet works because it reduces foods in the diet that cause inflammation, and conversely increases foods that reduce inflammation.

Specifically, he claims that biochemicals called prostaglandins play a primary role in the onset and relief of inflammation. One set of prostaglandins and other biochemicals (which he terms "antagonistic") increases inflammation, while a second set ("beneficial") suppresses or moderates it. Scala's diet strengthens the beneficial group when it is overpowered by the antagonistic group and restores the natural balance between the two.

According to Scala, the beneficial prostaglandins that are essential for arthritis sufferers are made from a fatty acid found in marine plants and fish called eicosapentaenoic acid (EPA). (EPA is not made by the fish, but rather by algae, plankton, and seaweed that fish eat.) EPA is one of three omega-3 fatty acids (the other two being alpha-linolenic acid [ALA] and docosahexaenoic acid [DHA]) which, in turn, are part of a larger group of polyunsaturated acids.

## Basic Nutritional Approach

Scala's Arthritis Relief Diet is directed toward rheumatoid arthritis, although its weight-control aspect also relieves the inflammation that accompanies osteoarthritis. The diet emphasizes lowfat protein (comprising 10 to 15 percent of total daily caloric intake) with the primary sources being fish, poultry, vegetables, and dairy products. It minimizes saturated animal fat and reduces polyunsaturated oil intake, specifically arachidonic and linoleic acids (the primary substances from which antagonistic prostaglandins are made); fat should comprise 20 to 25 percent of total calories.

Sixty to 70 percent of calories are consumed as carbohydrates, primarily complex carbohydrates. Scala's diet also includes 25 to 35 grams of fiber daily, or at least one ounce of dietary fiber with carbohydrate-rich foods and as fiber supplements. Dieters are urged to consume at least one gram of EPA each day in protein-rich fish and in capsules as food supplements, although 3 to 4 grams are preferable.

## Recommended Foods

Fish is central to Scala's diet because it provides the most protein for the least number of calories, and is an excellent source of EPA. Salmon, for example, delivers 67 percent of its calories from protein and 28 percent from fat with up to 1.5 grams of EPA.

High-EPA fish that Scala recommends include anchovy, herring, mackerel, salmon trout, catfish, tuna, and whitefish. Fish with lower levels of EPA include bass, cod, halibut, sole, and swordfish. Mollusks (oysters, clams), crustaceans (shrimp, crab), and cephalopods (squid, octopus) contain less EPA than fin fish — less than 1/2 gram per 3 1/2-ounce serving — and are not considered good sources.

According to Scala, frozen and canned fish (packed in brine, if possible) are acceptable alternatives to fresh fish; he recommends broiling, baking, and poaching as the best methods of preparation.

*Carbohydrates.* Scala emphasizes that consuming complex, natural carbohydrates is a crucial component in controlling arthritic inflammation. Good sources include rice, beans, grains, cereals, breads, vegetables, and fruits. He considers pasta an excellent source of both protein and complex carbohydrates, but urges people to read the ingredient list to make sure that the first ingredient is wheat, spinach (spinach pasta), or corn (corn pasta), and that if eggs appear (preferably not), they are far down on the list; ingredient lists go from maximum to minimum in content.

Scala suggests serving pasta with a fish, chicken, or clam sauce made with olive oil and no cream. If arthritis sufferers can eat tomatoes (which are in the "nightshade" class of foods, as explained later in this chapter), Scala considers tomato sauce "the choice for pasta," as it is low in fat and calories. Meat sauce, meatballs, sausage, or any animal fat should never be used, and Parmesan cheese should be used sparingly.

*Poultry.* Chicken, turkey, pheasant, guinea fowl, squab, and other birds are all low in fat and excellent sources of protein. Scala recommends eating only the breast and light meat of the leg, and avoiding dark meat and the wings. Duck and goose breast are also acceptable, as are chicken and turkey roll and canned chicken (light meat only). He advises removing the skin from all poultry before broiling, baking, or boiling.

*Fiber.* Scala's diet includes 25 to 35 grams (or at least one ounce) of dietary fiber each day, supplied primarily by fruit, cereal, grains, and vegetables. He specifically recommends soluble forms such as pectin, oat bran, and guar gum, which help bind and eliminate cholesterol and fat.

Scala recommends that dieters begin each day with a breakfast of high-fiber cereal such as All-Bran, bran buds, bran flakes, corn bran, oat bran, oatmeal, or barley. Breakfast cereals should be eaten with skim milk and fruit, and sugar used sparingly; preferable alternatives include brown sugar, honey, or maple syrup. Other fiber options include unprocessed bran in pancakes or waffles, fruit on cereals or pancakes, and high-fiber snacks such as high-fiber wafers, crackers, and cookies.

Fiber cannot perform its cleansing action without water, emphasizes Scala, which is particularly important for arthritis sufferers because waste materials can cause inflammation if not quickly eliminated. He urges dieters to drink eight glasses of water daily, preferably as pure water, although other beverages are also acceptable.

*Cereals and Grains.* According to Scala, arthritis sufferers cannot eat too much cereal and grain. In addition to breakfast cereals, as recommended above, he suggests the following as excellent sources of fiber, complex carbohydrates, and protein: barley, corn (including corn on the cob, cornmeal, and corn pasta), rice (including long grain, wild, and polished), wheat or wheat germ, and whole-grain bread (using spreads such as olive oil, peanut or sesame oil, and peanut butter or unsalted almond butter).

*Vegetables.* Scala advises dieters to eat one or two vegetables with each meal — except breakfast, which should always include fruit — together with a green salad. He does warn, however, that the "nightshade" vegetables (see Restricted Foods) may present a problem for some arthritics. The best way to prepare vegetables, he notes, is to lightly steam or stir-fry them (using only olive oil or Puritan oil). Vegetables should not be cooked in corn oil, butter, or animal fat. Frozen vegetables are permitted, although canned vegetables that contain excess salt and sugar are not.

Scala's recommended list of vegetables for arthritis relief includes: alfalfa sprouts, artichokes, asparagus, beets and beet greens, broccoli, Brussels sprouts, cabbage, carrots, cauliflower, celery, chard, corn, cucumber, eggplant, garbanzo beans, green beans (Italian and snap), kale, kidney beans, leeks, lentils, lettuce, lima beans, mushrooms, mustard greens, okra, onions, parsley, peas, bell peppers, pumpkin, radishes, scallions, snow peas, spinach, squash, sweet potatoes, turnip and turnip greens, watercress, and yams.

Beans are recommended because they provide protein, carbohydrate, and fiber, and contain no fat. Scala also cites research that has shown natural materials in garlic and onions can act as prostaglandins to some extent.

*Fruits.* Scala recommends that dieters consume fruit as dessert, snacks, and as a garnish for cereals, but cautions against dried fruit, which contain sulfite preservatives. Canned or frozen fruit should ideally be packaged in its own juices, while fruit juices should only be consumed if they are the whole juice (that is, whole frozen orange juice versus a clarified juice such as Hawaiian Punch, which contains only 10 percent juice).

*Beverages.* Scala recommends that arthritics should consume four to eight glasses of water daily, including mineral water that contains magnesium. He suggests that intake of coffee and other caffeine-containing beverages be limited to the equivalent of two cups of coffee daily. Four to six cups of tea, which is gentle on the stomach, are acceptable, as are occasional soft drinks (diet and caffeine-free).

## Eliminated Foods

Because Scala's diet attempts to eliminate as much arachidonic acid and saturated fat as possible, he strongly recommends avoiding red meat, including beef, pork, bacon, ham, veal, buffalo, and lamb along with organ meats and processed meats (such as sausage, frankfurters, bologna, liverwurst, salami, and most other sandwich or luncheon meats). Both rabbit (which is generally very low in fat) and venison can be eaten occasionally.

## Restricted Foods

Scala recommends that dieters restrict the following foods: animal fats, shortenings (except in baking), peanut butter, coconut oil, corn oil and corn oil products, palm kernel and safflower oil, hydrogenated soybean oil, sunflower and wheat germ oil, mayonnaise, butter, margarine made from corn oil, safflower or soybeans, and sandwich spreads such as Miracle Whip and those containing meat and cheese.

In addition, Scala believes that the nightshade foods (tomatoes, most varieties of white potatoes, eggplant, and green or red peppers), may induce arthritic attacks. Dieters are advised to try these foods, which provide essential nutrients, to determine if they have a sensitivity to them.

*Dairy Products.* Scala states that high-fat dairy products can cause inflammation, and his diet restricts high-fat ice cream and cheese, whole milk, lowfat (2%) milk, homogenized milk, evaporated and condensed milk, buttermilk, goat and soybean milk, yogurt or cheese made from whole milk, egg yolks, and butter. He suggests nonfat dairy products and dairy products such as cottage cheese and yogurt made from skim or nonfat milk. Lowfat, skim-milk, mozzarella, and ricotta cheese should be consumed sparingly, along with Parmesan cheese on pasta; all other cheeses are eliminated. Scala also urges people to experiment with egg substitutes whenever possible, including recipes that use the whole egg, such as scrambled eggs, omelets, and French toast.

## Vitamin and Mineral Supplements

Scala recommends that dieters take vitamin and mineral supplements to avoid any possible marginal deficiencies. Specifically, he suggests a daily supplement that provides 50 percent of the U.S. RDA for vitamins A, D, E, C, B6, and B12, folic acid, thiamin (B1), riboflavin (B2), niacin, biotin, pantothenic acid, calcium, phosphorus, iodine, iron, magnesium, copper, zinc, and selenium.

## Alcohol

Alcohol, according to Scala, has never been proven to alter the course of inflammation, although it does interact with some arthritis medications and can create problems. Excessive alcohol also interferes with fat metabolism. He urges people following the Arthritis Relief Diet to use caution and good judgment in consuming alcoholic beverages, and does not feel that drinking an occasional cocktail, or a glass of wine or beer, is detrimental.

## Physical Activity

Scala notes that exercise can promote healing and help restore tissues damaged by arthritis and diminished by inactivity because it improves blood circulation, increases joint flexibility, strengthens muscles, and improves mental alertness. He recommends starting with a minimum of fifteen minutes of exercise twice daily, provides basic limbering, stretching, and breathing exercises, and cautions against excessive physical exertion.

## Behavioral Modification

Scala strongly recommends that people with arthritis keep a food diary to help them monitor their daily reactions to certain foods and beverages, to learn which cause inflammation and which reduce it, and to then make appropriate dietary changes. The three essential behavioral modification components in making the food diary work, he notes, are being honest, keeping track of all foods consumed, and paying close attention to the results. He also urges people with arthritis to maintain normal blood sugar levels (to help avoid depression), adopt a positive mental attitude, make use of arthritis support groups, learn coping techniques, and set the goal of being a positive example for others.

## DR. GUS J. PROSCH'S DIET FOR ARTHRITIS

Dr. Gus Prosch is a specialist in clinical nutrition whose diet is included in the *Supplement to the Art of Getting Well: Proper Nutrition for Rheumatoid Arthritis*, published by the Rheumatoid Disease Foundation.

### Basic Nutritional Approach

In Prosch's observations and research, several findings struck him as quite significant in most patients with rheumatoid arthritis (RA):

- The great majority have bodily fluids (such as saliva and urine) that are too acidic.
- The great majority of these patients show signs and symptoms of a deficiency in free or ionic calcium.
- Most RA patients eat margarine instead of butter, and drink 2% or lowfat milk. They demonstrate a lack of vitamins A and natural D, as well as severe deficiencies of the essential fatty acids (EFAs).
- Vitamin and mineral supplementation helps shorten the recovery time by strengthening the immune system.

Prosch concluded that a diet consisting of high-alkaline foods (those high in potassium, calcium, magnesium, and sodium) should be consumed by those with RA, combined with the avoidance of acid-forming foods (those high in phosphorus, sulfur, or chlorine).

## Recommended Foods

Most vegetables (except corn) are highly alkaline and are an essential part of Prosch's diet. (The nightshade plants — those containing solanines — such as white potatoes, tomatoes, eggplant, and garden peppers should be avoided, however.) Prosch specifically suggests that vegetables be cooked in a wok or stir-fried in cold-pressed vegetable oil. Salad vegetables should be consumed daily, as well as fresh (not canned) vegetable juices. Prosch emphasizes the importance of preparing and serving as many foods in their raw and natural state as possible.

*Fruits.* According to Prosch, all fruits and fruit juices (except cranberries, plums, and prunes) are alkaline-forming and should be consumed at meals and as snacks.

*Protein-Rich Foods.* As a rule, Prosch states, most protein foods tend to be acid-forming since they contain phosphorus and sulfur. Animal sources of protein include lean meat (beef, lamb, veal), poultry, and eggs. With the exception of shrimp, most seafood is also extremely acid-forming. However, as these foods provide the building blocks for all bodily functions and processes, Prosch emphasizes that one of these proteins should be eaten with every meal, and balanced with alkaline-forming foods. (Pork should be limited, however.) He suggests cooking protein foods at low temperatures, as enzymes and trace minerals are reduced with excessive heat.

*Dairy Products.* Unlike Scala, Prosch argues that whole milk is an important food in his diet because it is high in calcium and also alkaline-forming. (He specifically recommends raw certified whole milk that, unfortunately, is available in very few states.) Prosch advises arthritics to consume at least two glasses of whole milk each day, and substitute butter for margarine. He also recommends plain yogurt as an excellent alkalinizing food that is easy to digest, and suggests combining it with fresh fruit such as raisins, dates, dried figs, and apricots.

## Eliminated Foods

Prosch's diet eliminates all processed and most canned foods, along with caffeine, sugar in all its forms, and simple carbohydrate foods that are immediately converted into sugar upon digestion. These include white-flour foods, crackers, many cereals, macaroni (pasta foods), white rice, and corn products. Ideally, both nicotine and alcohol should be avoided, along with any sweets, candy, soft drinks, pastries, and desserts.

*Nightshade Plants.* Prosch cites research published by Dr. Robert Bingham that found approximately one-third of arthritics are affected by solanines. He suggests eliminating all nightshade plants (white potatoes, tomatoes, eggplant, and garden peppers) from the diet.

*Processed and Hydrogenated (Hardened) Oils and Fats.* Most margarines, peanut butters, French fries, and potato or corn chips are prepared with processed or hydrogenated ("hardened") oils, and should be avoided. Prosch believes that sweet cream butter is better than other forms, and suggests using cold-pressed vegetable oils or Pam in home cooking. While most fats and fatty foods (such as butter, oils, sausages, and bacon) are neutral in acid-alkaline content, they should be limited because they contribute to excessive weight gain, which severely complicates arthritis symptoms. He recommends that those who are overweight limit all oily, greasy, fried, and fatty foods.

## Vitamin and Mineral Supplementation

Prosch believes that most arthritic patients have a free calcium deficiency, and to correct this, suggests consuming much larger amounts of vitamins A and D in their natural form than are recommended by the RDAs. He claims that the synthetic vitamin A and D preparations on the market do not work, and recommends Norwegian cod liver oil liquid as the ideal source (which seems to be even better than cod liver oil capsules and can be found in most health food stores).

Prosch has also found that none of the available inorganic calcium preparations is effective, but suggests that the compound calcium orotate (the naturally occurring calcium in plants that has been taken off the market by the FDA) enhances the body's ability to use and metabolize other forms of calcium consumed in food. Calcium chelate or calcium aspartate can be used as substitutes.

Prosch also prescribes magnesium orotate to balance the calcium/magnesium ratio and strengthen bone and cartilage structures in the body. However, as magnesium orotate has been removed from the market by the FDA as well, he recommends magnesium chelate and aspartate as substitutes.

Other vitamins and minerals he recommends for rheumatoid arthritis sufferers include vitamin B complex, vitamin C, zinc chelate, or zinc aspartate (as the FDA has removed zinc orotate from the market), selenium, beta-carotene, and vitamin E. These vitamin and mineral supplements, he claims, will not only help arthritis by stimulating the immune response system, but will also play an important role in counteracting the aging process and serve as a deterrent to some forms of cancer because many act as free radical and peroxide scavengers in the body.

## THE ARTHRITIS SURVEY DIET

The Arthritis Survey Diet was developed by Arthur C. Klein and Dava Sobel and outlined in *Arthritis: What Works*. The authors based their book on a nationwide survey of 1,051 people with osteoarthritis or rheumatoid arthritis, and on research of medical literature pertaining to arthritis. Many of the survey participants claim there is a connection between nutrition and arthritis, having found that a change in diet results in pain relief or a reduction of inflammation. And, as the authors point out, many researchers agree and are conducting studies that show how certain foods can aggravate arthritis, while others apparently ameliorate the symptoms. The authors' goal is to provide a diet that makes the most sense for the majority of arthritis sufferers.

### Basic Nutritional Approach

The Arthritis Survey Diet, which was developed in consultation with Kathleen Pratt, a registered dietitian, combines the participants' successful nutritional strategies with new research that indicates the important role dietary changes can make in treating arthritis, according to the authors. It is a lowfat, high-carbohydrate diet endorsed by researchers and physicians for the prevention or control of heart disease, diabetes, and certain forms of cancer. It provides a rich supply of the fish oils that have been shown to control arthritis symptoms, and also, despite the fact that the diet does not count calories, enables those following it to lose excess weight.

## Recommended Foods

The authors point out that foods low in fat generally have fewer calories and are more healthful and nutritious. Fruits, for example, contain almost no fat. They recommend choosing naturally lowfat items over fatty foods and snacks, and looking for lowfat alternatives to foods normally consumed. Examples include skim milk rather than whole milk, light margarine and sour cream, low-calorie mayonnaise, and tuna fish packed in water instead of oil. The authors also advocate reducing the amount of fat (oil, shortening, butter, or margarine) used in cooking.

*Vegetables.* Arthritics are urged to eat more vegetables, especially fresh ones and raw vegetables in salads. They should try to eat at least one meatless vegetable/pasta dinner per week.

*Fish.* The authors recommend that arthritics consume a minimum of three fish dinners per week and at least two fish lunches. If fresh fish is unavailable, frozen fish (unbreaded) is an acceptable alternative. People should pick varieties that have the highest content of omega-3 fatty acids, such as Norwegian sardines, Atlantic mackerel, lake trout, Atlantic herring, albacore tuna, anchovies, Atlantic salmon, bluefish, pink salmon, and Greenland halibut. When purchasing canned tuna, dieters should choose water-packed because the oil used in canning is vegetable oil, which contains no omega-3 fatty acids.

*Fiber.* The authors urge arthritics to eat a lot of fiber. The complex carbohydrates that have a high-fiber content, as well as important vitamins and minerals, are whole-grain breads and cereals, fruits, vegetables, and dried beans and peas.

*Beverages.* Everyone needs to drink about eight glasses of water a day, and medications may require arthritics to drink even more. The authors claim that milk is generally considered the best chaser for many arthritis drugs because of its stomach-coating action; they urge people following the Arthritis Survey Diet to drink at least two glasses a day for the calcium milk provides (if they are not lactose-intolerant).

If people are sensitive to citrus fruits, other fruit juice alternatives include apple, grape, apricot, and pear. In terms of hot beverages, if caffeine is irritating, options include decaffeinated coffee, herbal tea, and Postum (made from bran, wheat, and molasses).

## Eliminated Foods

Five percent of survey participants avoid one or all vegetables in the nightshade family — tomatoes, white potatoes, eggplant, and bell peppers of all colors. If people find their arthritis symptoms are irritated by these vegetables and they want to eliminate them from the diet, the authors warn them to be especially careful in reading labels on prepared foods because flakes of tomatoes, starch from potatoes, and pieces of peppers are common ingredients. They also point out that tobacco is a nightshade, so those who are sensitive should not smoke or chew it.

## Restricted Foods

The authors recommend eating less red meat, and substituting poultry and fish as often as possible. Pork should be avoided altogether. When preparing red meat, people should select the leanest cuts and remove the visible fat before cooking.

Those following the Arthritis Survey Diet should also restrict sodium intake by cutting down on lunch meats, salty snacks, and prepared processed soups and sauces. Various herbs and spices can be substituted for salt, such as rosemary on chicken, sage on cooked carrots, basil on peas or green beans, and fresh-squeezed lemon juice on broccoli. When shopping, people are urged to look for low-salt alternatives to foods they usually buy, such as low-sodium or low-salt cheeses, snack crackers, soy sauce, tomato sauce, and tomato paste.

The authors also advise using sugar in moderation and suggest sugar substitutes, such as low-sugar or no-sugar-added jams and jellies and canned fruit packed in its own juice instead of heavy syrup.

## Vitamin and Mineral Supplements

The authors state that a daily multivitamin and mineral supplement seems essential to fill gaps in the diet and compensate for some of the nutritional problems arthritis causes, from decreased appetite or cooking ability to incomplete absorption of some nutrients. If dieters have specific vitamin

## DAILY MEAL HABITS

1. Don't skip breakfast. Breakfast should supply one-quarter of the daily requirement for calories and nutrients.

2. Use lowfat cooking techniques such as broiling, baking, poaching, grilling, or stir-frying.

3. To keep as many vitamins in vegetables as possible, steam or microwave them instead of boiling in water. Vegetables can also be sautéed in a small amount of water and oil or in a low-salt broth.

4. When preparing chicken for cooking, remove the skin from the individual pieces; the skin contains much of the fat. You can prevent the meat from drying out by cooking in a covered dish or using a sauce for basting.

5. Identify your own food sensitivities and avoid those foods — whether chocolate, citrus fruits, or the nightshade vegetables, for example — at all costs.

6. Read food package labels to better select the most nutritious items. Ingredients are always listed in order of their concentration, with the most abundant ones first. Select items that have the least fat. Lowfat foods are also lower in calories because fat contains more than twice as many calories per gram as protein or carbohydrates.

7. Make it easy on yourself by stocking up on nutritious frozen foods for those days you are unable to cook. Frozen vegetables, for example, are almost as nutritious as fresh, and are already washed, peeled, and diced.

8. Enjoy your meals. The Arthritis Survey Diet is neither a starvation nor a fad diet. And while people need to eat nutritious foods such as those it contains, they also need to have some variety and enjoy their meals within sensible guidelines so the diet becomes a lifetime plan.

deficiencies, supplements can help them feel better. Surgery, for example, often increases the need for certain nutrients, including vitamins A and C and iron. Many arthritis drugs also create deficiencies by interfering with their absorption or speeding up their excretion — including aspirin (vitamin C), methotrexate (folic acid), penicillamine (copper and zinc), and steroid drugs (calcium). Some vitamins also play specific roles in relieving arthritis-related problems, such as vitamin C for the bruising common to rheumatoid arthritis, vitamin E for its possible anti-inflammatory action and relief of drug-induced tissue damage, and vitamin B6 for relief of some cases of carpal tunnel syndrome. For these reasons, the authors recommend that dieters take a multivitamin and mineral supplement.

## Physical Activity

According to the authors, the great majority of study participants exercise regularly, primarily a combination of stretching or strengthening exercises for their affected joints, along with some general fitness activity, such as walking or bicycling. Exercise relieves pain for many of the participants, increases their joint flexibility and range of motion, offers them some protection against deformity and disability, and improves their muscle tone. This in turn builds strength and guards against contractures and spasms. Some even find exercise helps them lose weight. The authors conclude that physical exertion can reduce arthritis symptoms, provided it is performed carefully with medical approval.

## Behavioral Modification

No matter what medications they take or other kinds of help they have received, many of the study participants considered their own positive outlook on life among their most potent weapons against arthritis. According to the authors, these people "complain little, although they have suffered much, and believe that their attitude helps them feel and function far better than they otherwise might." The authors therefore recommend that arthritics combine their diet with stress management, relaxation training, imagery, visualization, meditation, and self-hypnosis.

## RECENT RESEARCH

Robert Bingham, M.D., Medical Director of the Desert Arthritis and Medical Clinic in Desert Hot Springs, California, reports in *Alternative Medicine: The Definitive Guide* that yucca plant extract vaccines have proven highly successful in reducing arthritic infection and inflammation. The primary therapeutic agent in yucca extract is a high concentration of the steroid saponin, which improves circulation in the intestinal tract while reducing any abnormal fat content in the blood. One of the main benefits of this natural medicine, Bingham emphasizes, is that it has no harmful side effects, unlike many of the pharmacological medicines prescribed for arthritis.

Bingham's clinic has conducted several successful studies of yucca extract, finding that beneficial results are usually experienced within three weeks, and maximum effect experienced after four months. Yucca extract is safe enough to take for longer periods of time to prevent any recurrence of symptoms, and it can be purchased without a prescription. Yucca is already being used by more than three thousand physicians in the U.S. and is also available in Japan, Korea, England, Germany, and Canada.

# 17

## Diets for Coronary Artery Disease

More than 1.5 million people in the U.S. suffer from heart attacks every year, and 500,000 die as a result, nearly half of them women. In fact, more Americans die each year from cardiovascular disease — 44 percent — than from all other causes of death combined, including cancer, AIDS, infectious diseases, accidents, and homicides.

Cardiovascular is a general name for more than twenty different diseases of the heart and its blood vessels. Coronary artery disease (CAD), also referred to as coronary heart disease (CHD), is the most deadly of all heart disorders, accounting for approximately one out of every three deaths related to heart disease.

Most Americans are aware that the majority of coronary artery disease is caused by atherosclerosis (the condition in which fatty "plaques" block the coronary arteries), which often results from high blood cholesterol levels. A blood cholesterol level of more than 240 milligrams per deciliter of blood, for example, doubles a person's risk of developing coronary artery disease.

Because high cholesterol levels have been steadily linked with heart disease, the American Heart Association now recommends that everyone have their cholesterol levels measured annually. (Cholesterol levels are normally measured by taking a blood sample from a person's finger or arm.)

In addition to high blood cholesterol levels, the AHA pinpoints other major risk factors as being heredity, increasing age, high blood pressure, and cigarette smoking. Coronary heart disease can also result from contributing risk factors such as diabetes, obesity, physical inactivity, and emotional stress.

This chapter analyzes three authoritative diets for coronary artery disease: the Living Heart Diet, developed by the heart surgeon Dr. Michael Debakey, the American Heart Association (AHA) diet, and Dr. Dean Ornish's Diet for Reversing Heart Disease.

While the eminent authors whose books are described in this chapter are not in complete accord as to how best to prevent and treat coronary artery disease, they uniformly concur that high blood cholesterol levels are a primary causative factor contributing to this most deadly of heart disorders.

The authors also agree that a diet low in saturated fats and cholesterol can play a key role in lowering high cholesterol levels. They advocate the consumption of grains, fruits, and vegetables and the restriction or elimination of animal products (including red meat, eggs, and whole milk), which also tend to be high in calories. Stress reduction techniques and exercise are recommended as important adjuncts to diet, as are behavioral changes aimed at replacing habits that contribute to weight gain.

## THE LIVING HEART DIET

Dr. Michael Debakey is one of the nation's leading heart surgeons. His Living Heart Diet appears in his book of the same title. It is coauthored by Debakey's colleagues at Baylor College of Medicine: Dr. Antonio Gotto (scientific director), Lynne Scott (chief dietitian), and John Foreyt (director of Baylor College's Diet Modification Clinic).

### Basic Nutritional Approach

Debakey states that his diet has been clinically proven to prevent or reverse heart disease. The four basic goals of his diet are listed below:

Reduce the amount of fat consumed, especially saturated fat.
Substitute polyunsaturated fat for saturated fat in food preparation.
Decrease the amount of dietary cholesterol consumed.
Achieve and maintain ideal body weight.

To accomplish these goals, the Living Heart Diet contains:

- No more than 300 milligrams of cholesterol daily.
- 50 percent of calories as carbohydrates.
- 20 percent of calories as protein.
- 30 percent of calories as fat with
    a) less than 10 percent of fat calories from saturated fat;

b) up to 10 percent of fat calories from polysaturated fat; and
c) the remaining fat from monounsaturated fat sources.

## Recommended Foods

*Meat, Fish, and Poultry.* Debakey's diet limits meat consumption to six ounces daily, and recommends eating chicken (with the skin removed, which can cut fat content by three-quarters and total calories by nearly half), turkey, fish, and shellfish (except shrimp) often because they contain less saturated fat than beef, lamb, or pork, and are lower in calories. (All portions should be weighed after they are cooked.) When meats are preferred, people are urged to select the leanest cuts and trim off all visible fat before cooking. Acceptable meats are those containing 10 percent or less total fat.

*Beans and Grains.* Debakey's diet provides lowfat protein by combining beans, grains, and vegetables. Because most plant proteins lack one or more of the essential amino acids and are therefore incomplete, he recommends combining two or more plant protein sources at each meal to provide a complete protein. Examples include bean and rice casserole; wheat bread with baked beans; corn tortillas and beans; legume soup with bread; rice with sesame seeds; sunflower seeds and peanuts; sesame seeds in bean soup; sesame seeds and milk; pasta with milk and lowfat cheese; and cereal with skim or lowfat milk.

*Fruits.* Because fruits are an excellent source of vitamins A and C, and also provide other important vitamins and minerals, vitamin C–rich fruits should be eaten daily. Debakey suggests choosing fresh, frozen, or canned fruits, preferably without added sugar.

*Fiber.* Debakey recommends the consumption of 25 grams of dietary fiber daily. He warns that fiber should be added gradually to the diet, since the side effect of increased fiber is flatulence (which usually subsides after a few weeks). Sufficient amounts of fluid should be consumed as fiber is increased.

*Dairy Products.* Because dairy products are the richest sources of calcium, a nutrient that people of all ages require in varying amounts, Debakey recommends that skim-milk dairy products be used freely. Lowfat dairy products (including cottage cheese, yogurt, and ice milk) are also allowed.

*Vegetables, Bread, and Cereal Products.* Because the Living Heart Diet reduces one's consumption of meat and fat, the consumption of grain and cereal products (which provide protein, essential vitamins, minerals, and fiber) is increased to four or more servings daily as desired. For simplicity, Debakey combines starchy vegetables in the bread and cereal group, because they provide many of the same nutrients and are similar in calories. Starchy vegetables include potatoes, corn, lima beans, dried beans, and peas.

*Nonstarchy Vegetables.* Debakey explains that nonstarchy vegetables are lower in calories than the other food groups, although some carbohydrate and a small amount of protein are present. They are most nutritious when eaten raw or only lightly cooked (although sources of saturated fat, such as bacon or salt pork, should not be used to do so).

The Living Heart Diet includes a daily serving of a vegetable rich in vitamin A (such as spinach or sweet potatoes) and vitamin C (such as broccoli and red peppers).

## Restricted and Eliminated Foods

Foods that are restricted or eliminated in the Living Heart Diet are those that are high in cholesterol, triglycerides, and fat and contain large numbers of calories.

*Meat, Fish, and Poultry.* The Living Heart Diet recommends eliminating the following foods in this category: duck, goose, all "prime" graded meat such as rib eye steak, ground pork, and spare ribs, ground lamb and mutton, luncheon meat such as bologna, bratwurst, frankfurters, and salami, organ meats, commercially fried meat, fish, or poultry, and meats canned or frozen in gravy or sauce.

*Eggs.* Because egg yolk is the single-most concentrated source of cholesterol in the average American diet (one yolk contains 274 milligrams of cholesterol), the Living Heart Diet recommends that egg yolks be limited to a maximum of two per week, including those used in cooking. Cholesterol-free egg substitutes should be used for cooking, while egg whites (which contain no cholesterol) may be eaten freely.

In addition, Debakey advises dieters to eliminate from their diet cakes, cookies, batters, sauces, rolls, and other foods containing egg yolks, as well as eggnog, and other beverages containing egg yolks.

*Dairy Products.* The Living Heart Diet eliminates high-fat dairy products such as cheeses containing more than 12 percent butterfat (including American, cheddar, and swiss), butter, any tub margarine not listing safflower, sunflower, or corn oil as the first ingredient, chocolate, evaporated and condensed milk, half-and-half, ice cream, sour cream, yogurt made from whole milk, and whipping cream.

In addition, most dairy substitutes should not be used because they contain coconut oil, palm-kernel oil, or hydrogenated fat.

*Bread and Cereal Products.* Eliminated from the Living Heart Diet are bagels made with eggs or cheese, butter rolls, cheese and egg breads, canned biscuits, commercial doughnuts, muffins, sweet rolls, waffles and pancakes, croissants, cereals containing coconut or coconut oil, presweetened cereals, egg noodles, chow mein noodles, and snacks such as corn chips, potato chips, tortilla chips, and other commercial crackers.

In the dessert category, the following foods are eliminated: cheesecake pastries and commercial cakes, pies, cookies, fried pies, and cupcakes.

*Vegetables.* The Living Heart Diet eliminates the following: commercially fried vegetables (fried potatoes, French fries, onion rings, okra, eggplant), commercial vegetables (frozen or canned) that are packaged in a sauce or butter, and dried beans or peas seasoned with bacon fat, salt pork, or ham hocks.

## The Low-Calorie Living Heart Diet

The Low-Calorie Living Heart Diet is an adaptation of the Living Heart Diet for those who wish to reduce to their ideal body weight. It eliminates concentrated sweets, makes provisions for maintaining ideal body weight or losing weight, and utilizes food exchange lists to control the amount of carbohydrates, protein, fat, and calories eaten daily. Recommended foods are all low in cholesterol and saturated fat.

The authors contend that weight reduction plans should produce a loss of one to two pounds per week. Furthermore, although calories must be restricted for weight loss, it is not necessary to count them per se. By using the food exchange lists provided and eating the recommended number of servings from each food group, calorie control becomes easy. The key to losing weight, claim the authors, is staying full on the right kinds of foods.

Finally, they recommend moderate exercise as a valuable adjunct to any weight-loss program.

## Recipes

*The Living Heart Diet* features more than two hundred pages of recipes, each of which is prepared with ingredients low in cholesterol and saturated fat. Nutritional information is provided for each recipe, including total calories, grams of protein, fat, carbohydrate, saturated fat, monosaturated fat and polysaturated fat, and milligrams of cholesterol and sodium. The recipes, which encompass appetizers, entrées, meatless entrées, vegetables, salads and dressings, soups, sauces, and gravies, breads and desserts, are divided into two sections: Living Heart Diet Recipes and Low-Sodium Living Heart Diet Recipes.

In addition, the exchanges for meat, bread, dairy products, fat, fruit, and vegetables are provided. For example, one serving of lemon chicken breasts with mushrooms equals two meats, one vegetable, and one fat, while one serving of vegetable chop suey equals two vegetables and one fat.

## Alcohol

Debakey recommends no more than two servings of alcohol daily because it tends to increase weight and triglyceride levels and can replace the consumption of other more nutritious foods.

## Smoking

According to Debakey, cigarette smoking is one of the three major risk factors for heart attacks. Also, atherosclerosis is accelerated by smoking. Smoking has been correlated with low levels of HDL cholesterol, which he claims offers some protection against atherosclerosis. He discusses a variety of techniques and programs aimed at eliminating the smoking habit, including clinics, self-help programs, going cold turkey, and medications such as Lobeline.

## Physical Activity

Debakey states that while the link between exercise and the prevention of heart attacks has not been conclusively proven, a number of studies suggest that exercise reduces the risk of dying of an early heart attack. He therefore recommends exercise as a very helpful adjunct to diet, and encourages dieters, with the approval of their personal physician, to jog, play tennis, swim, jump rope, or cycle.

## Behavioral Modification

The author contends that for most people, dieting, exercise, medication, or combinations of these are usually unsuccessful over the long term. Therefore, he outlines an eleven-step behavioral modification program:

1. Keep a food record and track daily food intake to make you aware of when, where, and how much you eat.
2. Maintain a daily weight chart, weighing yourself each day at the same time.
3. Limit at-home eating to one place, preferably at the dining room table.
4. Eat more slowly, and lay down utensils between bites.
5. Reward yourself for improving your eating behavior, but never with food.
6. Control and eventually change your food consumption patterns, such as avoiding second helpings.
7. Control how you obtain and eat foods, such as distributing three meals throughout the day, and buying food once a week after your evening meal.
8. Control your eating cues by, for example, storing all food out of sight and having someone else scrape the dishes and put away leftovers.
9. Control indiscriminate eating by making a list of alternative activities in which you can engage, such as relaxation techniques.
10. Control eating habits away from home.
11. Maintain your goal weight.

## THE AMERICAN HEART ASSOCIATION LOW-FAT, LOW-CHOLESTEROL COOKBOOK

For more than forty years, the American Heart Association has educated the American public about the major risk factors associated with developing heart disease. The AHA's official diet for heart disease is detailed in *The American Heart Association Low-Fat, Low-Cholesterol Cookbook*. The book is coauthored by Dr. Scott M. Grundy, one of the foremost lipid specialists in the U.S., and Mary Winston, senior science consultant for the AHA.

### Basic Nutritional Approach

According to Grundy, most cases of high blood cholesterol are caused by diet, and like Debakey, his nutritional approach dramatically reduces fat intake, especially cholesterol and saturated fat. He recommends using polyunsaturated or monounsaturated fats (which do not contribute to increasing blood cholesterol levels), and consuming more complex carbohydrates such as fruits, vegetables, nuts, seeds, whole-grain breads, cereals, and pastas.

### Step-One and Step-Two Diets

The AHA has developed two diets, the Step-One Diet and the Step-Two Diet, both of which are based on a nutritious eating plan calling for reductions in saturated fat and cholesterol. As detailed below, the Step-One Diet is similar to the program the AMA recommends for the general public, while the Step-Two Diet is more restrictive and, consequently, will produce greater reductions in blood cholesterol levels.

People concerned about lowering cholesterol levels are first urged to follow the Step-One Diet for three months. If they do not reach their target level by this point, their doctor or dietitian may recommend the Step-Two Diet.

### Step-One Diet Nutritional Components

| Nutrient | Recommended Intake |
|---|---|
| Total fat | 30 percent or less of total calories eaten per day |
| Saturated fatty acids | Less than 10 percent of total calories |
| Polyunsaturated fatty acids | Up to 10 percent of total calories |
| Monounsaturated fatty acids | 10 to 15 percent of total calories |

| Carbohydrates | 50 to 60 percent of total calories |
| Protein | 10 to 20 percent of total calories |
| Cholesterol | Less than 300 milligrams per day |
| Total calories | To achieve and maintain desirable weight |

**Step-Two Diet Nutritional Components**

| Nutrient | Recommended Intake |
| --- | --- |
| Total fat | 30 percent or less of total calories eaten per day |
| Saturated fatty acids | Less than 7 percent of total calories |
| Polyunsaturated fatty acids | Up to 10 percent of total calories |
| Monounsaturated fatty acids | 10 to 15 percent of total calories |
| Carbohydrates | 50 to 60 percent of total calories |
| Protein | 10 to 20 percent of total calories |
| Cholesterol | Less than 200 milligrams per day |
| Total calories | To achieve and maintain desirable weight |

## Total Calories

The authors point out that severe obesity (more than 30 percent overweight) is a coronary risk factor in its own right, and recommend combining exercise with a modest reduction of 500 calories daily rather than severely restricting caloric intake, which can result in deficiencies of important nutrients. The only successful weight-reducing diet, they claim, is one that allows people to lose weight and monitor it.

Both the Step-One and Step-Two diets recommend a caloric intake that allows people to "achieve and maintain desirable weight." As a rule of thumb, a reduction diet for men contains approximately 1,600 to 2,000 calories, and for women, not fewer than 1,200 to 1,600. According to the authors, this should allow people to meet all their nutrient needs, minimize hunger, and promote healthy, lifelong eating patterns.

## Recommended Foods

Grundy, like Debakey, recommends that fat intake comprise no more than 30 percent of total calories — an amount recommended by the AHA for several years. He cites research indicating that fat restrictions of 10 to 20 percent of total calories are not necessary to produce adequate reductions in blood cholesterol as long as the diet is restricted in saturated fatty acids.

*Fish.* Although fish is not entirely cholesterol-free, it generally contains less cholesterol than red meat. Therefore, Grundy advises dieters to consume fish two to three times a week, especially fish high in omega-3 fatty acids (which may have cholesterol-lowering benefits). These include Atlantic and coho salmon, albacore tuna, club mackerel, carp, lake whitefish, sweet smelt, and lake and brook trout.

Shrimp, crab, lobster, crayfish, and most other shellfish are very low in fat, although the authors note that some varieties contain more cholesterol ounce for ounce than poultry, meat, or other fish. Even these, however, can be eaten occasionally within the recommended guidelines of less than 300 milligrams of cholesterol daily.

*Meat Products.* Grundy's AHA diet permits a total of six ounces of poultry, fish, or lean meat per day (in one or two portions), provided that it is reasonably lean and contains between 500 and 600 calories. Red meat (including beef, lamb, pork, and veal) is permitted, as long as it contains a minimum of visible fat, and all outside fat is trimmed before cooking.

Grundy states that poultry is a good substitute for red meat only if it is a lean variety and if the skin is removed before cooking. Chicken and turkey are preferable to goose or duck.

*Fruits, Vegetables, Grains, and Legumes.* These foods are recommended by Grundy because they contain no cholesterol, tend to be low in fat, and, in many cases, are high in fiber and vitamins. A few exceptions include coconut meat (which is high in saturated fatty acids), olives, and avocados. Grundy counsels dieters to check labels of processed foods made from vegetables, grains, or legumes for fats or cholesterol added during processing, and for excessive amounts of sodium. Generally, however, consumption of food in these categories need not be restricted except to avoid excess calories.

*Nuts and Seeds.* Although both nuts and seeds tend to be high in fat and calories, Grundy states they do not contain cholesterol, and most of their fat is unsaturated. Therefore, he recommends them as part of his diet, because they can replace high-protein, high-fat foods such as meat.

*Dairy Products.* The AHA counsels dieters to virtually eliminate whole milk and to choose instead 1% or skim milk, both of which are rich in protein, calcium, and other nutrients without containing too much fat. Also recommended is consuming only lowfat or skim-milk cream, ice cream, and cheese, and substituting margarine for butter.

The authors recommend that dieters limit egg yolk consumption to three per week on the Step-One Diet and one per week on the Step-Two Diet. Egg whites, however, contain no cholesterol and are a good source of protein. People can therefore consume as many egg whites as they wish and should substitute them for whole eggs in most recipes.

## Restricted Foods

Both the Step-One and Step-Two Diets restrict cholesterol and saturated fats found in animal products and in some plant products. According to Grundy, most Americans should reduce their daily saturated fat intake by about one-third to achieve recommended levels. The Step-Two Diet calls for further reduction in saturated fatty acids to less than 7 percent of total calories. This reduction, the authors note, applies to saturated fat only, not to all fats.

*Meat Products.* Processed meats that are high in fat and calories, including sausage, bologna, salami, and hot dogs, should be used only sparingly. Organ meats, including liver, sweetbreads, kidney, brain, and heart, are extremely high in cholesterol and should be restricted or eliminated.

*Bakery Goods.* Bakery goods such as pies, cakes, cookies, candy, and doughnuts are severely restricted on the AHA diet because they are typically high in calories and contain few beneficial nutrients. Baked goods made with egg yolks and saturated fats, as well as commercially produced baked goods, are the worst offenders. Home-baked goods prepared with unsaturated oils and egg whites rather than whole eggs are preferable.

*Fats and Oils.* All fats and oils that tend to harden at room temperature are eliminated from the AHA diet. These include butter, lard, and tallow from animal sources and palm, palm-kernel, and coconut oils from plants. Grundy advises dieters to use only oils that stay liquid at room temperature and which are high in unsaturated fats and help lower blood cholesterol, including corn, safflower, sunflower, olive, and rapeseed (canola) oils. Peanut oil has higher levels of saturated fatty acids, but can be used in cooking for flavoring. Margarines that have hydrogenated oil listed as a second ingredient can be used.

*Beverages.* The AHA suggests avoiding very high consumption (ten or more cups a day) of coffee and possibly tea because they are suspected of raising cholesterol levels. However, one to two cups a day does not appear to pose a risk. In addition, alcohol in moderation (one ounce daily) does not appear to be harmful, although the AHA does not believe it helps prevent heart disease.

## Recipes

The *AHA Low-Fat, Low-Cholesterol Cookbook* includes more than 225 recipes that have been analyzed by a computer to calculate the number of calories and the amounts of protein, carbohydrates, total fat, saturated fatty acids, polyunsaturated fatty acids, monounsaturated fatty acids, cholesterol, and sodium per individual serving. Salt is not used in most of the recipes, and where it is used, the amount is very small.

The recipes encompass appetizers and spreads, soups, salads, salad dressings, fish, poultry, meats, vegetarian dishes, vegetables, sauces, breads, desserts, basics, and techniques.

## Physical Activity

According to Grundy, there is growing evidence that regular, vigorous physical activity protects against heart disease. However, the authors caution that people who decide to begin an exercise program should consult first with their physician, especially if they are middle-aged or older and have not exercised for a long time.

## Behavioral Modification

Grundy states that the Step-One and Step-Two diets require not only nutritional changes but behavioral changes as well that will eventually become as firmly established as old patterns. He provides the following tips to help dieters adhere to their dietary program:

- Analyze your environment and eliminate those things that stimulate you to choose the overweight way of life.
- Either eliminate tempting foods or store them out of sight.

- Portion food onto plates in the kitchen rather than putting serving dishes on the table.
- Always eat in a designated place, and only eat while you are sitting down.
- Plan your meals ahead of time.
- Don't read or watch TV when you eat, and always eat slowly.
- Find friends and neighbors who support and encourage your new life-style changes.
- Set realistic goals and remember that people lose weight at varying rates. While you want lifelong changes, appreciate the smaller goals along the way.
- Concentrate on maintaining a gradual weight loss.
- Depriving yourself of special treats only makes you crave them. Plan to enjoy a small treat once or twice a week.
- Recording the food eaten daily (see Chapter 2) helps most people lose weight, especially in the beginning.
- Weigh yourself no more than once a week, preferably in the morning.

## DR. DEAN ORNISH'S DIET FOR REVERSING HEART DISEASE

The best-known diet program for lowering cholesterol and reversing heart disease is that developed by Dr. Dean Ornish, as detailed in his best-selling book *Dr. Dean Ornish's Program for Reversing Heart Disease*. The book details Ornish's Heart Disease Reversal Program, which, in one study, helped 19 of 24 patients achieve "some measurable average reversal of their coronary artery blockages." The group also experienced a 91 percent decrease in the frequency and severity of chest pain.

### Basic Nutritional Approach

Instead of asking people to follow a long list of do's and don'ts, Ornish provides them with a spectrum of choices based on their specific needs in two diet programs: the Reversal Diet (for those who have coronary heart disease and want to reverse it) and the Prevention Diet (for those who want to minimize their risk of developing coronary artery disease).

Ornish's nutritional therapy focuses on lowering high blood cholesterol levels, which form plaque and tear the linings of the coronary arteries. In addition to completely eliminating foods containing cholesterol, his vegetarian diet is low in saturated fat, which has a direct relationship to blood cholesterol levels.

Most people on the Reversal Diet, he explains, will be able to eat between 15 and 35 grams of total fat per day, or between 5 and 12 grams of saturated fat (compared to the typical American consumption of more than 100 grams daily).

In summary, Ornish's Reversal Diet

- is very low in fat and has almost no cholesterol
- has less than 10 percent of calories from fat, little of which is saturated

- excludes foods high in saturated fat (such as avocados, olives, coconut, cocoa products, nuts, and seeds)
- is high in fiber
- allows but does not encourage moderate alcohol consumption (less than 2 ounces per day)
- excludes all oils and animal products except nonfat milk and yogurt
- allows egg whites
- excludes caffeine, other stimulants, and MSG
- allows moderate use of salt and sugar
- is not restricted in calories

## Summary of the Prevention Diet

According to Ornish, his Prevention Diet is simpler and less restrictive than the Reversal Diet. Anyone whose cholesterol level is less than 150 (and who is not taking cholesterol-lowering drugs), or whose ratio of total cholesterol to HDL is less than 3.0, is probably following a diet that reduces the risk of developing coronary artery disease. Unfortunately, Ornish notes, many adults in the United States have cholesterol levels higher than 150, and therefore need to follow his Prevention Diet, which restricts fat intake (particularly saturated fat) to 20 percent of total calories.

Ornish suggests that most people can follow this diet by restricting or eliminating a relatively small number of foods that account for a disproportionate amount of daily cholesterol and saturated fat intake. These include meats, ice cream, butter, eggs, nuts, cheese, and oils.

In addition, he suggests taking the skin off chicken and eating more fish, avoiding oil-based salad dressings and all fried foods, substituting two egg whites for each egg yolk while baking, eating cereal instead of eggs for breakfast, and switching from whole milk to skim milk so as to further reduce saturated fat and cholesterol.

## Recommended Foods

People following either Ornish's Reversal or Prevention Diet are given an extensive list of vegetarian foods from which to choose. These include:

- Egg whites, nonfat milk, or yogurt (one cup per day).
- Whole grains: Amaranth, barley, buckwheat, bulgur, corn, millet, oats, quinoa, rice, rye, sorghum, triticale, wheat.
- Vegetables: Artichokes, asparagus, bamboo shoots, beets, broccoli, Brussels sprouts, cabbage (all types), carrots, cauliflower, celery, chili peppers, collards, cucumbers, eggplants, escarole, garlic, ginger root, Jerusalem artichokes, kale, leeks, lettuce (all types), mushrooms, mustard greens, okra, onions, parsley, potatoes, pumpkin, radishes, rutabagas, scallions, shallots, sorrel, spinach, sprouts (all types), squash (all kinds), sweet potatoes, Swiss chard, turnips and greens, watercress, yams, zucchini.
- Fruits: Apples, apricots, bananas, blackberries, blueberries, cantaloupes, cassaba melons, cherries, cranberries, currants, dates, figs, grapefruit, grapes, guava, honeydew melons, kiwi fruit, kumquats, lemons, limes, loganberries, mangoes, nectarines, oranges, papayas, peaches, pears, pineapples, plantains, plums, pomegranates, prunes, raisins, raspberries, strawberries, tangelos, tangerines, tomatoes, watermelons.
- Legumes: Azuki beans, black beans, black-eyed peas, brown beans, garbanzos, Great Northern beans, kidney beans, lentils, mung beans, navy beans, peas, pinto beans, red Mexican beans, soybeans (including miso, tempeh, and tofu), split peas.
- Beverages: Club soda, fruit juices (all kinds), grain coffees, herbal teas, mineral water, vegetable juices (all types).

*Fiber.* Fiber (comprising primarily complex carbohydrates and found in all whole grains, legumes, fruits, and vegetables) is highly recommended in the Reversal and Prevention diets in both soluble and insoluble forms. As Ornish notes, insoluble fibers (of which wheat bran is a major source) increase stool bulk and substantially decrease the amount of time it takes food to pass through the intestines.

Soluble fibers form gels that delay the absorption of certain foods, including cholesterol, and may lower blood cholesterol levels. Soluble fibers (that found in oat bran, rice bran, rolled oats, guar gum, beans, pectins, fruits, psyllium, Metamucil, and carrots) also increase the excretion of cholesterol in the bile and slow the absorption of carbohydrates, adds Ornish, so blood sugar levels remain more constant.

## Eliminated Foods

While Ornish admits that, for most people, his Reversal Diet is "a big change," he contends that as people eliminate the following foods from their diet, their palates will begin to readjust and the foods they once ate will begin to seem too rich or oily.

- All animal products (with the exception of nonfat milk, yogurt, egg whites, or products made from these), meats, poultry, seafood, and egg yolks.
- Vegetarian foods that are high in fat, including avocados, nuts, seeds, olives, and coconuts.
- All oils (except in very small quantities).
- Chocolate and other cocoa products.

## Recipes

Ornish's book provides more than 150 vegetarian recipes developed by nationally known gourmet chefs, including salads, dressings, condiments, and starters, vegetable side dishes, grains and legumes, pasta, soups, hearty vegetable dishes, tofu dishes, breads and pizza, breakfast foods, and desserts. Also included are general cooking instructions, recommended spices and nutritional analyses for fat, cholesterol, and protein content, as well as serving sizes and total calories — which make it easy for readers to customize a diet that meets their individual needs and tastes.

## Vitamin and Mineral Supplements

Although Ornish claims that both his Reversal and Prevention diets provide sufficient vitamins and minerals, he advises dieters to take a multivitamin supplement that contains B12, iron, and trace minerals each day.

## Alcohol

Although alcohol is not excluded from the Reversal Diet, Ornish does not recommend its daily use for several reasons. These include alcohol's direct toxic effect on the muscle of the heart, which, over time, can cause the heart to beat less effectively — a condition known as alcohol cardio-myopathy. Alcohol, he adds, is toxic to a number of other organ systems, including the liver, and is a major factor in most accidents at work and at home.

## Smoking

Ornish, who strongly urges all his dieters to eliminate smoking, cites a number of studies that have conclusively shown that even small daily amounts of nicotine can seriously damage a person's health. Furthermore, in addition to describing the negative effects of nicotine, he quotes a recent report from the Surgeon General that claims nicotine is far more costly and deadly on a national scale than heroin, cocaine, or alcohol.

## Physical Activity

Ornish was one of the first heart specialists to detail the medical benefits of exercise, especially for people at risk of developing coronary artery disease. He cites several clinical studies that document that moderate exercise (only thirty minutes of walking or similar activities once a day or an hour of walking three times a week) is enough to provide people with almost all of the health and longevity benefits without most of the risks of more intense exercise.

## Behavioral Modification

Ornish emphasizes that chronic emotional stress contributes to heart disease and many other illnesses. As he notes, "Anything that leads to the perception of isolation causes stress and, in turn, can lead to heart disease or other illnesses. Anything that enhances the perception of intimacy reduces stress, allowing the heart to begin healing and our lives to become more joyful." His book concludes by detailing a variety of stress reduction therapies that his program utilizes, including yoga, meditation, progressive deep relaxation, deep breathing, bellows breathing, alternate-nostril breathing, directed visualization, healing heart visualization, receptive visualization, inner teacher visualization, and inner heart visualization.

## RECENT RESEARCH

As reported in *The Alternative Health and Medicine Encyclopedia,* garlic contains sulfur compounds that work as antioxidants and help dissolve blood clots. A twelve-week study cited by H. Kieswetter in a 1993 issue of *Clinical Investigator* found that patients who took garlic-coated tablets significantly increased their ability to walk longer distances by the fifth week of treatment. This increase was accompanied by a simultaneous decrease in platelet aggregation, blood pressure, plasma viscosity, and serum cholesterol levels.

### Vitamin and Mineral Therapies

As cited in the May 20, 1993, editions of the *New York Times* and the *Wall Street Journal,* researchers at the Harvard School of Public Health and Brigham and Women's Hospital in Boston reported that people who take daily megadoses of vitamin E have a significantly reduced risk of heart disease, although they cautioned that it is still too soon to recommend widespread use. Separate studies of more than 120,000 men and women who took daily vitamin E supplements of at least 100 International Units — more than three times the current U.S. RDA — showed that they had a 40 percent lower risk of heart disease than those who did not use the supplement.

# 18

---

# Diets for Type I and
# Type II Diabetes

According to Shils, Olson, and Shike's *Modern Nutrition in Health and Disease,* diabetes mellitus, commonly called diabetes, is one of the three most serious diseases in the United States, following heart disease and cancer in total annual deaths. Its incidence is estimated to have increased tenfold in the past forty-five years, currently affecting more than 14 million Americans.

Furthermore, studies indicate there are 5 million adults in the United States with undetected diabetes, while another 20 million have impaired glucose tolerance that may lead to full-blown cases of the disease. And the National Institutes of Health report that undiagnosed diabetes is the reason that millions lose their vision.

Diabetes is now the number one killer of women in the United States. In 1993, for example, more than 90,000 American women died from the disease — almost twice as many as succumbed to breast cancer. In addition, diabetic women are twice as likely as nondiabetics to develop heart disease, and they face two to four times the risk of stroke.

Diabetes is a chronic, degenerative disease that, in simple terms, affects the way the body uses food. During normal digestion, the body changes sugars, starches, and other foods into a form of sugar called glucose. The blood then carries this glucose to cells throughout the body, where, with the help of the hormone insulin (which is made in the pancreas, a small organ located behind the stomach), glucose is changed into energy for immediate use by the cells or stored for future use. The process of turning food into energy is crucial because the body depends on food for every action, from pumping blood and thinking to vigorous physical activities.

While food is turned into glucose readily enough by people with diabetes, they are either unable to produce insulin, make too little of it, or have trouble utilizing it (or the latter two combined). When insulin is absent or ineffective, the glucose in the bloodstream cannot be used by the cells to make energy. Instead, glucose collects in the blood, eventually leading to the high sugar levels symptomatic of untreated diabetes.

There are two primary types of diabetes mellitus: type I and type II. James W. Anderson, an expert on diabetes, writes in *Modern Nutrition in Health and Disease* that insulin-dependent diabetes comprises about 10 percent of all cases. By far the most severe of the two types, it can occur at any age, but usually appears in childhood. Type I diabetics are unable to produce enough of the insulin hormone to metabolize food properly. They must follow both a dietary and medication regimen (including daily injections of insulin) for successful treatment.

Type I diabetes usually has a sudden onset, with symptoms that include frequent urination, extreme hunger or thirst, weight loss, weakness and fatigue, irritability and mood changes, and nausea or vomiting.

Approximately 90 percent of the diabetic population has type II (non-insulin-dependent) diabetes, and two of the three diets in this chapter are intended to treat it. It usually appears after the age of 40, and is characterized by resistance to insulin and poor utilization of the hormone rather than by lack of it. Type II diabetes is very strongly associated with obesity, sedentary lifestyle, and advancing age, and because it is currently increasing in the United States, some experts have termed it an epidemic.

The onset of type II diabetes is milder than with type I, and may include symptoms such as excessive thirst and urination, decreased libido, blurred vision, headache, itching, loose teeth, skin infections, slow healing, abscessed gums, tingling or numbness in the feet, weakness, and fatigue. In some cases, type II diabetes can develop without any pronounced symptoms.

The nutritional plan is the foundation for successful diabetes management. The basic treatment for diabetes involves the proper balancing and timing of food intake, exercise, and insulin dose — if necessary. Too much food and too little exercise or insulin can cause hyperglycemia, ketosis, and coma, while too little food and too much exercise may lead to hypoglycemia and insulin shock. In type I diabetes, replacement of insulin is usually necessary for life, and doses must be carefully timed and balanced with eating and physical activity. Type II diabetes can often be remedied by dietary management, exercise, and weight control — sometimes augmented with oral medications or insulin shots.

In treating both type I and type II diabetes, the primary goal is to stabilize blood glucose levels as close to the normal range as possible. Controlling blood glucose levels, in turn, reduces the risks for eye problems, atherosclerosis, hypertension, nerve degeneration, kidney failure, heart disease, strokes, loss of hearing, blindness, and even death.

## THE UCSD HEALTHY DIET FOR DIABETES

The diabetes diet developed at the University of California School of Medicine, San Diego, is outlined in *The UCSD Healthy Diet for Diabetes: A Comprehensive Guide and Cookbook,* coauthored by Susan Algert, Barbara Grasse, and Annie Durning. The authors are members of the staff of the University of San Diego Medical Center.

### Basic Nutritional Approach

The authors concur with the three primary nutritional recommendations of the American Diabetes Association (ADA):

- Maintain appropriate levels of glucose and fats in the blood.
- Maintain consistency in meal planning (nutrient intake and timing of meals) if you have insulin-dependent diabetes. Focus on weight management if you have non-insulin-dependent diabetes.
- Alter your diet to limit salt, fat, sugars, and alcohol while increasing the intake of complex carbohydrates (starch and fiber). The goal is to maintain a diet lower in total fat, saturated fat, and cholesterol and higher in polyunsaturated and monounsaturated fats than the typical American diet.

In addition, the authors' premise is that diabetics need not follow the bland diet previously recommended for treating this condition. Instead they offer culinary fare and flexible sample meal plans based on up-to-date and medically sound research, which will promote good health in both diabetics and nondiabetics alike.

Rather than ask people to make radical changes in their eating style, the authors provide more than two hundred recipes low in fat, salt, and sugar to make them compatible with the nutritional needs of diabetics. Because weight control is especially important for diabetics, the lowfat, high-carbohydrate recipes help dieters lose weight and maintain weight loss. This diet is less calorically dense and greater in bulk than some higher-fat diabetes diets, enabling adherents to eat a larger quantity of food for the same number of calories.

## Recommended Foods

Following the ADA's dietary guidelines, the UCSD diet recommends that protein comprise 12 to 20 percent of total calories; fat 30 percent or less (of which no more than 10 percent should be saturated); and complex carbohydrates 50 to 60 percent. A daily fiber intake of up to 40 grams is recommended (compared to the average intake of U.S. adults of 10 to 30 grams).

The UCSD diet does not require or recommend specific foods. It does, however, endorse the ADA's food exchange system. And it advises its dieters to follow the recommendations for a lowfat, low-cholesterol diet. Specifically, it advises consuming less animal protein and more plant protein, eating fish (not shellfish) at least three times a week in quantities of three to four ounces per serving, and drinking about eight glasses of water daily.

## Exchange System for Meal Planning

The authors advise dieters to follow the ADA's exchange system to make food selections and plan menus. This system groups foods into six lists called exchange lists, which are provided at the back of their book. Each list is made up of a group of measured foods of approximately the same nutritional value, so they can be substituted, or exchanged, with other foods in the same list. One exchange is approximately equal to another in the same group in terms of calories, carbohydrates, protein, and fat.

## Restricted Foods

The authors stress that diabetics should limit salt, fat, sugar, and alcohol in following the lowfat, low-cholesterol diet. Sodium intake, according to the ADA, should not exceed 1,000 milligrams per 1,000 calories — or a maximum of 3,000 milligrams per day. All sugars, including table sugar, honey, molasses, and maple syrup, should also be used in moderation — that is, up to one teaspoon per reasonable serving of food.

Commonly available caloric and noncaloric sweeteners offer an alternative to sucrose and other sugars. The authors counsel that the type of sweetener chosen should depend upon a person's caloric requirements, how well their diabetes is controlled, and the type of food they are consuming.

In terms of maintaining a lower-fat diet (30 percent of total calories or less), the authors contend that lowering the percentage of total calories

## HOW TO REDUCE FAT IN RESTAURANT MEALS

1. Request that salad dressings, butter, margarine, sour cream, and mayonnaise be served separately on a side dish. Use vinegar or lemon juice for a dressing or bring your own low-calorie dressing from home.
2. Order clear soups, such as broths or consommé, or vegetable-based soups (gazpacho) instead of cream soups.
3. Specify that no fat should be added to whatever type of chicken, fish, or red meat you order.
4. Ask that sandwiches be served without mayonnaise or margarine on the bread. Chicken, turkey, lowfat cheeses, and lean meats are recommended fillings.
5. Remove all visible fat from any cuts of poultry or meat.
6. Try to avoid bean salads, tuna salads, chicken salads, pasta salads, and potato salads made with mayonnaise. Choose a lettuce salad, plain vegetables, or sliced tomatoes.
7. Choose vegetables made without sauce or without added butter or margarine.
8. Avoid rich muffins, sweet rolls, and breads. Choose rolls or plain breads and lowfat crackers such as soda crackers, rye crackers, or melba toast.

derived from fat will increase the percentage of calories derived from other food groups. They also counsel diabetics to make sure that the types of fat they consume are either monounsaturated or polyunsaturated vegetable oils.

## Recipes

The authors' book contains more than two hundred recipes from around the world representing ethnic cuisines such as Chinese, Mexican, French, German, Italian, Indian, Middle Eastern, Far Eastern, and South American — as well as vegetarian dishes — all modified to meet the nutritional needs of diabetics. The dietary focus is on complex carbohydrates such as rice, beans, and pasta as main courses, emphasizing meat as a condiment rather than a main ingredient, and incorporating a far wider variety of seasonings than do traditional American recipes.

Just a few examples include black forest mushrooms, French onion soup, hearty lamb and barley stew, blueberry cobbler, ginger-lemon broccoli, frijoles refritos, spanish rice, snapper creole, party sushi rolls, melon with slivered almonds and ginger, shrimp and feta à la Grecque, veal Parmesan, cauliflower curry, beef teriyaki, Santa Fe blue cornmeal bread, and chocolate mousse pie.

The authors note that at least one-third of their recipes can be prepared and/or assembled in less than thirty minutes.

## Vitamin and Mineral Supplements

The authors state that many diabetic dieters can benefit from taking a vitamin-mineral supplement that helps them meet their recommended daily allowances for essential nutrients. They note that there is no scientific evidence that suggests that diabetics require extra amounts of any particular vitamin or mineral.

## Alcohol

The authors do not specifically recommend that diabetics refrain from drinking alcohol and, in fact, recipes in the "special occasions" section of their book are accompanied by an optional wine selection. An occasional drink of beer, wine, or hard liquor — taken close to or during a meal — isn't normally harmful and can be consumed without making meal plan substitutions or adjusting medication. However, to prevent hypoglycemia, the authors counsel diabetics not to omit any food from their meal plan when drinking and not to drink on an empty stomach.

## Physical Activity

The authors strongly advocate exercise as part of a successful insulin stabilization program for both type I and type II diabetes. They caution, however, that factors such as type of diabetes, current level of fitness, overall metabolic control, current nutritional status, age, and presence or absence of diabetic complications all have a significant impact on an individual's ability to exercise safely and effectively.

## Physical Activity and Insulin-Dependent Diabetes

According to the authors, because blood glucose levels are generally reduced during and after an exercise session, the potential exists for de-

## PRIMARY GOALS OF PHYSICAL ACTIVITY FOR DIABETICS

- To maintain or improve cardiovascular (heart and blood vessel) fitness in order to reduce the risk factors for coronary heart disease.
- To assist in the control of blood glucose levels.
- To help lose weight or maintain an ideal weight.
- To allow safe and enjoyable participation in sports and physical activities.
- To reduce stress and anxiety.
- To improve self-image.

creased insulin requirements due to increased sensitivity of the active muscle to insulin. They counsel type I and type II diabetics to consult with a physician to design a physical activity program tailored to their insulin profile and needs. The physician should conduct an exercise stress test, identify target heart rates, and monitor fluid intake and level of glucose.

The authors suggest that dieters should begin with lower-intensity forms of exercise, such as walking, climbing stairs, doing housework, or gardening, to allow the body to adjust safely to increased levels of activity over time. Once dieters become stronger and more flexible, regular aerobic activity, including bicycling, bowling, dancing, running or jogging, swimming, and tennis, is recommended four or five times a week.

## CONTROLLING DIABETES THE EASY WAY DIET

Dr. Stanley Mirsky, a board member of Joslin Diabetes Center, details his diet for diabetics in *Controlling Diabetes the Easy Way*.

Mirsky claims that he has developed "what to many is the simplest, easiest, most effective diet plan that has ever been proposed for controlling blood sugar. It is so easy, in fact, that you have only to remember just one rule and know how to count to 50 [50 grams of complex carbohydrates]."

### Basic Nutritional Approach

According to Mirsky, diet is the most important key to controlling diabetes. He states that his diet focuses not on calories (unless people want to lose weight), but rather on carbohydrates, and can be followed for a lifetime without difficulty. The only rule is that people avoid all refined sugar and eat 40 to 50 grams of complex carbohydrates at every meal. (Dieters who engage in strenuous exercise may need to consume more.)

This carbohydrate intake amounts to 50 to 60 percent of each dieter's daily food. The rest of the menu includes protein, fats, and water in whatever proportions dieters choose. If they are trying to lose weight, Mirsky advises them to control calories by adjusting their meat portions or incorporating the food exchange lists of the ADA.

## Recommended Foods

Mirsky explains that complex carbohydrates are a much better source of energy than fatty foods because they contain less than half the calories of fat and the same amount as protein, and often have substantially more vitamins, minerals, and fiber. In addition, complex carbohydrates are absorbed much more slowly than simple carbohydrates and, when eaten in certain amounts, will not raise blood sugar to abnormal levels.

Mirsky advises diabetics to choose their 40 to 50 grams of carbohydrates per meal from the food lists he provides on this basis: 10-gram fruits and desserts, 15-gram starches, 3 percent vegetables, and 6 percent vegetables.

He cautions that each meal must include two or more units, or at least 30 grams, from the starch list (the equivalent of two slices of bread) since this slowly absorbed carbohydrate provides essential energy between meals. Conversely, fruits and juices, because they raise blood sugar levels more rapidly, cannot be used as most or all of the food allotment.

Dieters are advised not to save carbohydrates from one meal to another, and to eat their full allotment at each meal, or they may experience low blood sugar levels. In addition, Mirsky warns diabetics who take insulin to eat the same amount of food every day, including the right amount of carbohydrate, spaced out in the same way, because their insulin doses are based on the foods they consume.

*10-Gram Fruits and Desserts.* Recommended items in this category (amounts are specified in Mirsky's food lists) include apricots, bananas, blueberries, blackberries or raspberries, cantaloupe, cherries, cranberry juice, nectarines, oranges and orange juice, peaches, pears, plums, strawberries, tangerines, tomato or vegetable juice, tomato sauce, watermelon, plain yogurt, ice cream, or ice milk. Other options include animal crackers, fortune cookies, ginger snaps, graham crackers, Triscuits, and Wheat Thins.

*15-Gram Starches*. Mirsky asserts that the easiest way to adhere to the 40 to 50 grams of carbohydrate per meal is to remember the equivalent of two slices of bread (or the required 30 grams of complex carbohydrate).

Recommended items (with amounts specified in his food lists) include bagels, cooked dried beans (such as lentil, mung, pinto, red, and garbanzo), bread (white, rye, pumpernickel, whole wheat, French, Italian), bread crumbs, bread sticks, corn, English muffins, French fries, French toast, cooked pasta, matzo balls, cold cereal, melba toast, mashed potatoes, cooked rice or barley, hamburger or hot dog rolls, and waffles. Evaporated milk, milk, and plain yogurt are other options.

*3 Percent Vegetables*. The following vegetables, which have only 3 grams of carbohydrate per 100 grams of weight, influence blood sugar very little. Consisting primarily of water and nondigestible fiber, they can be eaten raw as desired. If cooked, they should be limited to approximately one cup per portion.

The list includes fresh asparagus, bamboo shoots, bean sprouts, broccoli, cabbage, cauliflower, celery, cucumber, eggplant, endive, green or wax beans, green pepper, lettuce, mushrooms, parsley, radishes, sauerkraut, spinach, summer squash, Swiss chard, turnips, watercress, and zucchini.

*6 Percent Vegetables*. Six percent vegetables, which have six grams of carbohydrate for every 100 grams of weight, are usually restricted to 1/2 cup per meal. If dieters wish to eat more, Mirsky urges them to subtract equivalent amounts from their starch allotment.

The list includes artichokes, Brussels sprouts, carrots, green peas, kale, okra, onions, leeks, pumpkin, red peppers, tomatoes and tomato sauce, turnips, and winter squash.

*Fiber*. Mirsky recommends consuming high-fiber foods that are complex carbohydrates because fiber improves glucose tolerance. Water-soluble fiber foods, for example, such as pectin, guar, and oat bran, delay absorption of carbohydrates; this means that less sugar enters the bloodstream immediately after a meal. This kind of fiber also seems to lower blood cholesterol levels. He also recommends nonsoluble fiber foods such as cellulose, lignin, and wheat bran because they soften the stool and add bulk to it. Recommended fiber foods include whole-grain breads and cereals, especially whole bran or bran-containing foods; nuts and seeds; vegetables such as artichokes, broccoli, cabbage, cauliflower, Brussels sprouts, corn peas, peppers, beans, cucumber, and carrots; fruits such as strawberries, blueberries, grapefruit, and raw pears; and dried beans such as butter, haricot, kidney, and soybeans; and chickpeas.

## Restricted Foods

All foods containing simple carbohydrates (monosaccharides) are eliminated on Mirsky's diet. These foods, which have many calories but very little nutrition, include candy, pastries, and cookies, sugar-coated cereals, raisins, condensed milk, regular chewing gum, dried fruits, regular soft drinks, honey, any variety of sugar, jams, and jellies, sweet wine, marmalade and preserves, syrups, and molasses.

Other foods that diabetics should eliminate because they also raise blood sugar levels too quickly include apple juice, pineapple, apples, regular gelatin desserts, processed yogurt with fruit or flavoring, grape juice, instant breakfast or "diet" bars, sherbet, prune juice, maple-sugar-flavored bacon or sausage, and yams and sweet potatoes.

## Timing Meals and Snacks

Diabetics, especially those on insulin, according to Mirsky, should always add two or three snacks to their three meals so their carbohydrate intake is spaced out during the day and they do not experience high or low extremes in blood sugar levels. They also should eat at specified times and never skip a meal or a planned snack. If diabetics are dining out and know that dinner will be served later than their usual meal time, they should consume 30 grams of carbohydrate beforehand.

## Vitamin and Mineral Supplements

Upon the advice of their physician, Mirsky states that some diabetics will benefit from taking the following vitamin/mineral supplements: vitamin B1 (patients with diabetic neuropathy); vitamin B6 (pregnant women with diabetes); vitamin C (patients with diabetic retinopathy); vitamin E (may prevent some degenerative processes); calcium (dieters who do not drink milk, eat milk products, or get regular exercise; also postmenopausal women); magnesium; and zinc (patients with diabetic ulcers).

## Physical Activity

Mirsky stresses that exercise is particularly important for diabetics because it will help them lose excess weight, lower triglycerides and blood pressure, and decrease blood clots and atherosclerosis. Most importantly, it helps stabilize insulin levels and decreases their insulin requirements. Regular physical activity can also reduce the risk of developing diabetic eye changes (retinopathy) and other vascular diabetic complications.

Before beginning an exercise program, however, Mirsky is adamant that diabetics consult their physician because, in some cases, vigorous physical activity can actually aggravate the condition.

Mirsky advises diabetics to get approximately the same amount of exercise every day so they will know how much medication they need to take and what to eat. He also urges them not to make any insulin or food adjustments (such as taking less insulin or eating more food before exercising heavily) without consulting a physician.

Diabetics should always carry emergency rations of carbohydrate, and consume a small amount every twenty minutes during heavy exercise to boost their blood sugar. They should also drink plenty of water to replace fluids lost through sweating, Mirsky emphasizes. He also advocates exercising after a meal, if possible, as blood sugar levels are then rising. Before a meal, blood sugar levels may be very low.

## OUTSMARTING DIABETES DIET

The diet for type I diabetics developed by Dr. Richard S. Beaser is detailed in his book *Outsmarting Diabetes: A Dynamic Approach for Reducing the Effects of Insulin-Dependent Diabetes.* Beaser serves on the staffs of the New England Deaconess Hospital and Harvard Medical School and is chairman of the Patient Education Committee at the Joslin Diabetes Center in Boston, an internationally recognized diabetes research and treatment facility.

From the early 1980s through 1993, the Joslin Diabetes Center was one of twenty-nine centers participating in a major study called the Diabetes Control and Complications Trial, sponsored by the NIH. This long-term study involved 1,441 volunteers aged 13 through 39 with type I insulin-dependent diabetes. Its goal was to determine if normalization or near normalization of blood glucose levels would help delay or prevent diabetes complications such as eye problems, nerve degeneration, or kidney disease.

Half the volunteers used "conventional" diabetes management: they took one or two injections of insulin daily, monitored their blood glucose or urine once a day, were given dietary education, and saw their physicians and diabetes health care teams four times a year.

The other half used "intensive" therapy that involved three or more daily insulin injections or use of an insulin pump (with insulin adjusted on the basis of four or more daily blood glucose tests), intensive diabetes education, and dietary, exercise, and psychological counseling. They saw their physicians and diabetes health care teams every month.

Beaser states the differences between the two groups were "stunning." Those undergoing intensive therapy had a 76 percent reduction in the incidence of eye complications, a 56 percent reduction in kidney complications, and a 60 percent reduction in nerve complications.

However, the intensive therapy patients had three times more severe low blood sugar reactions than the conventional group (requiring assistance from someone or emergency room visits), and were about ten pounds heavier after five years.

Despite these disadvantages, and the fact that the intensive approach is more expensive than conventional therapy, Beaser claims it is a much better investment. He also feels that patients should be able to significantly reduce the risk of severe hypoglycemia and weight gain with proper training and follow-up, working with their physician, dietitian, and nurse educator.

## Basic Nutritional Approach

Since insulin-dependent diabetes prevents the body's cells from getting the fuel they need (in the form of glucose) because of a lack of insulin, the challenge facing type I diabetics is to replace that missing insulin in the right amount at the right time to provide energy for a given activity and metabolic needs. As Beaser admits, "This is truly a balancing act!"

He suggests that type I diabetics closely follow the basic nutritional guidelines outlined in the U.S. Dietary Goals:

- Eat a variety of foods every day.
- Maintain a desirable weight.

- Choose a diet low in fat, saturated fat, and cholesterol.
- Choose a diet with plenty of vegetables, fruits, and grain products.
- Use sugar in moderation.
- Use salt and sodium only in moderation.
- If you drink alcoholic beverages, do so in moderation.

Beaser emphasizes that without close attention to meal planning, no intensive insulin therapy is likely to succeed.

## The American Diabetes Association (ADA) Guidelines

Beaser endorses the 1994 guidelines released by the American Diabetes Association that recommend that meal plans and the distribution of calories and nutrients be individualized according to each diabetic's eating style and blood glucose and lipid (blood fat) levels. Recommendations that dictate a distribution of nutrients as a percent of total calories do not allow for individual variation and needs, he claims.

The current ADA guidelines recommend that protein contribute 10 to 20 percent of total calories, with saturated fat comprising less than 10 percent of total calories. The level of carbohydrate and unsaturated fats should be based on individual considerations.

*Carbohydrates.* Since carbohydrate is the food component that affects blood sugar levels the most, the amounts and types of carbohydrate should ideally be consistent for a specific insulin dose. That is, the more carbohydrate consumed during a meal, the higher the dose of regular insulin needed. Conversely, less insulin will be needed for less carbohydrate.

Beaser advises type I diabetics to keep daily records of all foods eaten, along with insulin taken and postmeal blood glucose values. With this information, they will be able to calculate how much premeal regular insulin their bodies require to bring their blood glucose back into a desirable range for carbohydrates consumed in a specific meal.

For this approach to allow successful insulin dose adjustments, Beaser cautions that type I diabetics need to accurately estimate the approximate carbohydrate content of a meal before eating. To do this, he suggests using the exchange lists developed by the ADA or the Joslin Diabetes Center.

*Sodium.* While sodium does not have a direct connection with blood sugar levels, some diabetics are affected by high salt levels that manifest themselves in the form of fluid retention or high blood pressure. Beaser recommends that sodium levels not exceed three grams per day.

*Fiber.* Fiber is an important component of any diabetic diet, according to Beaser, and the high-fiber fruits and vegetables in a typical meal plan will help people feel full and satisfied. He recommends consuming 20 to 35 grams of fiber daily — both insoluble (as found in bran cereals, whole-grain breads, whole fruits, and vegetables) and soluble (as found in oats, dried beans, whole fruits, and vegetables).

Insoluble fiber adds bulk to the diet, speeds up passage of foods through the intestines, and helps prevent and alleviate constipation. Because soluble fiber dissolves in water to form a gummy gel, it slows the passage of food through the digestive tract, and may help lower blood cholesterol levels.

## Vegetarian Diets

Beaser notes that a vegetarian diet low in fat and high in fiber may be beneficial for some diabetics because it satisfies requirements for calories, protein, vitamins, and minerals while lowering the risk of heart disease. However, the transition to a vegetarian diet — which is usually higher in carbohydrate content than a nonvegetarian diet — should be made gradually, with fiber content slowly increased to avoid bloating and cramping.

Beaser adds that foods high in fiber may raise blood sugar more slowly, so less insulin may be required for the same amount of carbohydrate at meal times. He suggests dividing meals into smaller meals and larger snacks to minimize glucose fluctuations after meals while still consuming adequate calories.

## Weight Gain and Intensive Therapy

Beaser postulates that the weight gain commonly experienced by people undergoing intensive diabetes therapy may result from improved caloric efficiency (that is, using all the calories consumed rather than excreting them in the urine), experimentation with new foods, increased frequency of hypoglycemic reactions that require extra food, and larger meals.

The insulin adjustment involved in intensive therapy makes overeating tempting, he admits, because insulin can be increased to cover extra foods and desserts. However, while consuming more food and more insulin may maintain desirable glucose levels, it also increases the number of calories that will be stored as fat. Therefore, Beaser advises diabetics to keep accurate lists of all foods consumed, and to be aware of their caloric content to help prevent weight gain.

### Meal Timing

According to Beaser, consistency of meal and snack times, while often less rigid with intensive diabetes therapy, is still important, as is coordinating the action of the insulin taken with daily food consumption. He suggests spacing meals and snacks at least two to three hours apart so they are readily digested. Blood sugar levels can then rise and fall again before more food is eaten. If snacks are consumed too close to a meal, blood sugar levels during and after a meal is eaten will probably be higher than desired.

### Snacks

Between-meal and evening snacks are an important feature of Beaser's diet because they help stabilize fluctuating insulin levels over long stretches of time or with increases in physical activity. Beaser suggests incorporating snacks into the meal plan at specific times, usually midmorning, afternoon, and evening, depending on the interval between meals and the action times of the prescribed insulin program.

Bedtime snacks that contain protein and carbohydrate prevent hypoglycemia (low blood sugar levels) during the night. Midmorning and afternoon snacks may help prevent drops in glucose levels if there are long intervals between meals.

### Alcohol

Certain alcoholic beverages such as sweet wines, cordials, and liqueurs contain high levels of carbohydrate that can cause blood sugar elevations. Beaser therefore advises diabetics to replace them with dry wines, light (or alcohol-free) beer, or hard liquors that contain less sugar and carbohydrate. He cautions, however, that alcohol should only be consumed when blood sugars are in good control, and even then in moderation.

### Physical Activity

Physical activity is especially important for diabetics, according to Beaser, because it is one of the three primary factors (along with insulin injections and food intake) that influences glucose metabolism. He notes that exercise has been shown to lower blood glucose levels, increase insulin sensitivity (so insulin works more effectively), and reduce the risk of vascular problems such as heart disease and hardening of the arteries. Furthermore, exercise reduces stress and helps improve self-image as people become more physically fit.

Beaser recommends that diabetic dieters starting an exercise program first be evaluated by a physician, who can help design a specific plan. He also suggests testing blood before, during, and after an exercise session to ascertain if blood glucose levels are low.

Beaser provides a list of recommended physical activities for people with diabetes, any of which should be performed for fifteen to twenty minutes per session. These include brisk walking, running or jogging, swimming, bicycling (including stationary), dancing, skipping rope, rowing, skiing (downhill and cross-country), badminton, skating (ice and roller), wrestling, golf (with brisk walking only), fencing, stair climbing, calisthenics, tennis, handball, squash, and racquetball.

Suggested team activities include soccer, volleyball, basketball, ice and field hockey, and lacrosse.

## Behavioral Modification

Beaser stresses that intensive diabetes therapy requires effort, thought, and discipline, and outlines a psychological profile of ideal patients. They must be highly motivated and willing to perform frequent blood tests and make frequent insulin adjustments. They must be able to set realistic goals and be prepared to cope with occasional setbacks. Individuals must be able to think independently and make decisions with confidence, yet have enough insight to know their limitations and call for help when needed. Finally, they must trust their health care team and follow through with whatever they undertake.

## RECENT RESEARCH

As reported by Jane Brody in the May 25, 1994, edition of the *New York Times,* a study directed by researchers at the University of Texas Southwestern Medical Center in Dallas suggests that a diet high in monounsaturated fats may be preferable to a high-carbohydrate diet for many people with diabetes.

Forty-two patients with type II (non-insulin-dependent) diabetes participated in the twenty-week study, consuming a diet deriving 55 percent of calories from carbohydrates and 30 percent from fats for six weeks. For another six weeks, the same number of calories were consumed daily, but monounsaturated fat in the form of olive oil contributed 45 percent of calories and carbohydrates provided only 40 percent. After following each of the diets for six weeks, patients then remained on the second diet they tested for another eight weeks.

On both diets, according to Dr. Abhimanyu Garg, who directed the study, levels of LDL cholesterol were similar. However, the diet high in monounsaturated fat produced lower blood levels of triglycerides, glucose and insulin changes that he said "should potentially reduce the risk of coronary heart disease in patients with adult-onset diabetes." The favorable changes persisted, said Garg, and were not merely temporary responses to a dietary change.

## Magnesium

Magnesium metabolism is altered in diabetics and may contribute to the development and progression of the disease. Not only is magnesium deficiency common, but low blood magnesium levels are associated with many complications of diabetes, including heart disease and high blood pressure. According to Elizabeth Somer, magnesium supplementation restores low blood and tissue levels in diabetics, helps correct glucose intolerance, produces a protective effect against heart disease, and may assist in the prevention of eye disorders associated with diabetes.

Researchers at the University of Messina in Italy, as reported in the July 1993 issue of *Clinica Terapeutica*, concurred that "the administration of dietary magnesium supplements can have a favorable influence on metabolic control (in diabetics), thus reducing insulin requirement and counteracting the progression of late diabetic conditions."

## Exercise

As reported in the June 1995 issue of *American Health*, UCLA researchers found in an eleven-year study of 652 people with type II diabetes that, in most cases, regular exercise and a stringent diet were enough to keep blood sugar in check, especially for patients in the early stages of the disease.

At the start of the study, two-thirds of the subjects were taking oral medication or injecting insulin to control their blood sugar; the rest took no medication. For three weeks, everyone followed a strict lowfat (less than

## EXERCISE AND DIABETES

Results of a new study reported in the May 1995 issue of the *University of California at Berkeley Wellness Letter* reinforce the link established by many experts, including the authors in this chapter, between exercise and the control — or even prevention — of diabetes. The study, part of the Honolulu Heart Program, examined 6,800 healthy men for six years and found that the most active men had a 50 percent lower risk of developing non-insulin-dependent diabetes than the least active.

10 percent of calories from fat), high-complex-carbohydrate diet and did at least forty-five minutes of aerobic exercise every day, including treadmill walking, cycling, and swimming.

After twenty-six days, the majority had lowered their glucose levels to the nondiabetic range. Seventy-one percent of the patients who had been taking oral medication and 39 percent of those injecting insulin were able to stop doing so. Of the 243 people not on any diabetes drugs, only five needed to be placed on medication at a later date. And subjects were able to stay off medication if they stuck to the regimen.

"If you go the standard medical route for type II diabetes — starting with oral medication and eventually moving on to insulin injections when the former is no longer effective — your chances of ever controlling the disease without medication are very, very slim," says study author and exercise physiologist R. James Barnard. "But this study and others like it show that making immediate lifestyle changes can turn diabetes around."

# 19

## Food Allergy Elimination Diets

I n the course of a normal lifetime, it is estimated the average person consumes several tons of foods and beverages, the vast majority of which are safe and usable by the body. Every person, however, consumes a small percentage of foreign proteins that are poisonous but which their body's immune system detects and eliminates. The gastrointestinal tract, for example, uses a variety of mechanisms to prevent the entry of foreign protein. The main immunologic barrier to foreign proteins is the secretion of secretory-IgA molecules into the gut lumen that bind with and quickly eliminate foreign proteins.

For most of us, the immune system's IgA mechanism works well enough to protect us against poisons. A small number of people, however, for reasons that are still not entirely known, overreact to foods that are ordinarily harmless. According to the American Academy of Allergy and Immunology, adverse food reactions can either be food *intolerances* or food *allergies* (food hypersensitivity). The development of food allergy is the result of an abnormal interaction between food allergens, usually a protein, and the immune system and/or the gastrointestinal tract. Reactions may occur within a few minutes or several hours after the food is eaten. One or several organ systems may be affected, including the skin (itchy rash or hives, swelling, or eczema), gastrointestinal tract (itching or swelling of the lips and tongue, nausea, vomiting, diarrhea, or cramps), and respiratory tract (sneezing, coughing, tightness in the chest, shortness of breath, and wheezing).

According to *Modern Nutrition in Health and Disease*, food allergies are, for the most part, incurable. They are, however, manageable if the allergens are identified and eliminated from the diet. Only a few foods have

## SYMPTOMS OF FOOD ALLERGY

| | |
|---|---|
| Puffiness under the eyes | Chronic noncyclic fluid retention |
| Dark circles under the eyes | Chronic swollen glands |

been documented to cause the majority of allergic reactions: eggs, milk, peanuts, soy and wheat in children and fish, shellfish, tree nuts, and peanuts in adults.

Diagnosis of a food allergy requires identification of the offending food and verification of immunologic involvement. Once the allergy is diagnosed and the allergen identified, treatment normally requires removing this food from the diet. Although Hippocrates first recorded an adverse reaction to food more than two thousand years ago, reliable testing for food allergens was only first developed in the 1970s. C. May introduced the use of double-blind, placebo-controlled oral food challenges (DBPCFC) in 1976, which really began the modern scientific treatment of food allergic disorders.

The usual method of identifying and treating a food allergy is an elimination diet. This chapter analyzes three food allergy diets that can help people identify those substances to which they are allergic. Together, the three diets provide an overview of the treatment of food allergies. Dr. Marshall Mandell was one of the pioneers of bioecological medicine. In the 1960s, along with Dr. Linus Pauling, Dr. Roger Williams, and Dr. Abram Hoffer, he argued that every tissue and organ of the body can react adversely to contact with a variety of chemicals in the environment, including poisonous or toxic foods. Every chemical, whether it impinges on the skin, is inhaled through the lungs, or is ingested into the gastrointestinal system, can elicit adverse reactions and affect the central nervous system. With regard to food, Mandell was one of the first to observe that psychological problems such as schizophrenia and psychosis could be triggered by food allergies. His book, *Dr. Mandell's Five-Day Allergy Relief System*, offered a message of hope for many sufferers.

Dr. James Braly's diet is the most recent and comprehensive extension of Dr. Mandell's pioneering work. It is notable for incorporating the latest scientific evidence on how vitamin and mineral supplementation can treat not only food allergies, but a number of other digestive disorders, including gallbladder problems, gluten sensitivity, herpes, hypoglycemia, iron deficiency anemia, irritable bowel syndrome, kidney stones, multiple sclerosis, osteoporosis, and viral infections. The third diet, that provided in *The Mayo Clinic Diet Manual,* is in fact a series of diets for different food allergies: corn, egg, fish or shellfish, milk, wheat, soy, and peanuts.

Each diet varies somewhat in how allergens are diagnosed and eliminated, how they recommend dieters restrict foods when planning meals, and how to ensure nutritional adequacy. More significantly, each diet recommends somewhat different vitamin and mineral supplements if needed, especially when multiple foods are omitted. Several also provide cookbooks, recipes, and daily meal plans.

## MAYO CLINIC ALLERGY DIET

The Mayo Clinic Diet for Allergies is presented by Jennifer Nelson in *The Mayo Clinic Diet Manual.* According to the *Manual,* foods most frequently reported to cause allergic reactions are cow's milk, eggs, peanuts, soybeans, wheat, corn, fish, and shellfish. Nelson notes that different allergies predominate in infants and young children, especially milk, eggs, peanuts, and soybeans. Milk and egg allergies generally disappear, while peanut and soybean allergies often persist into adulthood. Fish allergies are more prevalent in adults.

Nelson adds that food allergens may be "hidden" ingredients in other foods, especially in packaged or processed foods, which contain multiple ingredients. Therefore, it is especially important for people with allergies to carefully read food labels. The *Manual* provides several sections which present suggestions for managing various types of food allergies.

### Egg Allergy Elimination Diet

Many people are allergic to egg whites or egg yolks, and foods prepared with eggs, especially processed foods. Egg white contains the following allergens that may cause food sensitivity: ovalbumin, ovotransferrin (conalbumin), and ovomucoid. However, IgE antibodies can also be directed to egg yolk proteins, and cross-reactivity may exist between egg yolk and egg albumin protein.

*The Mayo Clinic Diet Manual* therefore recommends that both egg yolk and white be avoided by those with egg allergy. The goal of dietary management is to totally avoid egg consumption or to restrict it to a level the patient can tolerate.

## FOOD LABEL TERMS INDICATING THE PRESENCE OF EGG

Albumin
Egg, including egg white and egg yolk
Globulin
Livetin
Ovalbumin
Ovoglobulin

Ovomucin
Ovomucoid
Ovoviellin
Simplesse
Vitellin

Eggs may be present in beverages such as root beer (foaming agent), wine, and coffee (as a clarifier). Baked goods may not only contain egg but also may be glazed with egg whites. Any processed food should be checked to verify the presence or absence of egg.

Eggs are relatively easy to avoid, although the authors warn that many so-called egg substitutes also contain egg (minus cholesterol). They suggest that strict label reading is imperative, and that dieters consume only totally "egg-free" substitutes available from health food stores.

*Vitamin and Mineral Supplements.* The authors suggest that the following supplements may be necessary, although unlikely: vitamin B12, folate, biotin, pantothenic acid, riboflavin, and selenium.

### Fish or Shellfish Allergy Diet

Fish allergy, which is common in all age groups in Scandinavia, is the most common food allergy among adults in the U.S. The two most common allergens are bony fish and shellfish such as crustacean (shrimp, crab, lobster, crawfish) and mollusks (clams, oysters, scallops). *The Mayo Clinic Diet Manual* recommends that persons allergic to one crustacean avoid all the others because cross-reactivity is common.

Fish is typically not a hidden ingredient in other foods, and thus is relatively easy to avoid. Fish is, however, found in Worcestershire sauce which contains anchovies, Caesar salads, caviar, and roe. Foods such as French fries or fried foods, which are cooked in the same oil in restaurants as fish, should also be avoided. Many Asian foods include shellfish and must also be eliminated.

Any foods that supply the same nutrient-dense vitamins and minerals as bony fish or shellfish should be included in the diet, especially grains, fruits, and vegetables.

*Vitamin and Mineral Supplements.* Fish provides a source of high biological values — protein, niacin, phosphorus, selenium, vitamin B6, vitamin B12, iron, magnesium, and potassium. Dieters on a fish elimination diet should therefore consider taking supplements of these vitamins and minerals.

## Milk Allergy Elimination Diet

According to the *Manual*, persons of all ages may develop milk allergic reactions. The reactions can be varied and include gastrointestinal problems (diarrhea, vomiting, abdominal pain, bleeding, and malabsorption), respiratory problems (wheezing, coughing, nasal congestion), and skin problems such as uriticaria and eczema.

The most effective treatment for milk allergies is to eliminate all foods containing cow's and goat's milk. These foods can later be reintroduced on a very limited basis. The *Manual* notes that a milk allergy is usually caused by two common proteins found in milk (B-lactoglobulin and B-lactalbumin) and casein. Condensed, evaporated, dried, and pasteurized milk can be allergenic. Heated milk can also cause reactions because allergens are heat-stable. The protein in goat's milk is apparently closely related to cow's milk and should be avoided as well.

### RECOMMENDED FOOD ALTERNATIVES FOR PERSONS ALLERGIC TO MILK

| Nutrients | Alternative Sources |
| --- | --- |
| Vitamin B12 | Eggs, meat, poultry, fish |
| Vitamin D | Fish, liver, eggs |
| Pantothenic acid | Fish, legumes, meat, poultry, whole-grain cereals |
| Riboflavin | Poultry, meat, fish, leafy green vegetables |

## FOOD LABEL TERMS FOR FOODS
## CONTAINING SOY OR SOY PRODUCTS

| | |
|---|---|
| Bean curd | Lecithin |
| Miso | Soy, including soy albumin, flour, milk, nuts, oil (cold-pressed), protein, protein isolate, and sauce |
| Tempeh | Textured vegetable protein |
| Tofu | Soups, including vegetable broth, vegetable gum, and vegetable starch |

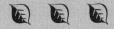

*Vitamin and Mineral Supplements.* Cow's milk is a major source of vitamin B12, D, riboflavin, and pantothenic acid, and the minerals calcium and phosphorus. Persons allergic to milk should consume alternative sources of these nutrients.

### Soybean and Peanut Allergy

Soybean and peanuts are the two most common legumes that cause allergic reactions. A reaction to them, however, does not mean that a person will necessarily be allergic to other legumes. Soy and peanut allergenic reactions include uriticaria, asthma, anaphylaxis, and gastrointestinal symptoms.

Foods that include soy and peanuts are relatively easy to avoid, and allergic persons may be able to tolerate other nuts, especially those grown on trees (walnuts, pecans, and almonds) that are not legumes. Most refined peanut oil is not allergenic, because its protein is removed during processing. Cold-pressed peanut oil, however, which is often used as a flavor enhancer in Asian foods, can cause reactions and should be avoided. All peanuts, soy, and peanut and soy oils and flavorings in Asian foods must be eliminated. Soybeans and the soy products are commonly added to many processed foods, and dieters should avoid them as well.

Dining out can be difficult because many fast foods contain soy extenders or expanders. Asian foods commonly contain soy sauce or tofu (soybean curd). In addition, any processed foods that contain "hydrolyzed vegetable protein" usually contain soy, and should be avoided. In all cases, careful label reading is essential.

*Vitamin and Mineral Supplements.* Soybeans provide calcium, folate, iron, magnesium, phosphorus, riboflavin, thiamin, vitamin B6, and zinc. Foods that contain substantial amounts of these nutrients should be substituted for soy and soy products, including grains, vegetables, and fruits. In some cases, an allergist or dietitian should be consulted to design a non-soy-based diet. Each person's individual intake of soy substitutes should be periodically assessed, and if they are found deficient, supplements should be taken.

Peanuts are important sources of chromium, magnesium, manganese, niacin, and vitamin E. They also provide lesser amounts of copper, folate, biotin, phosphorus, potassium, and vitamin B6. Since many foods, including grains, fruits, and vegetables also provide these nutrients, following a peanut substitute diet should not result in any nutritional deficiencies. However, an allergist or dietitian may prescribe supplements.

### Wheat Allergy Elimination Diet

According to the *Manual,* four constituents of wheat can be allergenic: gliadin, globulin, glutenin, and albumin. Gliadin, the alcohol-soluble component of gluten, can cause a gluten sensitivity as well. All proteins in wheat can stimulate an allergic response from the immune system, and hence all forms of wheat must be eliminated from the diet. In some cases, sprue and celiac disease can be caused by either gluten in wheat, or rye, barley, and oats.

Wheat is the major ingredient in many baked products, crackers, cereals, and pastas, and these foods must be eliminated by substituting other grains, including barley, corn, rye, rice, and oats. Dieters must make

---

### FOOD LABEL TERMS FOR FOODS THAT CONTAIN WHEAT

| | |
|---|---|
| Farina | Gluten: high-gluten flour, vital gluten, wheat gluten |
| Graham flour | High-protein flour |
| Wheat | Wheat bran, wheat germ, wheat gluten, wheat starch, whole-wheat flour |
| Malt | Cereal extracts |
| Gelatinized starch | Modified food starch |
| Vegetable starch | Vegetable gum |

sure that substitute foods, however, do not have wheat added in various amounts to provide bulk and must therefore read all labels carefully.

Foods that contain malt and certain alcoholic beverages, including beer, gin, and selected whiskey, must also be avoided.

Other recommended nongrain wheat alternatives include buckwheat, nut, seed or bean flours, potato flour, soy flour, and amaranth flour. Quinoa, which is similar to rice, is an ideal substitute for wheat noodles in casseroles and cold salads. Nelson recommends using the following thickeners in place of wheat flours: cornstarch, arrowroot, tapioca (quick cooking), rice flour, gelatin, and potato starch.

## Corn Allergy Elimination Diet

Corn allergies are extremely rare. Nevertheless, a corn elimination diet may be very difficult to follow, especially if patients have sensitivities to corn sugar, corn syrup, or cornstarch, which are widely used in processed foods. The difficulty is that corn is normally an important source of chromium, iron, niacin, riboflavin, and thiamin. These nutrients, however, can be consumed in noncorn nutrients substitutes such as grain products. Corn is used as a major ingredient in baked goods, beverages, candy, canned fruits, cereals, cookies, jams, jellies, lunch meats, snack foods, and syrups.

Recommended substitute sweeteners, thickeners, and leavening agents include fruit juice, beet or cane sugar, maple syrup, honey, aspartame, wheat starch, potato starch, rice starch, tapioca, baking soda, and cream of tartar. Baked goods and candies that contain no corn can also be consumed. Other grain products such as wheat, barley, oats, rye, and rice can be substituted for corn. Like other grain oils, corn oil is not restricted because the protein is removed in processing, and hence it does not usually cause an allergic reaction.

*Vitamin and Mineral Supplements.* Persons on a corn allergy elimination diet may need to take vitamin and mineral supplements to provide essential amounts of chromium, iron, niacin, riboflavin, and thiamin.

## DR. MANDELL'S FIVE-DAY ALLERGY RELIEF SYSTEM

Dr. Marshall Mandell, a clinical ecologist, was one of the first physicians and researchers to document how allergens could cause many forms of physical, mental, and psychosomatic disorders. His diet appears in *Dr. Mandell's Five-Day Allergy Relief System.*

## Basic Nutritional Approach

In Chapter 9 of his book *Controlling Your Food Allergies,* Mandell outlines his program for eliminating food allergies. He distinguishes two different types of food allergies: fixed allergies and cyclic allergies. With a fixed allergy, no matter how many months a person may avoid an exposure to the food or beverage to which they are allergic, they will still have a reaction once they are reexposed. Mandell details, however, several ways of controlling fixed allergies. Neutralizing doses which contain minute amounts of the allergen can also be administered sublingually (under the tongue) or taken before, during, or after meals. Fixed food allergies can also be treated by increasing doses of a special form of the food extract to desensitize allergic individuals so that the food may be eaten with mild symptoms or no symptoms at all.

Other methods of managing food allergies of this type include the use of nutritional supplements such as high doses of vitamins C and B6, desiccated liver, hydrochloric acid, sodium bicarbonate, and digestive enzymes.

Cyclic allergies, which constitute at least 50 percent of most food allergies, occur at varying times, depending on the frequency of exposure and the quantity of food ingested. Reactions vary in intensity — they are sometimes severe, at other times mild. If a number of potent food allergens are eaten at the same time, the combined effects can be severe.

To identify which kind of allergies they have, dieters must test all of the foods they eat, eliminate those to which they react for a period of six weeks, and then retest to determine if they have regained their tolerance. Mandell calls this elimination phase Diet for Life, Phase 1. Once dieters determine what forms of allergies they have, they begin following Phase II, an approach to diet planning that helps them avoid suddenly activating their dormant cyclic allergies.

Mandell advises dieters to consult a biologic classification of animal and plant foods that is provided in his book. He recommends working through the list: "If you're allergic to one food within a family, there is an increased chance you will be allergic to another food or foods within that family." He cautions that the only way for dieters to be sure their allergic reaction is caused by specific foods is to test them all and observe what kind of reaction, if any, they have.

## Vitamin and Mineral Supplements

Mandell strongly advises food allergy elimination dieters to consume all essential vitamins and minerals in fresh, organic substitute foods available from organic food stores in their geographic area. The only prepared foods that can be consumed are those packaged in glass jars or frozen foods packaged in cardboard containers. Mandell recommends health food store purchases, for if the foods have been organically grown and the meat comes from organically fed cows, chickens, sheep, and pigs, those foods are not treated with antibiotics, growth stimulants, or tranquilizers.

If dieters cannot avoid allergic foods and find natural food substitutes, Mandell suggests they take the Vitamin and Mineral Insurance Formula, developed by Dr. Roger Williams, the discoverer of pantothenic acid.

## Alkaline Salts

Mandell advises dieters to take alkaline salts if their food allergy symptoms become severe during the testing, rotation, and elimination process. He recommends dieters mixing two tablespoons of baking soda (sodium bicarbonate) with one tablespoon of potassium bicarbonate, and adding a teaspoon of this mixture to a large glass (16 ounces) of spring water. Aspirin-free Alka-Seltzer Gold is also helpful and has a pleasanter taste. He also suggests taking a gentle laxative such as citrate of magnesia or phosphosoda along with a sea salt or alkaline salts enema.

He cautions persons with kidney disease or heart disease to consult a physician before taking sodium-containing alkaline salts. Mandell also suggests that dieters consume 8 glasses of spring water, which is usually available in 5-gallon and half-gallon sizes. He advises dieters to avoid all food and nutrient products packaged in plastic because they often contain chemical pollutants.

The key to the success of his elimination diet, Mandell states, is that once dieters eat a particular food, they do not eat it again in any form for at least five days. Once they have completed the first five days on the Rotary Diversified Diet, they can begin substituting new foods in place of the ones tested.

## Eliminated Foods

Mandell's diet eliminates milk, wheat, chicken egg, tomato, and lettuce for the first six to eight weeks. Depending on reactions, these foods can be reintroduced once dieters have built up a tolerance for them. Mandell stresses, however, that reestablishing a tolerance for certain foods may take from three to six months. And it is critical during this period to determine if each food allergy is fixed or cyclic. If an allergy is fixed, the food cannot be eaten without producing allergic symptoms, unless there is special treatment to reduce or block these symptoms. By testing all potential foods, dieters can carefully observe and record all of their reactions in a daily food diary. The key is to separate the foods every day in the same family, note whether they caused identifiable reactions, and repeat all food for at least five days.

### Diet for Life, Phase II

In Phase II, dieters put together two foods that they have eaten from four to six times in rotation and seemed to tolerate, and observe the effects. They then should begin experimenting with combinations of three foods to observe their effect. It is essential that dieters keep detailed notes. Within a matter of days or weeks, dieters will develop a list of foods that are compatible with each other and may be combined to provide two- and three-food meals. Mandell stresses that his diet, combined with desensitizing treatments and vitamin and mineral supplements, is a more effective way of treating and eliminating food allergies than drug therapies.

### SAMPLE FIVE-DAY DIET FOR PERSONS ALLERGIC TO BEEF, MILK, WHEAT, CHICKEN, EGGS, TOMATO, AND LETTUCE

| Day | Breakfast | Lunch | Dinner |
|-----|-----------|-------|--------|
| 1 | Apple or pear | Squash or pumpkin | Lamb or goat |
| 2 | Orange/grapefruit | Lima beans or peas | Salmon or trout |
| 3 | Pineapple | Carrot or celery | Duck, goose, turkey |
| 4 | Cantaloupe or honeydew | Sweet potato or yam | Lobster, shrimp, crab |
| 5 | Banana | Cabbage, broccoli, beets | Pork |

## DR. MANDELL'S FASTING TIPS

1. Drink a gallon of water each day to eliminate food and chemical residues; bottled spring water available in glass containers is best.
2. Rest frequently and do not do vigorous exercises, because fasting induces rapid weight loss.
3. Make sure to stay warm, because fasting lowers the body's basal metabolism.
4. Avoid hot baths or showers or saunas, which may cause chills or fatigue.
5. Do not smoke or take medications except under supervision of a physician.
6. Do not eat *any* food — eating even the slightest amount of any type of food will disrupt the metabolism.
7. Do not use toothpaste or mouthwash, because they are absorbed like food: instead brush your teeth with sea salt or baking soda.
8. Breaking the fast: after fasting for five days, Mandell recommends that on the morning of the sixth day dieters gradually reinstate food. He notes that their perception should be especially clear, their minds alert, and they should be more able to record their reactions to each food.

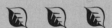

## Fasting

Like Braly's diet, Mandell's recommends that his dieters fast, because it's the quickest way for the body to cleanse itself of all food residues. Fasts, however, should be supervised by a physician or dietitian. He notes that persons with chronic addictive forms of food allergies may experience flareup symptoms on the second or third day of a fast as their body begins to undergo withdrawal from foods to which they are addicted. He recommends a two-tablespoon dose of unflavored milk of magnesia or a teaspoon of two parts baking soda (sodium bicarbonate) and one part potassium bicarbonate in a large glass (12 to 16 ounces) of spring water, which may relieve symptoms. He cautions persons with bronchial asthma, epilepsy, severe dizzy spells, psychiatric problems, and people who require medications to fast only under the supervision of a physician.

### Vitamin and Mineral Supplements

Mandell states that the best way to provide dieters with the unknown vitamins, minerals, and trace elements is to "eat as close to naturally grown complete foods as possible. Ideally, these foods should be grown in organic soil and be free of chemicals, additives, or enhancers." As noted, dieters who cannot consume their RDAs in organic foods should take vitamin and mineral supplements.

## DR. BRALY'S FOOD ALLERGY DIET

Dr. James Braly is a physician practicing in Florida who became an allergist to help those patients whose medical disorders seemed to be diet-related. He claims in his book *Dr. Braly's Diet and Nutrition Revolution* that his Food Allergy Diet has helped more than 10,000 patients.

Braly states that he has personally laboratory tested and treated "thousands of patients suffering from a wide variety of diseases related to food allergies including rheumatoid arthritis, epilepsy, migraine headaches, attention deficit disorder, hyperactivity, anxiety and panic attacks, addiction, asthma, chronic bronchitis, sinusitis, middle ear infection, eczema, hives, duodenal ulcer, and chronic fatigue syndrome."

Braly notes that the following emotional, mental, and behavioral symptoms are commonly caused by food allergens: inability to concentrate or to focus one's attention for any length of time, recurring mental fatigue, irritability for no apparent reason, inexplicable depression, free-floating anxiety, mood swings, hyperactivity, confusion, perhaps indirectly even an alcohol hangover, acute schizophrenia, bulimia, and some phobias. Frequent, recurring infections, especially in children, are common signs of associated food allergy. Chronic upper respiratory infections, such as sore throats, colds, and middle-ear infections, may be the result of reduced immunity due to food allergies.

Braly states that most food allergies form a vicious cycle in which improper diet (including eating undetected allergenic foods, overconsumption of alcohol, excess consumption of saturated and overly processed oils, and the improper metabolism or underconsumption of essential fats in the diet) cause profound digestive problems — the underproduction of secretory IgA, the easily destabilized gastrointestinal mast cell, the underproduction of hydrochloric acids, the malfunctioning of the pancreas, and the

## THE MOST COMMON ALLERGENIC FOODS

According to Dr. James Braly, the most common food allergies include:

| | | |
|---|---|---|
| Corn | Whole wheat | Milk |
| Eggs | Coffee | Chocolate |
| White potato | Malt | Beef |
| Yeast | Rye | Cheese |
| Soybeans | Citrus fruit (oranges) | Tomato |
| Various spices | Peanuts | Pork |

weakening of the mucosal barrier. This, in turn, can result in poor absorption of nutrients, penetration of undigested molecules into the bloodstream, and an assault on the entire body of released chemical mediators. Eventually the immune and digestive systems wear down from trying to destroy the toxic invaders and become less capable of processing food fully and breaking down their nutrients.

As long as allergenic foods remain in the diet, the damage is progressive. The system starts reacting to more and more foods, including previously nonallergenic foods that enter the system in conjunction with already allergenic foods. Eventually, weakened by such chronic stress and malnutrition, the immune system is overpowered.

Braly states that in the early 1980s the mechanism which causes allergies was first discovered. Even in healthy people, partially digested and undigested food from the digestive tract can pass through the paper-thin mucosal lining into the bloodstream. If large quantities of these incompletely digested foods get into the bloodstream, allergies can develop. The main difference between a food allergy sufferer and a nonallergic person is the amount of food that permeates the mucosal barrier and reaches their bloodstream.

Braly suggests that the most reliable test of food allergies is the Food-Specific Immune Complex test (FICA) developed at the University of Kansas Medical School. The test measures the actual presence of food-specific immune complexes and food-specific IgG antibodies in the blood. Results are read by computerized laboratory equipment, and if the blood serum contains a food-specific immune complex or an IgG antibody against a particular food, the anti-IgG antibody (subsequently introduced and radioactively labeled) will attach itself; if the measurement as determined by lab analysis is high enough, the person is considered allergic.

People who cannot take the FICA test have three at-home alternatives:

1. Food and Elimination Challenge. Eliminate from your diet foods you suspect to be allergens for five full days and then reintroduce each food one at a time to see if it provokes an allergic response.
2. Fasting and Challenge. Water-fast for five days to clear your system, and then eat the foods you want to test one at a time to see if allergic symptoms appear.
3. The Least Common Foods Test. Eat a full diet for as long as you can featuring foods that you rarely eat under normal circumstances. As with the other methods, after five days suspected allergens are then eaten to determine if they provoke symptoms.

### Required or Recommended Foods

After identifying allergic foods that should be eliminated, Braly outlines an Optimal Health Program Diet, which he believes prevents flareups. His diet consists of 60 to 70 percent complex carbohydrates, 10 to 20 percent protein, and 15 to 25 percent fats. These nutrient proportions are the best for optimal digestion, he suggests, and for the normal regulation of other body processes that depend on the consumption of a wide variety of foods.

*Fiber.* Braly strongly emphasizes that dietary fiber, ideally about 20 grams daily, is crucial to proper digestion and elimination. It also helps maintain a healthier level of serum cholesterol and may play an important role in the prevention of diabetes, hemorrhoids, varicose veins, colitis, diverticulosis, and appendicitis.

Bran is the best source of fiber, along with all whole grains, and most fruits and vegetables. He cautions, however, that some fiber-rich foods such as wheat, bran, and other grains can be allergenic.

### Restricted Foods

*Fats.* According to Braly, red meats and dairy products provide the wrong kinds of fat (saturated fats) and are often highly allergenic. In addition, he claims they are poorer sources of protein than some vegetables. Fish and poultry, beans, peas, vegetables, potatoes, and whole grains are better protein sources. Skim milk and yogurt are preferable to cheese and whole milk as dairy sources of protein. The best sources of protein, according to Braly, are foods that provide essential fatty acids: nuts, seeds, cold seawater fish, and other marine life. Salad and cooking oils should be cold-pressed oils from the same sources. Note *The Mayo Clinic Diet Manual* does not recommend cold-pressed peanut oil. Because the best fats are not always present in available foods, Braly stresses that most dieters will need to take essential fatty acids supplements, and he recommends evening primrose oil and marine lipid (MaxEPA) capsules.

*Refined Foods.* According to Braly, refined foods not only provide empty calories and dangerous additives, they often contain dozens of food allergens. Refined and packaged foods also tend to contain the same ingredients, either as preservatives or emulsifiers. Eating the same multiple ingredients can in itself lead to the development of allergies to those foods in allergy-prone individuals. Thus, Braly's diet eliminates all refined and packaged foods.

Braly also eliminates what he terms CATS — coffee, alcohol, tobacco, and sugar — which are, he notes, frequently associated with allergies. Coffee, alcohol, and sugar adversely affect the digestive tract and increase a person's allergic response to other foods and beverages consumed in conjunction with them.

*Cow's Milk.* Braly states that cow's milk and milk products are two of the three most allergenic foods, both in children and adults, and his diet eliminates them. Most milk products are also high in saturated fats, specifically arachidonic acid.

*Salt.* Braly's diet restricts foods high in salt, including bacon, sausage, pretzels, and potato chips. He advises dieters to use potassium and sodium chloride mixtures as salt substitutes.

## Vitamin and Mineral Supplements

Braly does not believe that even the most balanced and nutritious diet will provide all the essential nutrients, and he therefore advises that dieters take

## FINAL TIPS FOR FOLLOWING
## BRALY'S ROTATION DIET

1. Avoid caffeine, alcohol, tobacco, and sugar; avoid overconsuming caffeinated herbal teas, which can be toxic.

2. Be sure to consume a complete protein at two out of three meals, preferably during breakfast or lunch.

3. Eat a large salad daily and rotate oils and seasonings; select only unrefined, cold-pressed salad oils such as safflower, sunflower, soy, corn, sesame, chestnut, linseed, or walnut.

4. Drink several glasses of bottled water with each meal.

5. Take vitamin and other supplements with meals, except for iron and amino acid supplements, which should be consumed between meals.

6. Do not eat late at night and make sure that the last meal consumed during the day is low in calories, low in animal protein, and high in starchy complex carbohydrates.

7. Do not restrict caloric intake; instead, concentrate on eating healthy whole foods.

one or more of the following supplements, depending on their specific deficiencies, after consulting a nutritionist or dietitian:

**Vitamins:**
C: 1,000 milligrams crystal or powder twice a day with meals
B complex: 1 capsule twice a day with meals (children under eight, 1 capsule)
B3 (niacin): 25 milligrams twice a day with meals
B6: 100 milligrams twice a day with meals

**Minerals:**
Zinc: 25 milligrams once a day with meals
Magnesium: 200 milligrams once a day with meals
Calcium: 400 milligrams once a day with meals
GTF chromium: 25–50 milligrams twice a day with meals
Evening primrose oil: 3 capsules twice a day before meals
MaxEPA: 3 capsules twice a day before meals

Other digestive treatments Braly recommends include: correct the effects of hypochlorhydria with hydrochloric acid capsules and pancreatic

## SAMPLE MEAL PLANS FOR A STRICT
## DIAGNOSTIC ELIMINATION DIET

The following three-day sample meal plan for food allergy sufferers is recommended by the Food Allergy Network. It excludes eggs, wheat, milk, soybeans, fish, shellfish, peanuts, nuts, corn, beef, and chicken. FAN cautions that this diet should be started only with a physician's approval.*

**Day 1**
**Breakfast**
1 cup apple juice
1 cup plain puffed rice cereal
2 pork sausage patties
2 rice cakes with jelly
**Lunch**
1 broiled lamb chop
1 serving French-fried potatoes
1 serving cooked carrots
1 cup apple juice
**Dinner**
1 broiled pork chop
1 broiled potato
1 serving squash
1 serving canned pears
1 cup apple juice

**Day 2**
**Breakfast**
1 cup apple juice
1 cup plain puffed rice cereal
2 ounces grilled ham
2 rice cakes with jelly
**Lunch**
3 ounce ground lamb patty
2 slices egg-, milk-, and wheat-free bread
1 ounce potato chips
1 serving cooked carrots
1 serving applesauce
1 cup apple juice

## SAMPLE MEAL PLANS FOR A STRICT
## DIAGNOSTIC ELIMINATION DIET
### (continued)

**Dinner**
1 broiled pork chop
1 cup steamed white rice
1 serving cooked spinach
1 serving canned pineapple
1 cup apple juice

**Day 3**
**Breakfast**
1 cup apple juice
1 cup cream of rice cereal (without milk)
4 slices bacon
2 rice cakes with jelly
**Lunch**
2 slices ham
2 slices egg-, milk-, and wheat-free bread
1 ounce potato chips
1 serving canned pears
1 cup apple juice
**Dinner**
1 broiled lamb chop
1 baked potato
1 serving cooked broccoli
1 serving canned peaches
1 cup apple juice

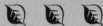

*Source: The Food Allergy Network, *Nutrition Guide to Food Allergies* (Fairfax, VA: Food Allergy Network, 1992): 19.

digestive enzyme supplements; stabilize the gastrointestinal mast cells with vitamin C in crystal or powder form before meals; assist the buildup of the gastrointestinal mucosal barrier with essential fatty acids, vitamins A, B, C, and zinc; and buffer the small intestine after meals with bicarbonates such as Alka-Seltzer Gold.

## Water Fasting

Braly suggests that water-fasting can sometimes be a useful way to self-test for food allergies. Fasting, he notes, also helps detoxify the digestive tract. Periodic short-term fasting may also be a beneficial adjunct to an anti-aging regime and serves to stimulate the immune system. Fasting, however, can be dangerous for certain individuals if undertaken without supervision. Athletes and exercisers should not fast because it depletes the glycogen energy stores they need for physical exertion and breaks down skeletal muscles and other essential tissues that provide alternative fuel sources.

## Food Diaries, Food Lists, and Rotation Diet Menus

In order to self-test for allergies, Braly states that it is necessary for dieters to keep an accurate food diary. He suggests that dieters make several photocopies of table 48 of his book, which lists food groups, along with his rotation diet planning form and diet diary form.

Using Braly's revised list of foods, dieters plan four days of breakfasts, lunches, and dinners, as well as a variety of meals and snacks. Each meal should use a different meat, grain, and vegetable. Even spices and sweeteners must be parceled out over the four-day rotation diet. In addition, each meal should include as few ingredients as possible. He notes that careful food planning is necessary to provide all the essential nutrients (especially protein, calcium, iron, and dietary fiber).

## Physical Activity

Braly, unlike Mandell or *The Mayo Clinic Diet Manual*, discusses the importance of exercise in his diet, although he does not state how exercise might directly help relieve a specific food allergy. He encourages dieters to perform aerobic exercise five to six times a week.

# 20

## Diets for Hypertension
## (High Blood Pressure)

Hypertension (excessive and sustained blood pressure against the walls of the arteries) is the most common stress-related disorder in the United States and a major cause of death, as reported in the *Alternative Health and Medicine Encyclopedia*. The September 1989 issue of the *Johns Hopkins Medical Letter* further states that approximately 60 million Americans suffer from hypertension (or high blood pressure), and half of them do not even know they have the condition.

High blood pressure results when the heart has to pump harder than normal because of an excess of fluid in the bloodstream combined with narrowed or constricted arteries, or to meet the increased demands of strenuous activity.

Two primary types of hypertension have been defined: that resulting from other medical disorders such as diabetes or brain tumors, called secondary hypertension; and "essential hypertension," for which the cause has not been fully established. Currently, 92 to 94 percent of all diagnosed hypertension is termed essential.

Long-term studies have shown that chronic high blood pressure typical of essential hypertension increases the risk of heart disease, stroke, atherosclerosis, and kidney disease. Anxiety, heart palpitations, increased pulse rates, or feeling "wound up" are not necessarily reliable indicators of high blood pressure. The only sure way to detect abnormal pressure and minimize the risk of hypertension (often a symptomless disorder) is to have an annual blood pressure examination.

A variety of factors has been tentatively linked to essential hypertension, including obesity, inactivity, prolonged stress, smoking, and drugs (including estrogens, indomethacine, phenylpropanolamine, amphetamines, and cocaine). Nutritional causes of hypertension include excessive salt, sugar, licorice, coffee, and alcohol intake.

Readers who think they might be suffering from hypertension will benefit by comparing the diets described in this chapter, as dietary considerations are now known to play a significant role in both causing and subsequently lowering high blood pressure.

According to Murray and Pizzorno in the *Encyclopedia of Natural Medicine,* dietary factors that have been linked with high blood pressure include sodium to potassium ratios, high cholesterol, and low fiber consumption.

A calcium deficiency may also play a role because people who decrease their calcium intake usually experience increased blood pressure. A high-calcium diet, on the other hand, appears to help counteract the harmful effects of a high-sodium diet. One reason for this is that sodium directly affects calcium metabolism. For maximum benefits, therefore, the diets discussed in this chapter recommend that people with high blood pressure adopt a diet low in sodium and high in both potassium and calcium.

## HOW TO CONTROL HIGH BLOOD PRESSURE DIET

Robert L. Rowan, M.D., F.A.C.S., is a clinical associate professor at New York University Medical School. He has contributed many scientific articles to medical literature and coauthored three books, including *How to Control High Blood Pressure without Drugs.*

### Basic Nutritional Approach

To minimize the chances of getting high blood pressure, or to reduce the risks if people already have hypertension, Rowan suggests:

- Develop eating habits that are nutritionally sound, and stick to foods that provide the basic daily requirements of vitamins, minerals, proteins, roughage, and carbohydrates.
- Count calories and carefully monitor weight.
- Control stress and anxiety, which can do irreparable harm to the body.
- Eliminate or at least greatly reduce consumption of tobacco and alcohol.

---

### EARLY SYMPTOMS OF HIGH BLOOD PRESSURE

- Nosebleeds
- Ringing in the ears
- Dizziness
- Fainting spells
- Morning headaches

- Depression
- Blurred vision
- Urinating at night
- A feeling of tenseness
- Flushing or redness of the face

---

- Reduce salt intake. (He specifically suggests avoiding especially salty foods such as potato chips, salted nuts, olives, pickles, soy sauce, corned and dried beef, canned crab meat, ham, and canned soups and vegetables, and reducing the use of processed foods with a high sodium content.)
- Exercise.
- Obtain medical care, if hypertension is diagnosed, and follow treatment exactly.

While Rowan admits that no clear evidence links obesity and hypertension, he feels it simply makes sense not to become overweight so as not to put additional strain on the vascular system.

For those who wish to reduce, he counsels that the simplest step is to reduce food intake by half. Not only is this effective, but the reduction makes the change to a nutritionally sound diet less difficult. Rowan further suggests that people count calories, and keep a record as they progress. "Dieting becomes simple once you develop the necessary self-control," he claims.

### Daily Menu Plan

Rowan's basic diet plan is based on low sodium intake; increasing carbohydrate consumption so it accounts for 55 to 60 percent of calorie (energy) intake; reducing total consumption of fat from approximately 40 percent to 30 percent; reducing consumption of saturated fats (which should account for only 10 percent of daily dietary intake); and reducing consumption of cholesterol to approximately 300 milligrams a day.

> ## HINTS TO ELIMINATE
> ## CALORIE-RICH FOODS
>
> - Don't go shopping for food when you are hungry.
> - Don't buy items on impulse.
> - Prepare in advance for that sudden craving to eat something while watching television.
> - Don't keep calorie-rich snack foods at home.
> - A food scale is an invaluable aid in controlling food intake, as many foods are acceptable if the amount consumed is limited.
> - Keep an accurate record of all you eat on a daily basis.
> - Weigh yourself each day and keep a careful record of your successes and failures while dieting.
> - As soon as you have maintained some weight loss for a week or so, have your clothing altered to fit.
> - Chew food slowly, and allow some time to pass before taking a bite and swallowing it.

## Recommended Foods

Any of the following foods are recommended, if consumed within people's caloric needs: vegetables such as broccoli, green and red peppers, zucchini, celery, lettuce, radishes, cucumbers, mushrooms, and spinach; fruits such as oranges, prunes, bananas, cantaloupes, strawberries, apples, grapes, and grapefruit; veal, chicken, and fish; beverages such as coffee, tea, skim milk, seltzer, and low-calorie, low-salt soda; pasta; whole-grain unsweetened cereals; unsalted nuts and raisins.

Additionally, foods that help supply carbohydrates include rice, potatoes, and sweet potatoes, spaghetti, bread, cereal, certain fruits such as bananas and oranges, all kinds of dried beans (lentils, lima beans, kidney beans), corn, and yams.

*Potassium-Rich Foods.* Because potassium may help protect against an increase in blood pressure caused by excess sodium, Rowan suggests that people whose diets may be deficient in this vital component include such foods as dried apricots, figs and dates, avocados, bananas, Brussels sprouts, chicken and goose, mushrooms, uncooked prunes, unsalted nuts such as Brazil nuts, filberts, and peanuts, oranges and orange juice, potatoes, and raisins.

## Restricted Foods

*Sodium.* Restricted foods on Rowan's diet include all foods that contain high levels of sodium, including:

- Baking soda (sodium bicarbonate), baking powder, brine (salt water), disodium phosphate (used in foods to aid "quick" cooking, such as Cream of Wheat).
- All vegetable salts.
- Seasoned salts such as vegetable salts, spices, and monosodium glutamate in combination.
- Monosodium glutamate (MSG). This is a form of sodium usually extracted from grains or beets that is added as a seasoning to many foods and is also present in bean curd and soy sauce.

*Sugar.* While Rowan recommends complex carbohydrates, he severely restricts foods in his diet that contain pure sugar. He suggests removing the sugar bowl from the table and avoiding sugar-filled soft drinks. He also urges dieters to avoid eating foods that contain dextrose, corn syrup, and sucrose.

## Eliminated Foods

Rowan's diet restricts fat consumption to 30 percent of total calories, because excess fat increases the danger of atherosclerosis by allowing the buildup of fat deposits in the blood vessels. Excess fat also increases the risk of cancer of the colon, breast, and prostate. Foods that have a high fat content, and which should therefore be eliminated, include red meats (particularly beef and pork), butter, lard, unsweetened chocolate (which is about 50 percent fat), nuts, peanut butter, bacon, luncheon meats, frankfurters, and doughnuts.

Because a diet high in saturated fat increases blood cholesterol by as much as 25 percent, Rowan counsels people to consume only 10 percent of daily calories as saturated fats. Instead, they should substitute polyunsaturated and monounsaturated fats found in safflower, corn, peanut, soybean, and cottonseed oil.

In addition, Rowan's diet reduces the consumption of cholesterol to approximately 300 milligrams per day, and substitutes high-cholesterol foods with safer ones such as fresh fruits, vegetables, grains, chicken, and fish. He limits or eliminates eggs, most cheeses, coconut and palm oil, and the high-fat foods listed above.

## Alcohol

Repeated scientific studies, according to Rowan, have confirmed that alcoholism is a cause of hypertension. The most reasonable explanation is that alcohol has an effect on the walls of the arteries. When alcohol is present in the bloodstream, it actually bathes the walls of the blood vessels, increasing their tension and thereby contributing to high blood pressure.

## Smoking

Because smoking can produce a significant rise in pulse rate as well as in systolic and diastolic blood pressure, Rowan counsels anyone with high blood pressure, and anyone who wishes to avoid having it, to stop smoking. Smokers who are not able to quit on their own are advised to contact the American Cancer Society or other associations that use peer support and behavior modification. Hypnosis seminars and acupuncture are other methods that have proven effective, as has nicotine gum.

## Use of Blood Pressure Medications

According to Rowan, new medications to treat hypertension have proven extremely effective. He advocates, however, that whenever possible, non-drug therapies such as sodium restriction, weight reduction, relaxation techniques, and exercise be used to lower blood pressure, especially for people suffering from mild hypertension.

## Physical Activity

A number of studies, including several cited by Rowan, have confirmed the importance of exercise in lowering blood pressure levels in both men and women. For example, a study of 15,000 men who attended Harvard University and were followed for six to ten years after graduation found that gaining weight increased the risk of hypertension. It also confirmed that hypertension occurred less often in those men who participated in vigorous sports than it did in sedentary men. The worst combination was excess weight coupled with lack of activity. Rowan concludes that simply keeping weight down is not enough; people must be physically active as well.

While adequate physical exercise results in a reduction in weight, blood pressure, and hypertension, Rowan believes the most important advantage is the feeling of well-being that ensues. (This sense of exhilaration results from an increase in opioid peptides, a kind of naturally occurring narcotic in the body.) If stress plays a role in causing hypertension, this feeling of well-being can only lead to a sense of ease that is beneficial in lessening the condition, he postulates.

However, Rowan warns, exercise is not advisable for people with hypertension secondary to tumors of the adrenal gland, diseases of the thyroid gland, kidney disease, or any disease that occurs within the brain or the aorta.

"Exercises that use large numbers of muscles are best for the person with essential hypertension," Rowan advises, and specifically recommends swimming, cross-country skiing, or jogging.

The key to exercise as a means of preventing and helping to control high blood pressure depends upon choosing exercises that are not too taxing, increasing them on a progressive basis, and doing them regularly so that no sudden or undue strain results.

Prior to any exercise program, Rowan suggests that people undergo a physical examination, including blood tests and urinalysis. "If your history reveals any potential illnesses or if your physical exam reveals any abnormalities, they should be evaluated and/or corrected before you start," he concludes.

## Behavioral Modification

Rowan contends that stress and how people react to it can help determine whether they will have high blood pressure. However, because the ways in which a person copes with stress is often learned behavior, he feels the stress-hypertension cycle can also be broken in a number of ways.

The key is rest (physical, emotional, or mental), which decreases the need for blood to pass through the vascular system and thus results in a drop in blood pressure. And rest can be obtained not only through sleep, but also through relaxation periods, meditation, biofeedback, the enjoyment of hobbies, and exercise.

## THE HIGH BLOOD PRESSURE DIET

The high blood pressure diet outlined in the book *High Blood Pressure* was developed by the doctors Neil B. Shulman, Elijah Saunders, and W. Dallas Hall. Shulman is associate professor of medicine at Emory University's School of Medicine and Grady Memorial Hospital in Atlanta, Georgia. Saunders is an associate professor of medicine, chief of the Division of Hypertension, and clinical director at the Center for Vascular Biology and Hypertension at the University of Maryland School of Medicine and Hospital in Baltimore. Hall is professor of medicine, director of the Division of Hypertension, and director of the General Clinical Research Center at Emory University's School of Medicine, the Grady Memorial Hospital, and Emory Hospital in Atlanta.

Together, the authors have treated more than 20,000 patients with high blood pressure, conducted more than fifty high blood pressure research trials, and lectured internationally to doctors, nurses, patients, and the general public.

### Basic Nutritional Approach

The two most important approaches to lower blood pressure, contend the authors, are losing weight and restricting salt intake. In fact, people who are overweight, or who gain too much weight, are two to six times more likely to develop this condition. However, even a small weight reduction — as little as ten pounds — can have a definite beneficial effect on blood pressure.

Although the authors admit that it is beyond their scope to cover weight loss in detail, they provide a sample 1,800-calorie diet from the American Heart Association to give readers an idea of the foods that are permitted. However, they warn, fewer calories — that is, 800 to 1,200 — might be necessary for effective weight reduction.

Besides losing weight, the most important thing people can do to help control blood pressure is to reduce their salt intake. In fact, as the authors point out, hypertension occurs most frequently among people who have a high level of salt in their diet, such as Americans and the Japanese. Conversely, people such as the Solomon Islanders of the South Pacific and those living in rural areas in Africa, who consume minimal amounts of salt, have very low rates of high blood pressure.

The authors suggest that reducing salt intake by 50 percent is usually

---

### SIMPLE WEIGHT-LOSS PRINCIPLES

- Eat less red meat. When you do eat red meat, choose leaner cuts, trim off the fat, and broil or bake instead of frying.
- Eat more fish and chicken. Broil or bake instead of frying, and consider taking the skin off.
- Avoid sugar and sweets. Cut down on the number of desserts you consume to perhaps one a week or one after every third meal. At other times, choose fruit.
- Pay attention to calories, and read the labels on foods you buy at the store.
- Eat smaller servings, and eat more slowly to give yourself time to feel full before you eat too much.

---

adequate to improve blood pressure, and provide a list of forty-three high-sodium foods that should be avoided, ranging from bacon to TV dinners.

### Recommended Foods

Similar to Dr. Rowan, the authors particularly recommend natural foods rich in potassium, and counsel against high intakes of calcium.

*Potassium-Rich Foods.* Although the role of potassium in high blood pressure has not been as thoroughly researched as the effects of sodium, studies suggest that high sodium intake is much more likely to cause hypertension if the amount of potassium in the diet is low. Furthermore, as the authors note, recent studies suggest that some of the damage done to the blood vessels of hypertensive people might be lessened by high-potassium diets.

However, the authors warn that people should be careful not to take extra potassium without first checking with a physician. It can be unsafe for some hypertensives with kidney damage, for example, or for those taking certain types of high blood pressure drugs.

Foods rich in potassium include bananas, raisins, oranges, grapefruit, potatoes, and spinach.

### Calcium

Although patients with high blood pressure are sometimes found to have a low dietary intake of calcium, the authors claim that a high dietary intake of calcium has not been proven to reduce blood pressure. Moreover, certain dairy products are rich in cholesterol and fats as well as calcium and can adversely affect fat and lipid levels in the blood.

## Cholesterol

According to the authors, while a high blood cholesterol level does not by itself cause high blood pressure, when it is present in a person with hypertension, the chance of having a heart attack is much greater because the cholesterol is more likely to deposit on the blood vessel walls and cause blockage.

Therefore, they suggest selecting foods that are low in cholesterol and saturated fats, such as lowfat dairy products, and eating fewer red meats and foods cooked with vegetable oils. The goal should be to decrease dietary cholesterol to less than 300 milligrams a day — compared to the typical American consumption of 400 to 450 milligrams.

## Alcohol

As the authors point out, people who drink excessive quantities of alcohol on a regular basis (more than two to three shots (four ounces) of 100-proof whiskey, two glasses (16 ounces) of wine, or four cans (48 ounces) of beer a day) have an increased risk of developing high blood pressure. In addition, if high blood pressure is already present, heavy alcohol drinking makes it more difficult to control, even with medication. Hypertensive patients are therefore advised to keep their alcohol intake well below the limits listed above.

## Smoking

According to the authors, smoking makes strokes more likely, as does high blood pressure. Therefore, people with high blood pressure are strongly urged not to smoke cigarettes if they wish to prevent a heart attack or stroke.

## Blood Pressure Medications

The authors believe that essential hypertension is a chronic condition, and that most people who have it "will need to take medication for life." They suggest, however, that people with mild hypertension may be able to control their blood pressure without medication by adopting lifestyle changes that restrict salt, alcohol, smoking, cholesterol, and fat, reducing stress, and increasing levels of exercise and the amounts of calcium and potassium consumed.

## Licorice

Licorice, either in candy or chewing tobacco, can cause the body to retain salt and consequently raise blood pressure. While this does not occur in every person who chews tobacco or eats licorice, the authors note, it can occur if a person uses large amounts and is predisposed to developing high blood pressure.

## Diet Pills and Recreational Drugs

The authors warn that an overdose of diet pills containing stimulants known as amphetamines can cause severe elevation in blood pressure and even stroke. Therefore, people with high blood pressure should not take any type of diet pill that has not been prescribed or approved by their physician.

Furthermore, the use of cocaine or street drugs (speed) can also cause extreme elevations of blood pressure, stroke, and heart attack.

## Physical Activity

Exercises such as running, swimming, and walking can lead to improved cardiovascular conditioning and generally are good for hypertensives. With sufficient time, the authors contend, consistent aerobic exercise can reduce the resting pulse (heart rate) and blood pressure, so medications can sometimes be reduced or even eliminated.

People with high blood pressure should have any exercise regimen approved by their physician, however, who will usually want the blood pressure controlled before approving certain types or levels of exercise. The authors conclude that exercises such as weight lifting are not advisable for most hypertensives because of the very high levels of blood pressure that can result.

## Behavioral Modification

Because stress plays a significant role in keeping blood pressure elevated, the authors suggest techniques such as biofeedback and meditation to lower it.

They also advise that spiritual healing, which may involve the "laying on of hands" practiced by many Pentecostal church groups, may be useful in treating some patients with high blood pressure, especially if coupled with a strong positive attitude.

The authors caution, however, that as with all treatments for high blood pressure, even when drugs are not used, a physician must be in charge to monitor blood pressure on a regular basis, and make sure that no harm is done by any form of therapy and that medications are not discontinued prematurely.

## LOWER YOUR BLOOD PRESSURE AND LIVE LONGER

Dr. Marvin Moser, a clinical professor of medicine at the Yale University School of Medicine, outlines a hypertension diet in his book, *Lower Your Blood Pressure and Live Longer*. He is also emeritus chief of the cardiology section at the White Plains (New York) Hospital Medical Center and a fellow of the Council for High Blood Pressure Research of the American Heart Association.

Moser has been actively involved in hypertension research for more than thirty years, and authored three medical texts and more than three hundred scientific papers in the field of cardiology and hypertension. In 1985, he received the National High Blood Pressure Education Program Award for outstanding contributions in the treatment of hypertension.

### Basic Nutritional Approach

According to Moser, "weight loss does not always bring blood pressure down to normal levels, but many hypertensive patients who lose at least some excess weight will also achieve reduced blood pressure."

However, acknowledging that it is counterproductive and perhaps even injurious to good health to go on an extremely restrictive diet for any length of time, Moser outlines a "common sense dietary approach that seems to work well for my patients" and "allows them to enjoy their favorite foods without feeling starved all the time."

As he emphasizes, a dietary regimen that ignores personal food preferences and asks for an abrupt change in lifelong eating habits simply doesn't work over the long term. Conversely, Moser contends that his approach, which takes into account what people now eat and then shows them how to modify it, will succeed.

Moser claims that reducing portion sizes is the best way for people to lower caloric intake without depriving themselves of their favorite foods. For this reason, he instructs patients to begin by cutting portions in half and limiting cakes, candies, cookies, and bread to a greater degree than fruits, vegetables, and other high-nutrition, low-calorie foods.

The rule he follows is that people can lose a pound of weight if they burn 3,500 more calories than they take in. Therefore, if dieters cut their intake by 500 calories a day, they will lose approximately one pound a week (500 x 7 = 3,500 calories, or one pound).

## Recommended Foods

According to Moser, the typical American diet tends to be high in calories, cholesterol, saturated fat, and sugar (or other refined sweeteners). His diet, on the other hand, recommends the following foods:

- Meats, fish, and poultry (fresh, unsalted, with all fat and skin removed): chicken, turkey, fish, and veal, as well as shrimp (once weekly), and low-sodium diet-packed salmon, shrimp, or tuna
- Vegetables: all fresh or frozen vegetables, excluding frozen peas and lima beans
- Fruit: all fresh, canned, or frozen fruit without preservatives, as well as sun-dried
- Fats: corn, soybean, sesame seed, and sunflower oils; unsalted, polyunsaturated margarine; and low-sodium mayonnaise
- Rice, pasta, and potatoes: all forms that do not have any added salt, cream, or butter, and that are cooked and served only with unsaturated vegetable oil or margarine
- Cereals: puffed wheat, puffed rice, shredded wheat biscuits, oatmeal, cream of wheat (not instant), Familia, muesli, and wheat germ
- Breads: regular whole-grain or enriched bread, unsalted melba toast, plain matzo, low-sodium bread and crackers, unsalted pretzels, and mayonnaise
- Salad dressings: lemon juice or fresh lemon, white or cider vinegar, or salt-free ketchup or salt-free chili sauce added to one of the above oils
- Eggs: two or three eggs per week; egg white and substitutes
- Milk: skim, lowfat, or evaporated skim milk
- Beverages: instant, regular, and decaffeinated coffee, tea, cocoa (without milk powder), seltzer, wine, alcoholic beverages in moderation
- Cheese: low-salt cottage cheese, farmer, pot cheese, skim-milk ricotta, and any other low-salt and low–saturated fat cheese

- Syrups, sugars, and candies: sugar, honey, pure maple syrup, pure jellies and jams, white or light brown sugar
- Desserts: fruit, tapioca, rice pudding, fruit or water ices, homemade pies, cakes, and desserts in moderation

Moser also recommends spices that can easily be substituted for sodium, including allspice, basil, bay leaves, caraway, chives, cinnamon, curry powder, dill, garlic, ginger, prepared horseradish without salt, lemon juice, mint, mustard (dry), nutmeg, onion, oregano, paprika, parsley, pepper, poppyseed, sage, thyme, and vinegar wine for flavoring. Saccharin and vanilla extract are suggested as flavoring substitutes for sugar.

*Potassium-Rich Foods.* Moser recommends that people include potassium-rich foods in their daily diet because it is essential to maintaining proper body chemistry. He cites research conducted by Dr. Louis Tobian of the University of Minnesota which has shown a low incidence of high blood pressure among populations that consume a high-potassium, low-sodium diet of mostly fruits, roots, grains, and other plant foods.

## Calcium

Moser does not believe calcium pills should be considered part of a treatment program, and warns that excess amounts of calcium may cause problems such as kidney stones. He recommends that people's diets provide 800 to 1,000 milligrams of calcium per day, the amount contained in two or three servings of milk (preferably lowfat) or milk products.

## Restricted Foods

Moser recommends that the following foods be used sparingly:

- Meats, fish, and poultry: all frozen fish fillets; canned, salted, or pickled fish such as herring, smoked salmon, or anchovies; canned, salted, or smoked meats such as bacon, bologna, franks, sausage, salt pork, corned beef, cold cuts, duck, turkey roll, heavily marbled meat, skin and fat from poultry, spare ribs, commercial frozen dinners, liver, and kidney. Shellfish should not be consumed more than three times weekly
- Vegetables: all canned vegetables or vegetable juices, frozen peas or lima beans, sauerkraut, pickles, and relish

- Fruits: maraschino cherries; canned, frozen, or dried fruits that contain salt or preservatives; glazed fruit
- Fats: butter, salted margarine, bacon fat, salt pork, meat fat, olives, products containing coconut or palm oils, lard or solid shortening, peanut butter, salted nuts
- Rice, pasta, and potatoes: creamed, scalloped, or fried in unknown fat
- Cereals: cooked cereals containing sodium; dried cereals other than those listed under recommended foods; cereals with coconut
- Breads: salted crackers, commercial cakes, muffins, pancake mixes, salted pretzels, potato chips, popcorn, corn chips, pizza, dark rye, and self-rising flour
- Salad dressings: all commercial salad dressings and mayonnaise
- Cheese: American, Swiss, Muenster, cheese spreads, and all other cheeses
- Milk: buttermilk, whole milk, chocolate milk, condensed milk, instant cocoa, nondairy cream substitutes, sour cream, cream, ice cream, aerosol whipped toppings, whole milk yogurt, sherbet, ice milk, creamed soups, half-and-half
- Beverages: all commercial soft drinks
- Syrups, sugars, and candies: dark brown sugar, molasses, candies containing salt or saturated fats, coconut
- Other foods: bouillon cubes or bouillon powders, baking powder or soda, canned soups, prepared mustard, horseradish, Worcestershire sauce, soy sauce, ketchup, chili sauce, celery, onion or garlic salt, cooking wine, meat tenderizer (or MSG), tomato paste, pickled relish

## Sodium

Moser states that while there is no doubt sodium plays a role in high blood pressure, it is not possible to definitively determine how important it is as a cause in each individual. In general, however, population groups that consume large amounts of salt have a higher incidence of hypertension than those with very low-salt diets.

He therefore recommends that hypertensives try sodium restriction before drug therapy to lower blood pressure. If their blood pressure is not reduced after six to eight weeks of following a low-salt diet, they should discuss other forms of therapy with their physician.

Frequently, Moser claims, the desired reduction in salt intake can be achieved by simple means, such as restricting the addition of salt to foods in the cooking process and at the table. "A good rule is first to try to cut salt intake in half, as you would the portions of food. If you can cut down to a little less than one teaspoonful (four grams) a day, you will probably see some decrease in blood pressure (if it is going to occur)."

Moser warns, however, that most of people's sodium intake is hidden in processed foods, including many that do not taste at all salty, such as soft drinks, ice cream, breakfast cereals, bread, and commercial pastries. Other foods high in sodium include many flavorings, additives, and preservatives.

## Salt Substitutes

Moser strongly urges his dieters to use salt substitutes in place of white table salt, most of which contain potassium chloride instead of sodium. These products, he cautions, can be tolerated by healthy people with normal kidneys, but can be dangerous for those with kidney damage or for people taking potassium-sparing diuretics. Therefore he advises dieters to check with their physician before using a salt substitute containing potassium chloride.

A better alternative, Moser suggests, is to use blended spices and herbs as salt substitutes, provided they do not contain monosodium glutamate.

## Physical Activity

Moser is more enthusiastic about the role of exercise which, he notes, may be helpful for some people in treating mild to moderate high blood pressure. However, he contends there is no proof that regular vigorous exercises such as running significantly lower blood pressure in the large majority of hypertensives. Rather he recommends moderate exercise in combination with a low-salt and, if appropriate, a reduced-calorie diet.

Suggested types of exercise include leisure-time walking, bicycling, tennis, golf, swimming, shooting baskets, and bowling. Exercises such as weight lifting that involve pushing or tugging (isometric exercises) should be avoided, as they raise blood pressure.

## Behavioral Modification

Moser states that high blood pressure usually requires lifelong treatment. Salt restriction, exercise, weight loss, and stress-reduction can produce a lowering of blood pressure in some people with mild hypertension. However, he has found that the number of patients who benefit from medication, biofeedback training, self-hypnosis, stress management, and other alternative nondrug treatments is not very great. Such approaches, Moser notes, may temporarily lower blood pressure but for most hypertensive patients, "they simply are not effective in maintaining the lowered blood pressures."

## RECENT RESEARCH

One excellent way of restricting table salt consumption is to use a mineral salt substitute. J. M. Geleijnse reports in the August 13, 1994, issue of *British Medical Journal* how Dutch physicians successfully treated one hundred men and women between the ages of 55 and 75 with mild to moderate hypertension. During the 24-week study, the intervention group received a low-sodium, high-potassium, high-magnesium mineral salt and foods prepared with it. The control group received common sodium salt and foods.

Follow-up studies on 97 of the 100 participants revealed that those receiving the mineral salt substitute experienced significantly lower blood pressure levels than the control group. The researchers concluded that replacing table salt with a mineral salt substitute "could offer a valuable nonpharmacological approach to lowering blood pressure in older people with mild to moderate hypertension."

### Dietary Fiber

Murray and Pizzorno argue in their book, *Encyclopedia of Natural Medicine,* that a high-fiber diet effectively prevents and treats hypertension. They recommend a diet high in oat bran, apple pectin, psyllium seeds, guar gum, and gum karaya. This diet reduces cholesterol levels and promotes weight loss, which helps lower blood pressure levels.

K. Eliasson reports a trial in the February 1992 issue of the *Journal of Hypertension* involving 63 patients with hypertension which confirm the benefits of fiber. In the trial, 32 patients were given fiber supplements, while 31 were given placebos. Eliasson notes that "body weight was significantly reduced in the fiber group. Dietary fiber significantly reduced diastolic blood pressure and fasting serum insulin. A dietary fiber supplement can lower diastolic blood pressure in mildly hypertensive patients independent of changes in body weight."

## THERAPIES FOR HYPERTENSION*

1. **Watch your weight.** An estimated 20 to 30 percent of hypertension cases directly result from excess body weight which, if lost, results in a commensurate drop in blood pressure.

2. **Reduce sodium intake.** Recent studies show that approximately half of those with hypertension can reduce their blood pressure by making a modest reduction in dietary sodium consumption.

3. **Reduce dietary fats to 20 percent of caloric intake.** Dr. Ornish's research proves that hypertension can be greatly reduced through a totally vegetarian diet with less than 20 percent of caloric intake consumed from fats.

4. **Increase calcium.** Increased calcium intake may slightly lower blood pressure.

5. **Increase potassium.** Potassium lowers blood pressure, although the benefit is modest.

6. **Reduce alcohol intake.** Curtailing alcohol consumption has corresponded to decreases in blood pressure in limited trials.

7. **Relaxation.** Relaxation techniques such as deep breathing, meditation, and progressive muscle relaxation relieve muscular tension and lower blood pressure.

8. **Stop smoking.** Nicotine constricts the arteries and increases blood pressure.

9. **Exercise.** Exercise helps to lower blood pressure.

*Adapted from James Marti and Andrea Hine, *The Alternative Health and Medicine Encyclopedia* (Detroit, Mich.: Gale Research Inc., 1994).

## Guava Fruit

R. Singh presents a novel thesis in the February 1993 issue of the *Journal of Human Hypertension:* that increasing consumption of guava fruit can decrease blood pressure. He conducted a trial in which 72 of 145 hypertensives were given a soluble fiber and potassium-rich diet containing 0.5 to 1.0 kilogram of guava fruit daily. The other 73 patients consumed their usual diet. Both groups consumed similar amounts of salt, fat, cholesterol, caffeine, and alcohol. Mean age, mean body weight, and male sex were similar along with other risk factors.

Singh found that increased intake of soluble dietary fiber and guava fruit was associated with a significant decrease in serum total cholesterol (7.9 percent) and triglycerides (7.0 percent), and an insignificant increase in HDL-cholesterol (4.6 percent), with a mild increase in the ratio of total cholesterol/HDL-cholesterol. He concludes, "It is possible that an increased consumption of guava fruit can cause a substantial reduction in blood pressure and blood lipids with a lack of decrease in HDL-cholesterol due to its high potassium and soluble fiber content."

# 21

## Diets for Hypoglycemia

The word "hypoglycemia" simply means "low blood sugar," yet the number of people diagnosed as hypoglycemic has grown to enormous proportions in the last few years — more than 20 million in the U.S. alone. And while the condition itself is not life-threatening, the symptoms can make the lives of sufferers miserable.

They may include general weakness, fatigue, inability to concentrate, listlessness, butterfly sensations in the stomach, subnormal temperature, rapid heart rate, shakiness and palpitations, sweating, and apprehension. As someone has described hypoglycemia, it is almost as if you have just been hit by a train.

Hypoglycemia is taken seriously and should be corrected as soon as possible. Not only is it a forerunner of diabetes and Addison's disease, it can also lead to other disorders such as cancer, heart disease, and brain dysfunction (due to reduced supplies of glucose to the brain). The only way to treat this condition is with diet.

The symptoms and causes of hypoglycemia vary with almost every individual. It can, however, be defined in simplest terms as the result of the failure of the stabilizing mechanisms of the body to maintain a proper blood sugar (glucose) level after a person has eaten. By way of comparison, when a normal person eats a simple refined carbohydrate such as white sugar, the blood level of sugar rises. The pancreas then secretes the hormone insulin, which soon brings down blood sugar to the fasting level. When the hypoglycemic person consumes the same amount of white sugar, however, the pancreas overreacts and secretes so much insulin into the blood that sugar is removed too rapidly, creating a glucose deficit. Most cases of hypoglycemia are usually caused by an excessive intake of refined carbohydrates — such as sugar, alcohol, and enriched white flour — over

## SYMPTOMS OF HYPOGLYCEMIA ATTACKS*

Symptoms of hypoglycemic attacks include:

- Inability to think straight, irritability, grouchiness
- Sweating, anxiety, trembling, fast heartbeat, or muscle weakness
- Hunger
- Headache
- Sleepiness

Hypoglycemic attacks can come on very suddenly, and people experiencing them should immediately eat some form of carbohydrate (sugar). For this reason, many hypoglycemics carry glucose tablets or sugar cubes with them at all times and take one at the first sign of a reaction. Hypoglycemics should contact their physician immediately if the attacks continue to occur.

*Source: Carol Barnett, *Life with Diabetes: Diabetes Defined* (Ann Arbor, Mich.: Michigan Diabetes Research Center, University of Michigan, 1987), pp. 15–17.

the course of many months or years by someone who is genetically predisposed to having the disorder.

Hypoglycemics need to regulate their blood glucose, keep daily records, and be able to instantly recognize and treat hypoglycemic reactions (or low blood glucose levels), which can occur if they are taking insulin or oral medications. Hypoglycemic attacks often occur when insulin action is at its peak, during or after strenuous exercise, or when a meal is delayed.

If a person starts feeling any symptoms or thinks his or her blood glucose levels may be too low, physicians advise patients to check blood level with a blood glucose test strip. If blood glucose is less than 70 milligrams per 100 deciliters of blood, one is probably experiencing a hypoglycemic reaction.

## CONTROLLING HYPOGLYCEMIA DIET

Dr. Stanley Mirsky is a distinguished specialist in metabolic disorders. He is a board member of Joslin Diabetes Center, Inc. His diet for hypoglycemia is outlined in his book *Controlling Diabetes the Easy Way,* coauthored with the health writer Joan Heilman.

## Basic Nutritional Approach

Dr. Mirsky argues that the only way to treat hypoglycemia, which he defines in general as "a blood sugar level below 50 milligrams that coincides with other symptoms," is with diet. Except in very occasional cases, no other treatments or medications are of any value, he claims, including injections and megavitamins.

Mirsky has found that the best diet for hypoglycemics is the same one he recommends for diabetics. This diet does not focus on restricting calories, and has only one rule: dieters must avoid all refined sugar and eat 40 to 50 grams of complex carbohydrates at every meal to keep their blood sugar levels within normal ranges. (Those engaging in strenuous exercise may need to consume more.)

This carbohydrate intake amounts to 50 to 60 percent of daily food, approximately the normal American diet. The rest of the menu should include protein, fats, and water in whatever proportions dieters wish. If weight reduction is not a goal, they may eat as much of these foods as they wish. People who are also trying to lose weight can moderate their calories by simply adjusting their meat portions. Mirsky suggests that hypoglycemics who adopt his diet may also wish to incorporate the food exchange lists of the American Diabetes Association to help them count calories.

## Recommended Foods

Mirsky suggests that the best foods for hypoglycemics are complex carbohydrates such as grains, starches, fruits, vegetables, and legumes. These foods are sources of high energy, contain less than half the calories of fatty foods and the same as protein, and often contain important vitamins, minerals, and fiber. Another advantage is that they help dieters feel full and more satisfied.

Additionally, complex carbohydrates are also absorbed much more slowly into the bloodstream than simple carbohydrates. If eaten in moderate amounts, they do not raise blood sugar to abnormal levels. Mirsky suggests that dieters who remain within his guidelines will maintain steady blood sugar levels of 199 milligrams percent two hours after a meal, which is just where they should remain.

To assist dieters in obtaining the 40 to 50 grams of carbohydrates per meal, Mirsky provides extensive food lists in his book, and suggests that they choose 10-gram fruits and desserts, 15-gram starches, 3 percent vegetables, and 6 percent vegetables.

*Vegetables.* Because vegetables contain important carbohydrates, Mirsky recommends incorporating those in the diet that contain three grams of carbohydrate per 100 grams of weight. Consisting primarily of water and nondigestible fiber, they influence blood sugar levels only slightly, in most cases, and may be eaten raw. If cooked, they should be limited to one cup per portion.

Examples include fresh asparagus, lettuces, bamboo shoots, bean sprouts, mushrooms, broccoli, parsley, cabbage, radishes, cauliflower, rhubarb, celery, sauerkraut, cucumbers, spinach, eggplant, squash, endive, Swiss chard, green or wax beans, turnips, green peppers, watercress, and zucchini.

Six percent vegetables, which have six grams of carbohydrate for every 100 grams of weight, should be restricted to 1/2 cup per meals. Examples include artichokes, pumpkin, Brussels sprouts, red peppers, carrots, tomatoes, green peas, kale, turnips, okra, winter squash, and onions.

*Fiber.* Mirsky feels strongly that fiber — indigestible, unabsorbable plant material that leaves the digestive system in much the same form it went in with virtually no caloric value — plays a number of vital roles in the digestive process.

For this reason, he recommends that fiber foods (whether eaten raw, cooked, frozen, or canned) be included in the 40 to 50 grams of carbohydrate allotted per meal. Examples include whole-grain breads and cereals, nuts and seeds, vegetables (see above section on vegetables), fruits such as strawberries, blueberries, grapefruit, and raw pears, and leguminous dried beans such as haricot, kidney, soy, lentils, or chickpeas. (For a more detailed description of Mirsky's recommendations about fiber foods for those with hypoglycemia and diabetes, see pages 304 to 308.)

## Restricted Foods

Foods that contain simple carbohydrates — the monosaccharides — must be avoided. Providing many calories but very little nutrition, these foods are too quickly absorbed into the bloodstream.

The simple sugars include candy, pastries and cookies, sugar-coated cereals, raisins, condensed milk, regular chewing gum and soft drinks, dried fruits, honey, all types of sugar, jams and jellies, sweet wine, marmalade and preserves, syrups, and molasses.

Other foods that hypoglycemics should avoid because they raise blood sugar levels too quickly include apples and apple juice, pineapples and pineapple juice, gelatin desserts, processed yogurt with fruit or flavorings, grape juice, instant breakfasts or "diet" bars, sherbet, prune juice, maple-sugar-flavored bacon or sausage, and yams and sweet potatoes.

## Daily Meal Planning

Mirsky suggests that the only way hypoglycemics can successfully adhere to the recommended 40 to 50 grams of complex carbohydrates per meal is to remember the equivalent of two slices of bread. (Dieters need this slowly absorbed carbohydrate to carry them over to their next meal or snack.) Two slices of bread are the equivalent of 1 cup of rice or pasta, 2 medium potatoes, 15 French fries, 1 English muffin, 2/3 cup of corn, or 1 cup of cooked cereal.

As long as hypoglycemics eat these equivalents at each meal and consume the rest of their calories in proteins and fats, they can go anywhere, eat in any restaurant, and be perfectly safe.

Hypoglycemics following Mirsky's guidelines are further counseled not to save carbohydrates from one meal to another, but rather to eat their full allotment at each meal. They should also spread out their carbohydrate intake throughout the day to avoid high or low extremes in their blood sugar levels.

Finally, Mirsky urges dieters to keep their meals well balanced and varied, eat at specified times, and never skip or delay a meal or a planned snack.

## Sample Menus

Mirsky does not restrict calories per se, and encourages dieters to be creative in their menu planning, as long as they avoid simple sugars and consume approximately 40 to 50 grams of complex carbohydrates (with at least 30 grams as starch) per meal.

*Breakfast.* For breakfast, Mirsky suggests one of the following: three ounces orange juice, 8 ounces tomato juice, or 1/2 cantaloupe. This accounts for 10 grams of carbohydrate. Then, adding another 30 grams, dieters can choose among the following:

- Two slices toast, two halves English muffin, two small corn muffins, two four-inch pancakes, or two slices of French toast. These total 15 grams each or 30 grams in all.
- Coffee or tea (preferably decaffeinated).

If hypoglycemics prefer cereal, they can substitute 3/4 cup (15 grams) plain cold cereal (the amount in the small packages) for the 30 grams of bread, and add 1 cup of milk (12 grams). For 3/4 cup of hot cereal, which totals 22 grams, they can add 1/2 cup milk.

People should feel free to add eggs or bacon, says Mirsky, unless they are concerned about weight or cholesterol reduction.

*Lunch.* For lunch, dieters might choose:

- Three ounces of meat (0 carbohydrate)
- Salad with lettuce and 1/2 cup tomatoes (6 grams carbohydrate), with French dressing (1 tablespoon or 3 1/2 grams)
- Two slices of bread (30 grams)
- 1/2 cantaloupe (10 grams)

*Dinner.* For dinner, dieters could select:

- Three to six ounces of chicken (0 carbohydrate)
- One ear of corn (30 grams)
- 1/2 cup of peas (6 grams)
- 1/2 grapefruit (10 grams)

A 10-gram fruit should always be included at dinner. And a piece of sponge, marble, or pound cake can be substituted for the bread allowance on special occasions, if the cake weighs the same as a slice of bread.

## Vitamin and Mineral Supplements

Although his balanced diet generally provides the RDAs of essential vitamins and minerals, Mirsky admits that taking supplements may be helpful for certain individuals. Vitamin B6 supplements, for example, are believed to increase glucose tolerance. Mirsky also recommends adding to the daily menu 50 milligrams of vitamin C, vitamin E (to improve circulation and help prevent some degenerative processes), calcium supplements (for anyone who does not drink milk, eat milk products, or get regular exercise), and zinc. He states that except in the price, there is no difference between natural and synthetic vitamins.

## Alcohol

Hypoglycemics, according to Mirsky, do not have to give up alcohol, although it is important to be a sensible drinker. In fact, he notes, alcohol in moderation may help raise high-density lipoproteins ("good" cholesterol) and decrease chances of atherosclerosis in some persons.

Mirsky offers the following guidelines for dieters who drink alcohol:

- Never drink on an empty stomach.
- Never have more than two drinks, even with food. Dieters may not be able to recognize a reaction or distinguish it from intoxication.
- Avoid sweet wines, stout, cider, ginger beer, port, liqueurs, and cordials, as well as sweet mixers such as tonic, unless they are sugar-free.
- A drink before dinner or a glass or two of dry wine with dinner is considered permissible for most hypoglycemics. Acceptable choices include Scotch, rye, whiskey, bourbon, tequila, brandy, rum, gin, and vodka.
- Remember to account for carbohydrates in the drinks consumed (eight ounces of beer contain about 10 grams, for example) against the total allotment for that meal, and omit other foods such as a slice of bread or a fruit.

## THE LOW BLOOD SUGAR DIET

Dr. Clement G. Martin is a hypoglycemia specialist whose diet appears in *Low Blood Sugar: The Hidden Menace of Hypoglycemia*.

According to Martin, hypoglycemia most often develops in people who are overweight or who slowly but steadily gain weight (which places a strain on the body's mechanisms that handle the digestion and use of food), and those who are predisposed to diabetes. Fatigue, either constant or in swings, is one of the most prominent symptoms. Fortunately, he states, he has helped hundreds of hypoglycemics reverse their condition with his diet.

## Basic Nutritional Approach

Martin's diet is high in protein and low in carbohydrates. The third element, fat, is usually found in the foods eaten as protein, and will therefore be automatically taken care of with protein intake.

The basic problem hypoglycemics have, claims Martin, is the need for quick energy, which is usually obtained through intake of carbohydrates or alcohol. Yet both of these dietary substances cause temporary sporadic increases of glucose in the blood which, in turn, result in the body's production of an excess of insulin. This creates a vicious cycle that Martin's diet — "which you must adhere to very rigidly and not moderate with your own desires at all," he warns — is designed to break.

## Recommended Foods

All fruits and vegetables are permissible. Fruit may be eaten cooked, canned, or raw, with or without cream, but without sugar. Lettuce, mushrooms, and nuts may be consumed as often as desired. Any unsweetened fruit or vegetable juice (except grape and prune juice) is allowed. Coffee substitutes and decaffeinated coffee or weak tea are permissible. If sweetening is needed, a sugar substitute, saccharin, or Sucaryl should be used instead of sugar.

Desserts can consist of any fresh fruit, unsweetened gelatin, or low-calorie gelatin and junket. Permissible beverages include club soda, dry ginger ale, and low-calorie sodas. Martin identifies the following foods as acceptable:

- Asparagus, broccoli, Brussels sprouts, cabbage, cauliflower, carrots, celery, corn, cucumbers, eggplant, lima beans, onions, peas, radishes, sauerkraut, squash, string beans, turnips, and tomatoes.
- Apples, apricots, berries, grapefruit, melon, oranges, peaches, pears, pineapples, and tangerines. Fruits may be eaten either cooked or raw, but sugar is not permissible — either added or as an ingredient in canned fruits.
- Lettuce, mushrooms, and nuts may be consumed as often as needed, and are ideal as snacks. However, they should be eaten in small amounts — no more than half an ounce at any one time.
- Any unsweetened fruit or vegetable juice except grape or prune juice.
- Weak tea, decaffeinated coffee, or coffee substitutes, sweetened with any sugar substitutes.

- Fruit desserts and unsweetened, low-calorie gelatin.
- Alcoholic and soft drinks such as club soda, low-calorie ginger ale, whiskey, and other distilled liquors.

## Eliminated Foods

Coffee, tea, and caffeine-rich soft drinks must be avoided — almost totally at first — because they stimulate production of excessive amounts of insulin. (If withdrawal symptoms such as a headache or feelings of weakness result, Martin suggests judiciously taking two aspirin tablets to relieve them.)

Alcohol in the form of wines, cocktails, and beer is not permitted, although one highball during the day made from distilled liquor is acceptable. And while Martin claims it is not necessary to stop smoking entirely, he recommends a considerable reduction — down to ten cigarettes a day or less.

Other eliminated foods include:

- Sugar, candy, cake, pie, pastries, sweet custards, puddings, ice cream, and all other sweets.
- Potatoes, rice, grapes, raisins, plums, figs, dates, and bananas.
- Spaghetti, macaroni, and noodles.

## The Rigid Diet: Two-Week Plan

This diet, called the Harris Diet because it was first developed by Dr. S. Harris, who first detected hypoglycemia, should be followed for several weeks to allow the body to stabilize. Quick-energy foods such as starches, caffeine, and alcohol are the primary substances to be avoided.

*Daily Meal Planning.* The object of this rigid diet (which need only last two weeks in most cases) is to give hypoglycemics a level intake of energy. Crucial to its success, Martin notes, is the proper mid-meal snacks: dieters must have them available or their symptoms may reappear. If one cocktail a day is desired, it should be consumed before either lunch or dinner.

**On arising**
A medium orange, four ounces of juice, or half a grapefruit
**Breakfast**
Fruit or four ounces of juice, one egg (with or without two slices of

**363**

ham or bacon), one slice of bread or toast with butter, and a beverage

**Two hours after breakfast**
Four ounces of juice

**Lunch**
Fish, cheese, meat or eggs, salad, a large serving of lettuce, tomato, or apple salad with mayonnaise or French dressing, vegetables if desired, one slice of any bread or toast, and a beverage

**Three hours after lunch**
Four ounces of milk

**One hour before dinner**
Four ounces of milk

**Dinner**
Soup if desired (not thickened), vegetable, a liberal portion of meat, fish, or poultry, one slice of bread, dessert, and a beverage

**Two to three hours after dinner**
Four ounces of milk

**Every two hours until bedtime**
Four ounces of milk or a small handful of nuts

## The Final Diet

After a few weeks on this diet, which is fairly close to a normal diet, Martin suggests that hypoglycemics may be able to go back to a fully normal diet. However, he cautions, three absolute and permanent modifications remain.

- Never, at any time, consume an undue amount of sweets, candy, or desserts.
- Avoid caffeine completely, whether from coffee, tea, or colas.
- A bedtime snack of one of the types described below is crucial each and every night.

**Daily Menu Planning**
**Breakfast**
One serving of fruit or juice
Cereal (dry or cooked) with milk or cream
Optional: one egg and two slices of ham or bacon
One slice of bread or toast, heavily buttered
Beverage

**Lunch**

Meat, fish, cheese, or eggs

Salad: lettuce, tomato, mixed greens; with mayonnaise or other oily dressing

Vegetables, buttered if desired

One slice of bread or toast, heavily buttered

Dessert: crackers and cheese

Beverage

**Mid-afternoon snack**

Eight ounces of milk

**Dinner**

Soup if desired (not thickened with flour)

A liberal portion of meat, fish, or poultry

Two servings of vegetables

One serving of potatoes, rice, noodles, spaghetti, or macaroni

One slice of bread, if desired

Dessert: crackers and cheese

Beverage

**Bedtime snack**

Milk, crackers and cheese, and a sandwich or fruit

## Vitamin and Mineral Supplements

According to Martin, if a diet consists of too many canned, frozen, or preserved foods, hypoglycemics will have to take vitamin and mineral supplements. He recommends a low dose or "maintenance" type of vitamin-mineral capsule once a day, with meals, is probably the best insurance hypoglycemics can have of nutritional adequacy.

## Physical Activity

Dr. Martin considers regular exercise desirable and necessary — particularly rhythmic activities combined with an emphasis on adequate breathing such as walking, jogging, swimming, running, skating, and skiing.

However, he cautions that hypoglycemics should not start an exercise regimen while they are following his first rigid diet. And he warns dieters to discontinue their exercise program if they become shaky, excessively sweaty, or nervous. These are symptoms, he notes, that more sugar is being burned up than their bodies can replace quickly.

Martin recommends that hypoglycemics exercise on a daily basis, with a goal of 10 to 15 minutes, although 30 minutes is even better. When beginning an exercise program, he advises that 5 minutes of interval training are adequate for the first week. This can be increased during the second week to 7 or 8 minutes, and to 10 minutes during the third week.

Exercise is just as important to any diet routine as food, Martin asserts. A minimum exercise program such as the one he outlines will greatly speed up the return of hypoglycemics to normal, he claims, and give them the full level of mental and physical functioning to which they are entitled.

## Behavior Modification

Nutrition and diet, Martin believes, are crucial to treating hypoglycemia, but diet alone cannot be successful. Dieters need to feed themselves "mentally" with positive thoughts as well. He concludes that his non-weight-producing diet, in which people consume small balanced meals and snacks throughout the day, can pour essential new vitality into their bodies and give them a new mental outlook that prevents them from relapsing into old dietary habits.

## THE AIROLA HYPOGLYCEMIC DIET

Paavo Airola, Ph.D., N.D., was a nutritionist, naturopathic physician, educator, and award-winning author. He was a visiting lecturer at many medical schools, including the Stanford University Medical School. Now deceased, his diet is included in *Hypoglycemia: A Better Approach.*

## Basic Nutritional Approach

Airola strongly critiqued the high-protein, low-carbohydrate diet. While such a diet can control the symptoms of hypoglycemia, patients complained of fatigue, constipation, headaches, skin disorders, and physical and mental sluggishness, Airola claimed. Also, on a prolonged basis, he believed, such a high-protein diet can be extremely harmful, and may contribute to the development of arthritis, cardiovascular disorders, osteoporosis, periodontal disease, and even cancer.

The "safer and more effective dietary program" that Airola recommends is a low-protein, high-natural-carbohydrate diet that controls the symptoms of hypoglycemia, helps correct the condition, and eventually facilitates a complete restoration of health. It does so, stated Airola, by normalizing the functions of the pancreas, adrenals, and other vital organs and glands, and by contributing to the betterment of the total health and well-being of the patient.

## Recommended Foods

The basic diet for hypoglycemics, according to Airola, should be made up of three food groups: grains, seeds, and nuts; vegetables; and fruits.

*Grains, Seeds, and Nuts.* These are the most important and potent health-building foods of all, Airola contends, and their nutritional value is unsurpassed. Eaten mostly raw and sprouted, but also cooked, they contain all the nutrients essential for human growth, health maintenance, and prevention of disease.

Airola feels that sprouting increases the nutritional value of seeds and grains, and recommends that hypoglycemics eat as many sprouts as possible — wheat, mung beans, alfalfa seeds, and soybeans among them.

Not only are seeds, grains, and nuts excellent sources of protein, but they are also the best natural sources of essential unsaturated fatty acids. They are an excellent source of lecithin (a key substance for the proper functioning of the brain, nerves, glands, and arteries), as well as important vitamins, minerals, and trace elements.

Airola particularly recommends sesame seeds (an excellent source of calcium), brown rice, millet, buckwheat, flaxseeds (which contain essential fatty acids), chia seeds, pumpkin seeds, almonds, peanuts, and hazelnuts.

All seeds and nuts, Airola counsels, should be eaten raw, while grains should either be cooked (as in breads or cereals) or sprouted.

*Vegetables.* Vegetables, which Airola ranks as the next most important food group in his diet, are "extraordinary" sources of minerals, enzymes, and vitamins. Among those he considers specifically beneficial are leafy green vegetables, garlic, onions, avocados (which actually suppress insulin production and therefore lower blood sugar levels), string beans, and Jerusalem artichokes.

Airola recommends that most vegetables should be eaten raw in the form of green salad. Others such as potatoes, yams, squashes, spinach, rhubarb, asparagus, cauliflower, cabbage, and green beans should be cooked, steamed, or baked.

*Fruits.* Airola ranks fruits last in importance in his diet because they contain high amounts of quickly assimilated sugars that can cause a rapid increase in blood sugar levels if consumed in quantity. Fruit juices, especially, must be consumed in strict moderation, he warns, and in small quantities at a time.

Preferable fruits for hypoglycemics are those that are not excessively sweet, such as sour apples, cherries, strawberries, papayas, grapefruit, lemons, limes, and pineapples. Dried fruits, grapes, grape juice, and dates should be largely avoided. The best way to eat fruit, contends Airola, is raw, in season, and preferably in the morning for breakfast.

He specifically recommends lemons for hypoglycemics because they stimulate the liver, an organ that helps maintain a proper sugar balance in the body.

*Milk and Milk Products.* Airola states that milk and milk products can play an especially important role in the hypoglycemic diet, particularly when meat is not eaten, as a source of vegetable protein, minerals (particularly calcium), and essential fatty acids. However, he recommends only uncontaminated, raw, unpasteurized milk from healthy animals, such as that sold in health food stores.

The best way for hypoglycemics to consume milk, he explains, is in its soured form (which is very easily assimilated): yogurt, kefir, acidophilus milk, buttermilk, or plain clobbered milk. Natural, cultured cheeses are also recommended, as is cottage cheese, especially homemade kvark.

*Cold-Pressed Vegetable Oils.* Airola recommends moderate quantities of high-quality, fresh, cold-pressed, crude, unrefined, unheated, and unprocessed vegetable oil as a regular addition to the diet. However, he warns that these oils are extremely perishable.

Airola favors olive and sesame seed oil, but cautions that vegetable oils should never be used for cooking or frying.

*Honey.* Natural, raw, unrefined, unfiltered, and unheated honey is the only sweetener allowed in Airola's diet, but it should be used only moderately — one teaspoon a day, one-half teaspoon at a time — as a sweetening for herb teas or food.

*Brewer's Yeast.* Airola considers brewer's yeast an extremely useful supplementary food in the hypoglycemic diet. It is an excellent source of high-quality proteins and B-complex "anti-stress" vitamins. In addition, he describes it as an "unmatched source" of the trace minerals that are specifically involved in sugar metabolism: selenium, iron, zinc, and chromium.

Airola recommends using brewer's yeast as a snack food mixed, for example, with pineapple or grapefruit juice. He counsels that it should not be taken during or immediately before or after meals, as it requires a plentiful supply of hydrochloric acid to be effectively digested.

*Water.* As Airola emphasizes, hypoglycemics should make sure to incorporate naturally mineralized or distilled water (augmented with plain sea water or sea water concentrate) into their diet. Not only are minerals in natural water well digested and assimilated by the body, but natural water is a good source of chromium — a trace mineral that is essential for proper sugar metabolism.

## Eliminated Foods

The following foods and drinks should be completely excluded from the diet:

- white sugar and everything made with it, including ice cream, pastries, cookies, candies, breakfast cereals, soft drinks, and commercially baked breads
- other forms of sugar, such as brown, raw, turbinado, and fruit sugars. Honey can be used as a sugar substitute, but only in strict moderation
- white flour and all white flour products, including bread, packaged breakfast cereals, cookies, pastries, pies, and gravies

---

### DR. AIROLA'S HEALTH-PROMOTING HABITS

- Eat only when hungry.
- Eat slowly in a relaxed, unhurried atmosphere.
- Eat several small meals during the day rather than two or three large meals.
- Do not mix raw fruits and raw vegetables in the same meal.
- When protein-rich foods are eaten with other foods, eat protein-rich foods first.

---

- all soft drinks (even sugar-free soft drinks), root beers, and all juice drinks
- coffee and caffeine-containing soft drinks such as colas
- alcohol and tobacco
- excessive amounts of sweet fruit or vegetable juices, including carrot, grape, apple, and orange juices, all of which contain large amounts of sugar
- all processed, canned, refined, and denatured supermarket-sold foods, including TV dinners and breakfast cereals
- an excess of protein, especially meat. While a moderate amount of meat or fish is allowed, perhaps once a week, it is not necessary that it be included in the food plan.

### Daily Meal Planning

Airola's suggested menu for a daily diet consists of three main meals and three to four snacks eaten between meals throughout the day. In most cases, he does not specify the quantity of food to be consumed, but rather suggests that people consume sufficient amounts to satisfy their hunger. If weight is a concern, dieters should simply eat smaller portions. All vitamin and mineral supplements should be taken with the three main meals. No liquids, including water, juice, or tea, should be consumed with meals, unless specified.

### Vitamin and Mineral Supplements

Airola's hypoglycemic diet should be supplemented with the following adult daily doses of vitamins, minerals, and other supplements. Airola recommends dividing the supplements equally and taking them with the three main meals. Also, if at all possible, dieters should use only 100 percent natural brands.

- Vitamin C: 2,000 to 3,000 milligrams
- 100 percent natural B-complex vitamins made from yeast concentrate: four to six tablets
- Vitamin B6: 50 to 100 milligrams
- Pantothenic acid: 100 to 200 milligrams
- Vitamin E, natural, mixed tocopherols: 600 to 1,200 I.U.
- Vitamin B12: 25 to 50 micrograms
- Magnesium-calcium supplement: two to three tablets

- Bone meal: three tablets or 1/2 teaspoon powder
- Potassium citrate: 300 to 500 milligrams
- Vitamin A and D supplements: one or two capsules (10,000 units of A and 400 units of D per capsule)
- Brewer's yeast: three to four tablespoons of powder or the equivalent in tablets
- Lecithin: two teaspoons of granules
- Kelp: two tablets or 1/2 teaspoon of granules
- Sea water: one to two tablespoons a day or 1/2 teaspoon of concentrate

## Botanical Supplements

On the basis of his own research, Airola suggests that the following herbs (most commonly taken in the form of herb teas) are beneficial in the treatment of hypoglycemia. He makes no recommendations, however, in terms of dosages.

- Juniper cedar berries (*Juniperus sabina pinaceae*)
- Capalchi, or Copalquin (*Croton niveus*), also known as Quina Blanca in Mexico
- Licorice root (*Glycyrrhiza glabra*)
- Mexican wild yam (*Dioscorea villosa*)
- Golden seal (*Hydrastis*)
- Lobelia (*Lobelia inflata*)

Other beneficial herbs, Airola claims, which are of more general value but are also useful for hypoglycemia, include dandelion (root and leaves), garlic, horsetail, American helebore, chicory, wahoo, and cornsilk.

## Physical Activity

Dr. Airola, who emphasizes that oxygen is the most important nutrient that every organ and cell in the body needs, counsels that the only sensible solution is to "get out in the fresh air and exercise." Furthermore, he claims, "if you do not exercise regularly and vigorously, you will never enjoy good health."

Airola warns, however, that hypoglycemics must not overexert themselves when they first take up exercise. Rather, they should eventually graduate to walking and jogging intermittently. Also recommended are gardening, yoga, tennis, basketball, swimming, bike riding, and other vigorous exercises and/or games.

## RECENT RESEARCH

*Alternative Medicine: The Definitive Guide* recommends the following vitamins and minerals to help stabilize blood glucose levels and prevent hypoglycemia: niacinamide, pantothenic acids, adrenal glandular, vitamin C with bioflavonoids, vitamin B complex, vitamin B6, zinc, protein supplements such as amino acids (especially alanine), calcium, magnesium, and multitrace minerals. People should consult with their physician or nutritionist, however, before adding any of these supplements to their diet.

The same book also suggests that botanical medicines such as burdock, licorice, and dandelion may be beneficial for some hypoglycemics. Again, they should be only taken at home under appropriate professional supervision.

Balch and Balch report in *Prescription for Nutritional Healing* that injections of B complex, as well as pyridoxine and liver, have proven helpful in treating hypoglycemia in clinical trials. Injections, they counsel, should be administered twice weekly for three months, then decreased to once a week for two months or more. Some hypoglycemics have found fasting once a month with a series of lemon juice enemas to be beneficial. They note that in order to prevent a low blood sugar reaction while fasting, one should take spirulina or protein powder supplements.

# 22

## Diets for Irritable Bowel Syndrome

Irritable bowel syndrome (IBS) is a chronic disorder that may be prevalent in as many as 22 million Americans, according to *The Mayo Clinic Diet Manual.* Reportedly afflicting twice as many women as men, IBS ranks close to the common cold as a leading cause of absenteeism from work due to illness. It has been described as the most common chronic gastrointestinal disorder in the Western world, and accounts for 40 to 70 percent of referrals to gastroenterologists.

People suffering from IBS usually complain of abdominal pain and changes in their bowel habits; they may also experience excessive gas, bloating, indigestion, constipation or diarrhea, or an alternation between the latter two (which makes elimination extremely painful). Symptoms usually occur after a meal and may be temporarily relieved by bowel evacuation. Other symptoms include dysmenorrhea, nausea, cramping, and fatigue.

IBS is not life threatening, and apparently it does not lead to other serious diseases. However, it can cause considerable discomfort, can be extremely debilitating, and can interfere with work and other activities. IBS affects all age groups, particularly adults between the ages of 20 and 50.

According to *The Mayo Clinic Diet Manual,* IBS may be caused by food intolerances, significant gut motility disorders of the small and/or large intestine, stress, and psychiatric disorders. Most people suffering from this condition have irregular muscular contractions of the intestines that interfere with the movement of waste material through their bowels. The result is often an excess of mucus and toxins in the bowels and the bloodstream.

Even though surveys have indicated that between 8 and 24 percent of Americans experience some IBS symptoms, fewer than 50 percent actually present their complaints to physicians. According to Dr. Phillip Mac of

Stanford University, writing in the introduction to Deralee Scanlon's book *The Wellness Book of I.B.S.*, the financial cost of IBS, as well as the cost of suffering and loss of quality of life, is staggering. Treatment can involve expensive medical testing, an overwhelming amount of medication to control symptoms, and many visits to physicians. Yet, according to Mac, many people suffering from IBS can manage the condition by being aware of the important role that food and diet play.

Other experts agree that with proper attention to diet, stress management, and prescription medications (if needed), most people with IBS can keep their symptoms under control.

## RELIEF FROM IBS DIET

Elaine Fantle Shimberg, a member of the American Medical Writers Association, suffered from IBS and developed a treatment regimen to relieve her symptoms. This regimen is presented in her book *Relief from IBS*.

### Basic Nutritional Approach

Shimberg contends that while food doesn't cause IBS, eating can be a trigger for its symptoms because it induces movement in the colon — called gastrocolic reflex. For those who have IBS, this motor response not only continues after eating but also gradually gets stronger.

She notes that although studies have thus far shown no specific food intolerance unique to IBS patients, about 20 to 40 percent of them have a lactose intolerance — an inability to digest lactose, the main sugar found in milk and other dairy products. In fact, she states, approximately 30 percent of those people who see a physician with symptoms of IBS discover they have a lactose intolerance.

Shimberg therefore suggests that IBS sufferers first eliminate all milk and dairy products (including cheese and butter) to determine if their symptoms subside. Dairy products, she cautions, may also hide in bread, cakes, cookies, and many ready-to-eat foods, so all labels should be checked carefully.

Other foods known to trigger symptoms in many IBS patients include wheat, corn, citrus fruits, onions, beans, Brussels sprouts, cabbage, and fatty foods such as pork, bacon, and fried foods.

And, although fiber is important in treating IBS, some people react badly to extra fiber, especially if they attempt to add it too quickly to their diet. Shimberg believes that any discomfort associated with the additional fiber (such as gas) tends to dissipate in four to six weeks, when the intestine becomes accustomed to the extra bulk.

She asserts that laxative overuse is a major trigger of IBS symptoms, along with antibiotics, high blood pressure medications, nicotine, narcotics, diuretics, and alcohol.

## Food Diary

The triggering of IBS symptoms by particular foods is a highly individualized problem, Shimberg admits, and is further complicated by the fact that a specific food may trigger symptoms only when other internal or external stimuli (such as fatigue or stress) are present.

For this reason, she recommends keeping a detailed "detection diary" in which each day's diet, mood, fatigue level, and other variables such as medications, mealtime locations, and even any added spices are recorded. These should be filled out at mealtimes, as well as when sufferers feel any symptoms, in order to help people with IBS identify and eliminate those foods and situations that present problems for them.

Shimberg states that for most people IBS is irreversible — they must monitor symptoms for life. However, as with all chronic disorders, cure is not really the issue, she claims. Rather, it is the gaining of further knowledge and the development of coping strategies that produce a sense of personal control over the condition.

## Recommended Foods: Fiber

Because her book focuses on how stress and psychological factors, along with diet, contribute to IBS, Shimberg does not recommend specific foods or food groups. She does, however, agree with most experts that daily fiber intake is absolutely essential to help regulate bowel function.

Eating bran, especially unprocessed bran or "miller's bran," is an easy way to increase fiber intake. She also suggests that IBS sufferers consume high-fiber foods for snacks, including sesame bread sticks, Fig Newtons, date or prune bars, breads, and oatmeal-raisin cookies.

Recommended high-fiber foods include:

- Vegetables: broccoli, carrots, cabbage, beets, Brussels sprouts, celery, corn, cauliflower, and potatoes
- Fruits: prunes, apricots, raisins, blackberries, strawberries, pears, oranges, bananas, peaches, cantaloupes, and apples

- Additional sources: cereals (especially those containing bran, wheat, and oats), nuts, brown rice, popcorn, peas, lentils, kidney beans, dark breads such as whole-wheat and pumpernickel, and graham crackers

## Eliminated Foods

According to Shimberg, most people with IBS tend to have more troublesome symptoms after eating fatty foods, including those that are greasy or fried. This is because the hormonal system releases chemicals to help digest the fat. These chemicals, particularly cholecystokinin (known as CCK), trigger additional abnormal movement in the colon. For this reason, she suggests avoiding them.

## Eating Habits

The physical and psychological environment in which IBS sufferers eat is extremely important. Many IBS sufferers, for example, report experiencing pain, bloating, and diarrhea shortly after eating any meal, but especially breakfast, regardless of what they have eaten. In addition, many admit that breakfast is often a "meal on the run." Shimberg therefore suggests that IBS dieters get up thirty minutes earlier in the morning and practice a relaxation technique before breakfast.

*Regulating Mealtimes.* Shimberg warns that eating at odd hours places additional stress on the digestive tract. She advises IBS sufferers to eat meals at the same time each day, especially on the weekends and during emotionally straining holidays.

## Professional Therapy

Shimberg rightly cautions people about diagnosing their own nutritional requirements and recommends that all IBS sufferers consult with a physician or local hospital for the name of a registered dietitian or qualified nutritionist. These trained professionals can help analyze people's detection diaries and advise them on how to avoid problem foods or situations, add fiber, and decrease fat while still enjoying a balanced diet.

## Medications and Other Therapies

While Shimberg advises that it's always a good rule to try to use as little medication as possible, she concedes that, because IBS is a chronic disorder, sufferers sometimes need medication to ease their discomfort. Drug therapy avenues currently available include anticholinergic prescription agents and other antispasmodics for pain, antidepressants for the depression that often accompanies IBS, antidiarrheal drugs for diarrhea, and bran and commercial bulking agents for constipation.

Shimberg notes that while physicians disagree as to the overall effectiveness of medications in treating IBS, most agree that short-term use when discomfort is most acute can be useful.

*Peppermint Oil.* Oil from the peppermint plant, coated and in capsule form to prevent its being absorbed before reaching the colon, is often given to IBS sufferers, particularly in Europe. According to Shimberg, the capsules inhibit gastrointestinal smooth muscle activity and consequently reduce both pain and gas. Available at many health food stores, they seem to have few side effects, but should be taken only under a physician's guidance.

## Physical Activity

Shimberg strongly recommends exercise for IBS dieters, primarily because it relieves stress and reduces the fatigue which she believes contribute to the disorder. She specifically recommends aerobics, basketball and baseball, cycling and climbing, dancing, fencing, golf and gymnastics, hiking, handball and racquetball, swimming, water skiing, tennis, volleyball, and walking. She emphasizes that dieters should exercise at least three times during the week for twenty to forty minutes. It's a good idea to undergo a physical examination before starting the program and to vary one's form of exercise to prevent boredom.

## Behavioral Modification

Shimberg outlines a comprehensive behavioral modification program for controlling some of the factors that trigger IBS symptoms and relieving them. "Since IBS symptoms are triggered by stress and emotions," she writes, "you're obviously going to have to develop ways to reduce stress so IBS doesn't affect you so greatly."

Methods she describes to cope with stress and emotional situations include making a personal commitment to create certain lifestyle changes, keeping progress charts or a journal, visualizing success, thinking positive thoughts, focusing on feeling healthy, seeking counseling from a clergyman, psychiatrist, or mental health professional, taking a self-assertiveness

## COPING WITH IBS

The International Foundation for Bowel Dysfunction (IFBD) suggests that IBS sufferers follow several simple rules:

- If your physician has made a definite diagnosis, stop worrying about whether it is "something else" (like early cancer); it isn't.
- Avoid things that you know make you worse, such as particular foods.
- Use medication to avoid crises; for example, take an antidiarrheal agent before leaving home if you are worried about being somewhere and facilities are absent. Avoid constipation by using bulking agents (provided they don't upset you). There are also effective medications available that relieve the pain and improve changes in bowel habits. Discuss with your physician which medication may be appropriate for your symptoms.
- Look for the sources of stress in your life, and see if you can do something about them.
- With professional help, try to sort out which problems in your life you are trying not to face, and do something about them.
- Learn to relax — you probably do not know how. Exercise, yoga, acupuncture, and meditation may be useful, but nothing is as useful as a better understanding of yourself.
- Above all, make up your mind who is running your life. Life is much easier once you make up your mind that you are in charge.

course, developing effective coping skills, resolving family issues that trigger symptoms, sharing anxiety with others, discovering the magic of laughter, and utilizing relaxation therapies such as yoga, meditation, progressive relaxation, biofeedback, water immersion baths, and massage.

## THE IBS WELLNESS DIET

Deralee Scanlon is a registered dietitian and diet counselor who frequently appears as a nutritional authority on radio and television. She also writes about health and nutrition for magazines and newspapers, and teaches nutrition and weight-loss classes at Emeritus College. Barbara Cottman Becnel is author of *The Co-Dependent Parent and Parents Who Help Their Children Overcome Drugs*. Their diet for IBS appears in *The Wellness Book of*

*I.B.S.: How to Achieve Relief from Irritable Bowel Syndrome and Live a Symptom-Free Life.*

## Basic Nutritional Approach

The authors explain that their book is intended to provide a therapeutic dietary strategy that, coupled with a diligently followed stress management program, will enable IBS sufferers to control this chronic disorder and its symptoms.

To augment their diet, they also strongly recommend stress-reducing techniques, including biofeedback, progressive relaxation, differential relaxation, deep muscle relaxation, imagery, hypnotherapy, laughter, and exercise.

## Recommended Foods

The Scanlon IBS diet is low in fat and high in protein and fiber foods which can be digested easily and do not produce gas, bloating, or gastrointestinal discomforts. Because reactions to different foods can vary substantially among individuals, the authors caution that their list of recommended foods should only be used as a starting point.

By food groups, their recommended foods include:

- Vegetables: cooked tomatoes, carrots, and mushrooms, raw vegetable juices, creamed baby foods such as corn, puréed or well-cooked spinach, and shredded zucchini
- Seafood and skinned poultry
- Beverages: spring water and decaffeinated teas
- Dairy products: lowfat or nonfat cottage cheese and lactose-free milk (Lactaid)
- Fruits: cooked or stewed bananas, grapes, apples, raisins, avocados, and blueberries
- Cereals/grains/starches: rice, potatoes, corn flour, arrowroot, tapioca, millet, and well-cooked brown rice
- Spices/condiments: common spices cooked with sherry or white wine (the alcohol will burn off but leave the flavor)
- Sugar substitutes such as honey
- Nuts: wheat germ

## Eliminated Foods

Foods eliminated on Scanlon's diet include:

- Raw vegetables: celery, onions, garlic, broccoli, Brussels sprouts, corn on the cob, spinach, zucchini, green or red bell peppers, tomatoes, carrots, artichoke hearts, black or green olives, lettuce, water chestnuts, cabbage, dried peas and beans, and mushrooms
- Beverages: apple juice, prune juice, mineral water, citrus juices and all alcoholic beverages, coffee, carbonated beverages, and black teas
- Protein: tofu, ham, red meat, smoked or processed fish, and deli meats
- Whole-milk dairy products
- Fat: saturated fat, butter, coconut oil or any partially hydrogenated oil, all fried, creamed, or scalloped foods, and foods cooked au gratin
- Raw fruit: bananas, grapes, apples, raisins, avocados, strawberries, blackberries, raspberries, and cantaloupe
- Cereals/grains/starches: wheat products, barley, refined flour products such as white bread and pastries, and whole-grain products
- Spices/condiments: pepper, cinnamon, nutmeg, chili powder, fresh parsley, capers, Tabasco, tamari soy sauce, cloves, mustard seed, and grated orange rind
- Sugar substitutes, including Mannitol and Sorbitol
- All nuts

The authors eliminate all red meat from their recipes because seafood and skinned poultry provide as much protein and contain much less fat and cholesterol. They also caution against frying, scalloping, or au gratining because these cooking methods increase either fat or lactose intake.

Finally, they urge IBS sufferers to avoid raw fruits and vegetables because they are high in fiber and therefore may be difficult to digest. Instead, they recommend puréeing or juicing them and, in the case of citrus juices, diluting them with water (half and half).

## Food Sensitivities

The authors cite research published by the Clymer Health Clinic that suggests that the stomach wall is an imperfect barrier to large molecules (antigenic material) which can find their way into the bloodstream before digestion has broken them down completely. In reacting to these "invader" antigens, the body creates a defense system that is retriggered whenever antigens of the same foods are introduced into the stomach and thus the stomach becomes sensitive to those foods.

Foods that are commonly thought to cause sensitivities or allergies include (listed in descending order): milk and dairy products, colas, chocolate, corn, eggs, legumes (soybeans and peanuts), citrus fruit and related fruits, tomatoes, wheat, cinnamon, pork, beef, onions, garlic, white potatoes, fish, coffee, shrimp, bananas, walnuts, and pecans.

## Food Intolerances

Food intolerances occur when a person's body lacks specific enzymes needed to break down a particular food substance. Lactase, for example, is the enzyme for lactose (the sugar found in milk). Anyone with a deficiency in lactase will develop an adverse physical reaction to milk or milk products and may experience typical reactions such as gas, diarrhea, nausea, or bloating after drinking fluid milk or consuming milk products.

## Recipes

The authors provide more than fifty recipes especially created for IBS sufferers featuring main dishes, side dishes, soups, breads, and desserts. Each recipe is analyzed for its nutritional content, including calories per serving, and percentages of protein, carbohydrates, and fat.

## Thirty-Day Basic Comfort Meal Plans

The authors also provide daily meal plans that can be easily digested during periods of distress. Incorporating all of their fifty recipes, the meals are balanced to include the basic food groups.

Each day is divided into six reasonably sized meals in order to prevent overeating at any one time. Snacks are recommended for 10 A.M., 3 P.M., and 9 P.M.

### Sample Meal Plan (An asterisk indicates one of the authors' recipes.)
**Breakfast (293 calories):**
3/4 cup cooked cereal
1/2 bagel
1 pat margarine
1/4 cup applesauce
1 teaspoon jelly

Snack (185 calories):
1 toasted bagel
1 tablespoon jelly
Lunch (377 calories):
1 turkey meat loaf sandwich with mustard on 2 slices whole-wheat bread*
1 slice tomato
1 dill pickle
1 cup decaffeinated tea or spring water
Snack (190 calories):
1 medium baked potato with creamed spinach
1 pat margarine
Dinner (610 calories):
1/2 cup fruit nectar
1 serving broiled filet of sole with lemon wedge*
1 cup brown rice
1/2 cup crookneck squash
1 plain baked apple
1 pat margarine
Snack (114 calories):
2 canned peach halves
2 graham crackers

Total daily calories: 1,769

## Vitamin and Mineral Supplements

The restrictive nature of an IBS diet during periods of distress can result in an inadequate intake of certain essential vitamins and minerals. Thus, the authors recommend certain vitamin and mineral supplements to increase supplies of vital nutrients and promote healing of irritated areas of the gastrointestinal tract. They caution, however, that dieters should consult their physician before beginning any supplementation program.

Commonly used supplements — which the authors warn should not replace food on a long-term basis — include:

- Pantothenic acid: 500 milligrams per day
- Lactobacillus acidophilus or lactobacillus bifidus: 1 gram, four times a day
- Metamucil: 1 tablespoon once a day in an 8-ounce glass of water

- Oat bran: 2 tablespoons three times a day in soup, stew, cereal, or juice
- Vitamin B6: 1 to 2 tablets of 50 milligrams once a day
- Vitamin A: a maximum of 25,000 units per day, starting with 5,000 units per day and increasing only with a doctor's approval
- Hypoallergenic vitamin B complex: 1 tablet daily
- Buffered vitamin C: 500 milligrams once a day
- Calcium lactate: 1 to 2 tablets a day taken between meals
- L-Arginine: 2 to 10 grams daily

## Medications

Although the authors believe that IBS symptoms can be relieved with dietary and lifestyle changes, they acknowledge that medications may be necessary in some cases. All of the following medications, they caution, should only be prescribed by qualified physicians: tranquilizers, bulking agents, anticholinergics (antispasmodic drugs), antidiarrheal agents (narcotic and nonnarcotic).

## Eating Habits

How people eat is often as important, the authors suggest, as what they eat. Therefore, they outline basic eating habits which have proven helpful in reducing IBS symptoms, including eating slowly and chewing thoroughly in order to break down food into smaller pieces. People are also encouraged to take a brief walk after meals, which helps to relieve tension and increase energy expenditure. Most importantly, IBS sufferers are cautioned against overeating, which overburdens an already weakened digestive system.

## Physical Activity

The authors contend that developing an exercise program is fundamentally essential to the maintenance of good health, especially for IBS sufferers. They do warn that exercise, like diet, should be tailored to fit the physiological requirements of each individual. Also, all dieters should consult a physician before beginning any exercise regime.

## GASTROINTESTINAL HEALTH DIET

The Gastrointestinal Health Diet is presented by Dr. Steven R. Peikin in his book *Gastrointestinal Health*. Dr. Peikin is professor of medicine and director of gastroenterology at the University of Medicine and Dentistry of New Jersey, Robert Wood Johnson Medical School at Camden, Cooper Hospital/University Medical Center. He has been a fellow at Massachusetts General Hospital and Harvard Medical School and a clinical associate at the National Institutes of Health.

## Basic Nutritional Approach

As Peikin emphasizes, "by far the best approach for the long-term management of IBS symptoms is diet," particularly one high in fiber.

In his practice at the Jefferson Digestive Disease Service at Thomas Jefferson University Hospital, he developed (with the help of dietitians) a nutritional program designed to treat the full spectrum of common digestive disorders, including IBS.

The six principles underlying his program include:

- High fiber
- Low fat
- Low lactose
- Low spice
- Low gas-forming legumes
- Low calories

Peikin notes that in the standard American diet, 35 to 45 percent of daily calories come from fat, 12 to 20 percent from protein, and 40 to 50 percent from carbohydrates. His Two-Week Master Program, incorporating the six principles listed above, shifts the emphasis so that less than 30 percent of daily calories come from fat, 12 to 20 percent are consumed as protein, and 55 to 60 percent as carbohydrates.

## Two-Week Master Program

Peikin claims that the self-help diet he developed is a breakthrough in the treatment of digestive problems because it doesn't depend on drugs or on severe restriction of many foods. Rather, it is a high-fiber, lowfat, totally balanced diet that works in harmony with the digestive tract. Also, it takes into account people's appetites and their cravings for "comfort" foods, and regulates the delicate biochemical balance between the brain and the digestive system so that dieters feel satisfied and gratified. Finally, it recognizes that foods are chemicals and that certain ratios must be maintained to soothe the digestive system, satisfy hunger, and meet nutritional needs.

*Fiber.* Peikin notes that a diet high in fiber is now recommended by the National Cancer Institute, the Food and Nutrition Board, and the National Academy of Sciences.

He describes fiber as a "near miraculous protector of the intestinal tract." Fiber both relieves constipation by making the stool bulkier and softer and stops diarrhea by absorbing excess water in the stool.

While a high-fiber diet is not a cure-all for IBS, Peikin says that it helps most patients, especially those with constipation. In some people, however, a high-fiber diet may make symptoms of diarrhea or bloating worse. Usually this will not occur if grains and vegetables, which are naturally high in fiber, are gradually introduced into his diet.

*Vegetables.* Vegetables, as Peikin comments, are an excellent source of fiber, help a wide range of gastrointestinal disorders, and play a vital role in preventing other diseases. A few of them, however, particularly cabbage, are known to aggravate some GI symptoms.

*Water.* Since Peikin's IBS diet is high in fiber, and fiber absorbs considerable amounts of water, he recommends that people following his Two-Week Master Program drink eight 8-ounce glasses of water each day for every 2,000 calories consumed. Drinking water will not increase the body's fluid retention, he notes, nor will it make dieters feel heavy or bloated.

## Restricted Foods

*Fat.* The primary goal of Peikin's nutritional program is to decrease total fat in the diet. Not only are all kinds of fats minimized, but only 21 to 28 percent of calories are derived from fat each day — less than the amount recommended by the National Cancer Institute.

As Peikin observes, fats can be reduced by decreasing the amount, eliminating the fats entirely, or using cooking methods that do not require fats. Those included in the Master Program are usually derived from vegetable oils; if a recipe calls for a saturated fat such as butter, only a very small amount is used.

Peikin also recommends omega-3 fatty acids, found in salmon, tuna, herring, sardines, halibut, trout, and mackerel.

*Spicy Foods and Spices.* Spicy foods and spices may aggravate preexisting digestive disorders such as IBS and exacerbate their symptoms, particularly if consumed on an empty stomach. For this reason, Peikin suggests avoiding chili pepper, black pepper, mustard seed, cloves, and nutmeg.

Those spices least likely to irritate the stomach include cinnamon, allspice, mace, thyme, rosemary, basil, sage, paprika, and caraway seed.

Overall, Peikin recommends a low-spice regimen to alleviate IBS symptoms. Therefore, most of the recipes in his nutritional program do not include spices. The herbs listed above may be added to suit dieters' own tastes and sensitivities.

*Gas-Forming Legumes.* Some foods, especially beans, legumes, and cruciferous vegetables such as cabbage and broccoli, can produce excessive gas for IBS sufferers. Therefore, the recipes Peikin developed substitute whole grains (such as bulgur wheat and kasha) and other vegetables for gas-producing beans and legumes.

## Recipes

The recipes included in the last section of Peikin's book are designed to be nutritionally balanced, varied, and quick and easy to prepare. He notes that on many days, dieters will consume animal protein only once, while meal portions will be smaller than those they are usually accustomed to.

Peikin's Master Program recipes intentionally avoid the Spartan and often monotonous fare that normally characterizes nutritional treatment of GI disorders. The best part of this program, he notes, is that it comprises foods everyone else eats. As one of his patients commented, "I'm finally eating real food again!"

## Meal Plans

Peikin notes that some people with IBS, especially those who have an exaggerated, almost uncontrollable urge to move their bowels after a meal, do much better if they break three standard meals into smaller units and eat several times a day. Under no circumstances should dieters eat fewer than three meals daily, he counsels.

## After Two Weeks

The Two-Week Master Program provides dieters with the macronutrient values (for protein and carbohydrates) as well as fiber and calorie values for each recipe and meal plan. After two weeks, dieters are encouraged to choose recipes that personally appeal to them and suit their particular nutritional requirements. They can also design their own recipes using the guidelines Peikin provides.

Overall, Peikin's nutritional program is so "normal" that people will be able to easily incorporate it into their family's lifestyle. The tenets, he suggests, are good for people of all ages: reduced fat and cholesterol and increased complex carbohydrates.

*Sample Daily Menu.* The menu for Day 7, for example, contains 1,778 calories, 53 grams of fat (27 percent of calories), and 24 grams of fiber. (An asterisk indicates one of his recipes.)

**Breakfast:**
Granola Cereal*
1/2 cup strawberries
1 cup 1% lowfat milk
1 slice whole-wheat toast
1 teaspoon margarine or butter
**Lunch:**
Tuna Patties* on hamburger roll
1 peach
2 plums
**Dinner:**
Oriental Barbecued Chicken*
Veggie Stir-Fry*
2 slices Easy Cornbread*
1 Peanut Butter Bar*

## Vitamin and Mineral Supplements

According to Peikin, everyone needs approximately forty vitamins and minerals to maintain health, most of which can be obtained from food. For the most part, he states, vitamin and mineral supplements are usually unnecessary — and potentially dangerous if dosages are abused.

He contends that his Two-Week Master Program supplies all necessary nutrients for the majority of people with GI problems. However, if IBS dieters are attempting to lose weight and their caloric intake is less than 1,200 calories a day, he suggests they take a calcium supplement and a multivitamin supplement that includes iron. Calcium supplements may also be of value for women at risk for osteoporosis.

## Alcohol

Alcohol is one of the dietary factors most frequently associated with gastrointestinal disorders such as IBS, according to Peikin. While many people can tolerate small amounts on a daily basis without adverse effects, he warns that alcohol can aggravate IBS symptoms. He does not include it in his nutritional program.

## Caffeine

Peikin claims that large amounts of caffeine can cause intestinal secretion and diarrhea and promote the secretion of acid in the stomach. And the tannins in tea can cause constipation. He therefore recommends that his dieters drink grain-based coffee substitutes such as Postum, Pero, or herbal teas.

## Smoking

While Peikin admits that the effects of smoking on nutrition have not been thoroughly researched, he warns that tobacco use hinders calcium metabolism and may accelerate osteoporosis. And, because smoking also increases the urgency to defecate, it further complicates the symptoms of IBS.

## Physical Activity

Peikin is a strong advocate of exercise, which, he says, is the most efficient way for people to elevate their metabolism to burn fat. Furthermore, exercise can help IBS and constipation sufferers because it improves bowel function, produces a remarkable sense of well-being, and generally makes them feel better. Exercise also helps reduce stress, which is a key aggravator of most GI problems. The best exercises for helping the digestive system, he claims, are swimming, walking, and bicycling.

## Behavioral Modification

According to Peikin, if people have IBS or any other digestive disorder, excessive stress increases their risk of an attack and is likely to aggravate their symptoms. Stress tends to be most dangerous when it is cumulative, he warns, although even one significant stress event can trigger a reaction within twenty-four hours (if not immediately).

He offers several suggestions to relieve stress. These include overcom-

---

**DIETARY RECOMMENDATIONS FOR IBS***

1. Identify food allergens, sensitivities, or intolerances.

2. Avoid offending foods as needed, including milk and dairy products (lactose intolerance), gas-forming foods and beverages, foods containing high amounts of fructose and raffinose, and dietetic foods containing Sorbitol.

3. Eat regular, small, lowfat meals.

4. Gradually increase dietary fiber to 15 to 25 grams daily.

5. Limit caffeine and alcohol intake.

6. Exercise regularly and practice stress reduction techniques.

7. Drink 8 or more cups of water or fluid a day.

*Source: Jennifer Nelson, *The Mayo Clinic Diet Manual: A Handbook of Nutrition Practices, Seventh Edition* (St. Louis, MO: Mosby-Year Book, 1994).

---

ing harmful habits that undermine health (especially smoking, drug or alcohol abuse, and binge patterns of eating), seeking professional counseling or therapy, and planning time for relaxation and pleasure. For example, he recommends a daily walk or an afternoon nap, daily relaxation exercises (including yoga, meditation, and deep breathing), regular workouts, and balanced, well-timed meals, all of which can add harmony to life and keep moods more balanced.

## RECENT RESEARCH

Murray and Pizzorno, in the *Encyclopedia of Natural Medicine,* cite one clinical study in which enteric-coated peppermint oil significantly reduced the symptoms of IBS. The study concluded, "Peppermint oil appears to be an effective and safe preparation for symptomatic treatment of the irritable bowel syndrome."

European physicians, according to *Alternative Medicine: The Definitive Guide,* have successfully used enteric-coated peppermint oil to treat IBS as well. Ginger also has a long history of use in relieving digestive complaints, including IBS, according to *Alternative Medicine.* Herbs such as chamomile, rosemary, balm, and valerian also have antispasmodic effects on the intestines.

Balch and Balch suggest in *Prescription for Nutritional Healing* that lobelia, pau d'arco, rose hips, and cascara sagrada may be effective in treating

IBS. They also note that alfalfa tablets containing vitamin K (needed to build the intestinal flora for proper digestion) may be helpful in treating mild symptoms of this disorder.

Balch and Balch further recommend that IBS sufferers eat daily amounts of acidophilus to replenish friendly bacteria. Some patients may also benefit from drinking 1/2 cup of aloe vera juice three times a day on an empty stomach. The juice is now available in products which taste like spring water and acts as a general colon cleanser. Aloe vera juice, they suggest, keeps the colon walls clean of excess mucus and slows down food reactions.

In addition, garlic aids in digestion and destroys toxins in the colon. Primrose oil, which supplies essential fatty acids, is also beneficial. Free-form amino acids may be included in the diet because they are necessary for the repair of the mucous membranes of the intestines. Finally, proteolytic enzymes (use brands low in hydrochloric acid and high in pancreatin) help the body digest protein and cleanse the bloodstream of undigested foods.

# 23

## Multiple Sclerosis Diets

D
r. Deepak Chopra relates in *Quantum Healing* the remarkable story of Jacqueline du Pré, the celebrated British cellist who died when she was 42 of multiple sclerosis (MS). Du Pré was stricken with the disease when she was only 28, and her musical career ended very quickly because she lost the ability to coordinate her arms. A year passed, during which time she had no contact with the cello. One morning, however, she awoke to find that her muscular coordination had returned intact. She was rushed to a studio where she recorded beautiful performances of music by Chopin and Franck. Unfortunately, her remission lasted only four days, and she then returned to her former state.

The inexplicable advent and remission of du Pré's MS point to the baffling nature of the disease that scientists still do not fully understand, and for which there is no cure. According to the National Multiple Sclerosis Society, more than 350,000 Americans are affected by this disabling disease of the central nervous system that is believed to be caused by an immunological malfunction. In MS, the body seems to mistakenly attack the protective myelin sheath that insulates nerve fibers in the brain, spinal cord, and eyes. The deteriorated myelin is subsequently replaced by patches of scar tissue that impair the ability of nerves to transmit messages between the brain and muscles that control bodily function.

The resulting symptoms, which can occur very suddenly — as in du Pré's case — include fatigue, loss of balance, double vision, slurred speech, stiffness, tremors, loss of bladder or bowel control, impairment of memory, difficulty in walking, and loss of muscle coordination.

Early in the disease, remissions tend to be quite complete and often develop soon after the exacerbation or attack. As MS progresses, remissions are slower to develop and less complete. Later, remissions fail or nearly fail to occur. MS leads eventually to advanced permanent disability.

While diets have not proven successful in preventing or reversing MS, several have proven helpful in alleviating its symptoms (especially when they are initiated in the early stages) and even in slowing the progression of the disease and determining whether or not disability will develop. This chapter reviews MS diets developed by Dr. Roy Swank, Dr. Kurt Donsbach and Dr. H. Rudolph Alsleben, and Judy Graham, a founding member of the Action for Research into Multiple Sclerosis, a self-help group for MS sufferers in the United Kingdom.

## THE SWANK LOW-FAT DIET

Perhaps the best-documented diet for MS is that developed by Dr. Roy Swank, Professor Emeritus of Neurology at Oregon Health Sciences University, who began investigating MS in 1948. His *Swank Low-Fat Diet*, first published in 1972, was followed by a more comprehensive book, *The Multiple Sclerosis Diet Book: A Low-Fat Diet for the Treatment of MS*, in 1977. Substantially revised and expanded in 1987, Swank's text was co-authored by Barbara Brewer Dugan, a research associate in the Department of Neurology at Oregon Health Sciences University.

### Basic Nutritional Approach

Since undertaking MS research in 1948, Dr. Swank claims to have examined approximately 3,500 MS patients throughout the United States and Canada, and maintained contact with 2,000 of them for ten to thirty-six years. He has also tracked numerous nutritional studies conducted around the world that confirm a strong correlation exists between fats of animal origin and the frequency of MS. The Swank Low-Fat Diet is based on decreasing saturated fats and increasing unsaturated oils in the diet, while eliminating various types of canned, frozen, and processed foods.

To obtain maximum benefit from treatment, Swank and Dugan advocate its application as early as possible — that is, while MS symptoms are transient and before a major disabling attack. The authors claim that the degree to which the diet is adhered to, as well as the avoidance of fatigue and nervous stress, will determine the rate at which the disease will progress and whether or not disability will develop.

## Recommended Foods

The authors classify recommended foods as "permissible in any amount" and "permissible in limited amounts" as follows:

*Dairy Products.* Permissible in any amount are nonfat milk, skim milk, buttermilk (without cream or butter bits added), evaporated skim milk, nonfat dry milk powder, rinsed lowfat cottage cheese, dry-curd cottage cheese, 99 percent fat-free cheeses, and nonfat yogurt. Permissible in limited amounts are dairy products containing 1 percent butterfat (but never to exceed 1 gram of fat per serving). Dieters are allowed one serving daily.

*Fats and Oils.* Permissible (but not to exceed 10 teaspoons per day) are safflower oil, sunflower seed oil, corn oil, cottonseed oil, soybean oil, sesame oil, wheat germ oil, linseed oil, peanut oil, and olive oil.

*Commercial Mixes.* Permissible in any amount are prepared mixes (indicating 0 to 1 gram of fat) made without hydrogenated oil, lard, butter, margarine, palm oil, coconut oil, or egg yolks. Permissible in limited amounts are all dry soup mixes (one cup per day).

*Commercially Canned Foods.* Permissible in any amount are all canned fruits and vegetables and sauces containing no hard fat (hydrogenated or processed oils, palm oil, or coconut oil).

*Chips, Crackers, Breads, Cereals, and Pasta.* Permissible in any amount are all varieties of whole-grain breads, enriched wheat bread, sourdough bread, pumpernickel bread, raisin bread, English muffins, bagels, French bread, melba toast, RyKrisp, all pastas, all grain cereals, matzo, pretzels (made only from flour, water, and salt), and rice. Permissible in limited amounts (2 to 3 per day) are saltines, graham crackers, wheat and vegetable thins, vanilla wafers, lemon and ginger snaps.

*Pastry.* Permissible in any amount are angel food cake and any commercially prepared pastry made without hydrogenated vegetable oil, coconut oil, palm oil, or lard.

*Fruits and Vegetables.* Permissible in any amount are all fruits and vegetables (except as indicated below), all fruit and vegetable juices, and all frozen or canned vegetables without butter or high-fat seasonings. Permissible in limited amounts are avocados (1/8 daily), ripe olives (3 medium), and green olives (6 medium).

*Eggs.* Three whole eggs are allowed per week, but no more than 1 egg daily. Egg whites are allowed in any quantity.

*Sugar Products.* Because sugar tends to increase nervousness in MS patients, the authors suggest that intake be minimal and for taste only. The following can be eaten in minimal amounts: sugar, jam, jelly, marmalade, honey, molasses, maple syrup, corn syrup, gelatin and desserts made with egg white, and rice, tapioca, or cornstarch puddings made with skim milk. Plain chocolate syrup can be used for making cakes, brownies, frosting, or chocolate milk; dieters are allowed 1 tablespoon per day.

*Beverages.* No more than three cups combined of caffeinated coffee, tea, and cola are allowed per day. In terms of decaffeinated products, unlimited herb tea is allowed, as are four cups daily of decaffeinated coffee. Because of their high sodium content, cola products should be limited to 16 ounces per day.

A moderate amount of alcohol is allowed, although the authors note that in general, MS patients tolerate about 50 percent as much alcohol as they did before the onset of the disease, and suffer unusually severe hangovers after consuming relatively small amounts of it.

*Poultry.* White meat of chicken and turkey with the skin removed before cooking is permissible in any amount, as it contains only small amounts of saturated fat.

*Fish.* For the same reason, any amount of the following is permissible: cod, abalone, halibut, snapper, smelt, flounder, sole, sturgeon, tuna canned in water, shark, mahi mahi, haddock, perch, and pollock. In the shellfish category any amount of the following is permissible: clams, crab, lobster, oysters, scallops, and shrimp. The authors counsel that patients with elevated cholesterol levels should eat shellfish infrequently, and they warn those watching their weight to restrict serving sizes to no more than 4 ounces.

The following can be eaten only in limited daily quantities because of their high unsaturated fat (oil) content: tuna canned in oil but not drained (2 ounces), tuna canned in oil but rinsed and drained (3 ounces), Chinook salmon (1 ounce), coho salmon (2 ounces), trout (2 ounces), sardines canned in oil (1 ounce), and herring and mackerel (1 ounce).

*Meats.* The Swank Low-Fat Diet does not allow any red meat, including dark meat of chicken and turkey, for the first year. Following the first twelve months, 3 ounces of red meat are allowed once a week, although the authors discourage the intake of red meat except on special occasions. Meat should be weighed after cooking.

Three ounces of the following lowfat beef, poultry, and game contain the equivalent of 5 grams of saturated fat: leg of lamb, liver (beef, calf, chicken, turkey, or pork), kidney (pork, veal, or lamb), heart (calf or beef, lean portion only), calf tongue, rabbit, horsemeat, venison and elk, and chicken gizzards.

Two ounces of the following medium-fat beef, poultry, and game contain the equivalent of 5 grams of saturated fat: lean beef or ham, lamb (rib, loin, or shoulder), lean pork, veal, lamb heart, beef kidney, beef tongue, chicken or turkey (dark meat, skin removed), heart (chicken and turkey), turkey gizzard, pheasant, and squab (skin removed).

## Eliminated Foods

The authors term the following foods "forbidden" and completely eliminate them from the Swank Low-Fat Diet:

*Dairy Products.* Whole milk, cream, butter, margarine (including those made from safflower or corn oil), sour cream, ice cream exceeding 1 percent butterfat, ice milk, cheese exceeding 1 percent butterfat, creamed or partially creamed cottage cheese, and imitation dairy products containing palm, coconut, or any hydrogenated oil.

*Fats and Oils.* All margarines, butter, shortening, lard, cocoa butter, coconut oil, palm oil, and all oils that have been hydrogenated (processed).

*Commercial Mixes.* All packaged commercial mixes for cakes, cookies, pastries, pancakes, biscuits, and dessert bread products containing saturated fat (hydrogenated or processed oils, palm oil, or coconut oil).

*Commercially Canned Foods.* Chili, soups, spaghetti and meat sauces, stews, pork and beans, hash, canned chicken and turkey, and sandwich spreads.

*Chips, Crackers, Breads, Cereals, and Pasta.* All commercially prepared chips (including potato), as well as fancy and flavored crackers, chow mein noodles, commercially prepared biscuits, and sweet muffins.

*Pastry.* Commercially prepared pies, pastries, doughnuts, cookies, and cakes.

*Sugar Products.* Chocolate and all products containing chocolate and fresh or flaked coconut.

*Meats.* Because of their high fat content, spareribs, goose, duck, bacon, lunch meats, salami, frankfurters, ground turkey or chicken, wieners (including chicken and turkey), and all sausages.

## Vitamin and Mineral Supplements

Although the authors contend that intake of vitamins on a well-balanced diet is quite adequate, they do recommend the following daily vitamin supplements: 1 teaspoon cod liver oil or 4 capsules, 1 therapeutic-type multiple vitamin and mineral, 1,000 milligrams of vitamin C, and 400 IU of vitamin E.

## Recipes

*The Multiple Sclerosis Diet Book* contains more than 350 recipes for breakfast, lunch, dinner, and even the cocktail hour. These include muffins and breads, appetizers, soups, salads and dressings, stuffing for meat, poultry, and fish, fish and seafood, poultry, beef, Oriental cuisine, meatless cooking, sauces, vegetables, pies and cakes, cookies, desserts, icings and dessert sauces, and candy. Sample menus for one week are also provided, as are tips for eating in restaurants or at other people's homes, traveling abroad, shopping, equipping the kitchen, using herbs and spices, and cooking methods.

## Physical Activity

The authors state that patients in different stages of MS have different physical limitations that determine the types of physical activities they can tolerate. If this tolerance is exceeded to the point of exhaustion, the patient does not benefit and may be harmed.

Patients who ambulate normally can engage in a wide variety of activities — such as jogging, aerobic exercises, walking, swimming, calisthenics, or bicycling — but are warned to avoid deep or continuing fatigue.

Patients who ambulate with mild or severe difficulty are still able to walk, swim, exercise lightly, perform stretching exercises such as yoga, or use a stationary bicycle. The authors note that most MS patients will find swimming several times a week satisfying, although the temperature of the pool should not be warmer than 82–84 degrees Fahrenheit.

For MS patients who are no longer ambulant, active exercises are usually limited to the upper extremities, and upper back and neck. The authors also recommend passive manipulation of all joints through a full range of movement to prevent pain and the atrophy of the adjacent muscles. Daily massage of the skin with lubrication solutions such as baby oil or glycerine is further advised to prevent breakdown of the skin and subsequent ulceration.

### Behavioral Modification

The authors are very cognizant of the behavioral aspects of MS and its treatment, and structure *The Multiple Sclerosis Diet Book* so patients can most readily adopt a new eating regimen to ensure optimal health and longevity. They advise patients that the Swank Low-Fat Diet be accompanied by adequate rest (including a one- to two-hour midday nap to prevent fatigue) and a reduction of stress. Equally important is adopting a mental attitude that fosters optimism and a satisfying life within the limitations of the disease.

## THE JUDY GRAHAM SELF-HELP MS DIET

The MS diet developed by Judy Graham is described in *Multiple Sclerosis: A Self-Help Guide to Its Management*. Ms. Graham was diagnosed as having MS at the age of 27 in 1974, and was a founding member of Action for Research into Multiple Sclerosis (ARMS), a self-help group for MS sufferers in the United Kingdom that funds its own research on topics such as diet, physiotherapy, and hyperbaric oxygen treatment. Graham admits she has been a "guinea pig" for several ARMS-funded researchers exploring new treatments for MS including evening primrose oil capsules and a diet high in essential fatty acids. And, while she still has

## WATCHING YOUR WEIGHT
## AND EXERCISE*

Weight is an important issue for people with MS, counsels the National Multiple Sclerosis Society, because being overweight adds to problems of mobility and strains the respiratory and circulatory systems. The additional weight can also increase fatigue and make people avoid exercise.

The National MS Society further warns that skin breakdown or irritation can occur more easily in overweight people who are fairly inactive, while being underweight may decrease resistance to infection and — if people are sedentary — may increase the risk of pressure sores.

Besides helping people with MS control their weight, increased activity provides the following benefits:

• Makes the most of potential muscle strength.

• Increases endurance.

• Maximizes joint range-of-motion and flexibility.

• Strengthens the heart.

• Protects bone mass.

• Reduces problems of elimination.

• Makes MS sufferers feel better about the world — and themselves.

*Source: *Food for Thought: MS and Nutrition,* the National Multiple Sclerosis Society, 1993.

MS, Graham's condition has stabilized, and she has had no MS attacks since first being diagnosed. In addition, Graham works as a part-time television producer and as a freelance writer, while raising a very active young son.

Graham challenges the conventional view that there is no known cause, cure, or recognized treatment for MS, and believes there are several treatments to help sufferers recover their health and well-being. These treatments or management programs also suggest strongly that the progression of MS can be slowed down, halted, or even reversed. Graham's book, which she describes as a self-help guide, is intended to strengthen the immune system without resorting to drugs, and to suggest a healthy way of life.

## Basic Nutritional Approach

Graham defines the essential points of her nutritional therapy for MS as follows:

- Cut down drastically on saturated fat — found in animal fats, dairy produce, and hard fats.
- Increase intake of polyunsaturated fats considerably to provide essential fatty acids — not just in spreads and oils but also in foods such as fish, liver, and green leafy vegetables.
- Find out to which foods and substances you personally are sensitive or allergic (most commonly milk for MS sufferers), and eliminate them completely.
- Eat the most nutritious diet possible by eliminating junk foods and convenience foods, consuming fresh rather than processed and packaged foods, and cutting down on foods such as sugar that only give empty calories.
- Take supplements of evening primrose oil and fish oils to guarantee a good intake of the essential fatty acids needed for many vital bodily processes.
- Take supplements of certain vitamins, minerals, and trace elements that work with the essential fatty acids.

## Recommended Foods

The diet Graham describes was developed by Michael Crawford, Professor of Nutrition at Nottingham University, and studied for three years by ARMS. At the end of the study, researchers concluded that patients who carefully followed the dietary advice did not deteriorate, whereas those who did not stick closely to the diet deteriorated significantly.

This essential fatty acid diet is characterized by the following recommendations:

- Choose lean meat, and trim all fat off the meat before cooking.
- Use polyunsaturated margarine and oil, making sure that these have not been processed and hydrogenated.
- Eat at least three fish meals a week.
- Eat organ foods, particularly liver (1/2 pound of liver per week is recommended).

- Eat a big helping of dark green leafy vegetables every day.
- Eat some linseeds (which are a good source of alpha-linolenic acid) or products made with linseeds daily.
- Eat a salad of mixed raw vegetables each day with a French dressing made of polyunsaturated oil.
- Eat as much fresh food as possible rather than processed foods.
- Eat some fresh fruit each day.
- Eat whole foods rather than refined foods, particularly whole-grain cereals and bread.

As Graham explains, this diet is designed to provide a balance among the different food groups, as well as a balanced nutrition in terms of vitamins, minerals, and trace elements. It is also high in fiber and accords with recommendations made by nutritional organizations in recent years.

*Dairy Products.* As the fat in whole milk is almost all saturated (about 97 percent), Graham recommends skim milk or semiskim milk (1% or 2%), although the latter still contains some cream. Rather than high-fat milk products, she suggests lowfat (or nonfat) yogurt, curd cheese, lowfat cottage cheese, and other cheeses that are low- or medium-fat. Soft cheeses such as Brie and Camembert can be eaten occasionally. Three or four eggs a week are also allowed.

*Meat.* Lean meat, according to Graham, is an excellent source of arachidonic acid for MS patients. She specifically recommends lean pork, ham, beef, lamb, chicken, turkey, and rabbit, all of which should be trimmed of any fat before cooking.

Organ meats such as liver, kidneys, brains, and sweetbreads are especially rich in arachidonic acid, and Graham advises MS patients to consume at least one-half pound of fresh liver a week. Liver and kidneys are also very good sources of vitamin B12, which is important for the nervous system, and contain iron, zinc, folic acid, and vitamins A, B1, B2, and B6. Dried or desiccated liver tablets cannot be eaten as a substitute for fresh liver, she warns, because many of the nutrients are destroyed in processing.

*Fish.* Fish high in essential fatty acids is highly recommended — including shellfish and oily fish such as mackerel, herring, kippers, whitebait, tuna, crab, lobster, sardines, mussels, cod roe, sprats, squid, prawns, and shrimp.

These are also rich in docosahexaenoic acid, which is an essential nutrient for the brain, Graham notes.

Also recommended are white fish such as cod, flounder, and haddock, as well as freshwater fish like salmon and trout. Fresh fish is preferable, followed by frozen and then canned (with the oil drained off).

*Vegetarians.* Graham states that strict vegetarians with MS cannot follow this diet because meat and fish are very important components of it. However, it is possible for vegetarians to work out a modified version of the diet by replacing the meat and fish with legumes and nuts, although these do not provide the same essential fatty acids as meat.

*Fruits and Vegetables.* While all vegetables are recommended, Graham suggests that green vegetables are better because they are an excellent source of alpha-linolenic acid and vitamin E. Specifically suggested are spinach, broccoli, kale, green pepper, parsley, green beans, and sprouted beans. Other recommended vegetables for salads (using a French dressing made with a linoleic-rich oil) include tomatoes, carrots, beets, red peppers, and red cabbage. Fresh fruits and vegetables are preferable to frozen ones.

*Nuts and Seeds.* Nuts and seeds are a good source of essential fatty acids, vitamins, and trace elements, and can be eaten on their own or in salads, in bread, or on breakfast cereals. Graham recommends sunflower seeds, pumpkin seeds, sesame seeds, almonds, Brazil nuts, hazelnuts, walnuts, chestnuts, and linseeds, which are the best source of alpha-linolenic acid.

Nut oils are allowed on the diet as well, as long as they do not contain butter or other animal fats. The products should be pure and natural, and not hydrogenated.

*Breads and Cereals.* Graham counsels that unrefined cereals and whole-grain bread are better than refined cereals and white bread in terms of the essential fatty acids, vitamins, minerals, and trace elements they contain, and also recommends whole-wheat pastas and brown rice.

This diet, she notes, recommends extra bran so the roughage content of the overall diet is high. This is because bran helps prevent and relieve constipation — a common complaint of MS sufferers. A maximum of three tablespoons daily is suggested, which should be spread over the whole day while drinking a lot of fluid to bind the bran in the bowel.

## REDUCING BLADDER AND
## BOWEL CONCERNS*

MS sufferers who find urinary tract infections a problem, according to the National Multiple Sclerosis Society, may benefit from drinking more fluids that increase urinary acidity — because high acid levels in the urine provide an environment unfriendly to bacteria. These include cranberry, apple, apricot, and prune juice.

Conversely, foods should be avoided that make urine alkaline (the opposite of acidic): citrus fruit (such as oranges and grapefruit), tomatoes, milk and milk products, potatoes, lima beans, and antacids that contain sodium bicarbonate.

Because constipation can be caused or worsened by too little fluid in the diet, the National MS Society suggests an increased intake of fluids, as well as fiber from fruit, vegetables, and grains. Also recommended are prune juice, unprocessed bran, and whole-grain breads. (Approximately 30 grams of fiber and two quarts of fluid are necessary each day to promote good bowel function.) Consumption of chocolate, nuts, and hard cheeses should be restricted as these foods may cause constipation.

*Source: *Food for Thought: MS and Nutrition*, the National Multiple Sclerosis Society, 1993.

*Legumes.* Legumes — including peas, beans, and lentils — are recommended as their fat content is low, and the fat contained is polyunsaturated. Legumes are also a good source of protein, alpha-linolenic acid, and vitamin C.

*Fats and Oils.* Graham counsels those with MS to use sunflower seed oil, safflower seed oil, olive oil, sesame seed oil, soybean oil, cottonseed oil, or corn oil in cooking, as they all contain linoleic acid. These oils should be pure, ideally cold-pressed oils available in health food stores. Whichever oil is chosen, people should be sure not to heat it to the point of smoking, and not to use the oil more than once. The best way to consume these oils is unheated, as in salad dressing.

### Eliminated Foods

Graham suggests that people with MS follow Dr. Roy Swank's guidelines in terms of eliminated foods (see pages 392 to 396).

In addition, she recommends that the following foods be avoided:

- Whole milk (with about 97 percent saturated fat), as well as all milk products high in fat — such as all kinds of cream, hard cheeses, and creamy yogurts.
- Manufactured meat products such as Spam, luncheon meat, pâtés, pork pies, meat pies, sausages, and hamburgers.
- Deep-fried fish.
- Sugar and sugary foods — because they fill people up without providing much nutritional benefit.

## Vitamin and Mineral Supplements

Graham disagrees with ARMS — which states that vitamin and mineral supplements are not necessary if MS patients adhere to its EFA diet. She notes that in its own research, ARMS found that more than one-third of people with MS did not comply with the dietary advice they were given.

Graham strongly recommends that MS patients take the following supplements:

- Evening primrose oil capsules
- Fish oil capsules
- Vitamins C, E, B complex, B6, and B12
- Minerals and trace elements: zinc, magnesium, manganese, and selenium
- Lecithin
- Freeform amino acids
- Organic germanium
- Coenzyme Q10
- Acidophilus (or a similar product)

## Physical Activity

According to Graham, studies have now proved that physical therapy and exercise have real benefits for MS sufferers, and should be started as early in the disease as possible before permanent damage has occurred.

If MS patients cannot do exercises on their own, Graham recommends that they see a physical therapist. Otherwise, possible forms of physical activity include walking, swimming, dancing, stretching, and gentle aerobic exercise classes and rebounding (mini-trampoline). Whatever exercise is chosen should be done regularly — ideally, every day.

Not only will exercising make a noticeable difference in strength, stamina, and endurance but, Graham claims, it can make the difference between standing and walking or becoming wheelchair-bound.

### Behavioral Modification

In addition to discussing the importance of nutrition and exercise in coping with MS, Graham also explores a more all-embracing approach to the disease that includes yoga (which calms the mind and energizes the body, and may even slow down or halt the disease process), meditation, self-help therapies, counteracting depression, improving self-esteem, visualization, and counseling.

## THE MS DIET BY DR. KURT DONSBACH AND DR. H. RUDOLPH ALSLEBEN

The MS diet developed by Dr. Kurt Donsbach and Dr. H. Rudolph Alsleben is detailed in their book *Multiple Sclerosis, Muscular Dystrophy and ALS*.

Dr. Donsbach began his career in the health field as a chiropractic physician. He served as chairman of the board of the National Health Federation for fifteen years, founded the Donsbach University School of Nutrition, the Hospital Santa Monica in Rosarito Beach, Mexico, and the Institut Santa Monica in Poland. Donsbach is cofounder of the Health Restoration Institute in Tijuana, Mexico, and has authored more than fifty books and booklets on nutrition-related subjects.

Dr. Alsleben, well known for his work in the field of preventive medicine, has opened many clinics in the United States and abroad and has treated more than 65,000 patients. He pioneered the use of intravenous chelation therapy, ion extractor therapy, and oral-sep immune therapies, and he is cofounder of the Health Restoration Institute in Tijuana, Mexico.

Drs. Alsleben and Donsbach jointly developed immune modulator blueprints (ultraspecific vaccine-type DNA modifiers) for the treatment of arthritis and cancer.

### Basic Nutritional Approach

Donsbach, who terms Dr. Swank "one of the most respected individuals in MS research," concurs with his conclusion that all saturated fat is bad for MS patients and should be avoided. He also cites the benefits of wheat germ oil and gamma-linoleic acid concentrate, available in both tablet and capsule forms, in treating the disease.

Donsbach further recommends that MS patients supplement their diet with Oral Chelating Formula, vitamin E, free amino acid complex, oat bran wafers, and flaxseed oil on a daily basis.

## Recommended Foods

Alsleben, who provides specific food recommendations in the second half of the book, claims that his diet is easy to follow and will enhance the health of MS sufferers. His suggestions include:

- Eat a bowl of oatmeal or other whole-grain cereal every morning.
- Consume four cups of vegetables daily — half raw and half cooked — and be sure to eat a wide variety.
- Eat one cup of fruit daily, preferably raw.
- Eat only the following fats: butter, olive oil, and peanut oil.
- Eat only whole-grain, freshly baked breads and rolls.
- Eat the heaviest meals at breakfast and lunch, with a light meal at night.
- Eat a minimum of five servings of chicken, fish, or turkey each week, and consume beef or pork only occasionally. Vegetarians should be sure to consume sufficient amounts of seeds and nuts to supplement their diet.
- Eggs and dairy products may be used sparingly.
- Do not combine fruits or fruit juices with concentrated proteins such as meats, dairy products, or eggs as this will produce gas and discomfort.
- Use seasoning salts such as those made from kelp as flavor enhancers.
- Be positive and happy when eating to enhance the functioning of the digestive system.

## Eliminated Foods

Alsleben agrees with Swank that fats should be eliminated from the diets of people with MS. He also counsels that the following foods be avoided:

- All bleached flour products.
- Products containing hydrogenated or hardened oils, including crackers and baking mixes, frozen pies or prepared pie crusts, all margarines and

many of the peanut butters, French fries and potato chips prepared in oils or fats containing hydrogenated compounds, and fried foods.
- Unsaturated oils in cooking.
- Soft drinks, candy, and pastries high in sugar.

## Restricted Foods

Alsleben strongly advises MS sufferers to eliminate coffee, if possible, or to restrict consumption to one cup or less a day. If used, it should be refrigerated and never reheated. Drinking a noncaffeine herbal tea or coffee substitutes such as Postum and Pero is preferable.

## RECENT RESEARCH

### Polyunsaturated Fatty Acids (PUFAs)

As previously noted, Swank found in his clinical trials conducted between 1949 and 1984 that MS patients often have low levels of linolenic and linoleic acids, essential fatty acids that are important in maintaining myelin production.

In *Therapeutic Claims in Multiple Sclerosis*, Dr. William A. Sibley cites three scientifically controlled, sizable studies that suggest "dietary supplementation with linoleic acid or natural oils containing PUFA appears to slow progression and reduce the severity and duration of MS exacerbations without affecting their frequency." While he cautions that "the effect is apparently a very modest one," Sibley concludes that MS patients with minimal disability may benefit from taking PUFA in terms of experiencing less increase in disability than those who do not.

### Additional Therapies

Balch and Balch claim that massage, exercise (especially swimming), and an effort to keep mentally active are "extremely valuable" in bringing about remission of MS symptoms. However, exercises that increase body temperature can decrease the function of the nerves involved and make symptoms worse. They recommend exercises in cool water (which help by supporting the body's weight), as well as stretching exercises that help to prevent muscle contractures.

Balch and Balch also urge MS sufferers to avoid extremely hot baths, showers, and overly warm surroundings, as these may trigger an attack. They also note that a two-year multicenter study reported in the January

1993 issue of the *Archives of Neurology* found that exacerbations of MS can be relieved by spinal injections of natural human fibroblast interferon.

## Vitamin B12

As discussed, specific vitamins, minerals, trace elements, and amino acids (including vitamin C, beta-carotene, B complex, zinc, magnesium, calcium, selenium, and the amino acid glutathione) are often recommended to compensate for deficiencies and act as cofactors for the efficient metabolism of essential fatty acids. According to *Alternative Medicine: The Definitive Guide*, vitamin B12 has also proven highly effective in decreasing symptoms of MS, especially when they are associated with mercury poisoning.

One cited practitioner prescribes B12 doses as high as 12,000 micrograms once a week by intravenous infusion, usually with other essential nutrients. However, intramuscular doses are commonly between 4,000 and 8,000 micrograms once a week. *Alternative Medicine: The Definitive Guide* reports several cases in which high doses of intravenous vitamin B12 relieved MS relapses within thirty minutes of administration.

# 24

## Cancer and Chemotherapy Diets

O ne out of every five Americans is likely to develop cancer during his or her lifetime, and of those, one person in five is likely to die from it. According to *Modern Nutrition in Health and Disease*, the estimated number of annual deaths is slightly more than 500,000 in the United States. In 1991, for example, it was 514,000. Approximately one-third of all cancers are caused by cigarette smoking and other forms of to-bacco use. It is estimated that 80 percent of all cancers could be prevented if people ate nutritious lowfat foods, did not smoke, and limited other unhealthy behaviors.

One of the most promising fields of research in medicine today is that of chemoprevention: the use of micro- or macronutrients, often found in foods, that can prevent, retard, or reverse the process of cancer development. In 1993, the National Cancer Institute conducted more than forty studies in the area of how nutrition involving fiber, fat, micronutrients, and vitamins might play a role in preventing and treating various cancers.

The three cancer diets reviewed in this chapter represent a broad spectrum of nutritional approaches to prevention, recovery, and coping with chemotherapy and radiation treatment. The Simone Diet outlines a ten-point dietary plan to *prevent* cancer. The Nixon Diet presents excellent dietary guidelines to help people who are *recovering* from cancer. The Bruning Diet, developed by a woman who was diagnosed with breast cancer, presents very helpful food suggestions for patients undergoing chemotherapy.

### NUTRITION AND CANCER

Shils writes in his article "Nutrition and Diet in Cancer Management" (in *Modern Nutrition in Health and Disease*), that cancer is "many diverse con-

## NATIONAL CANCER INSTITUTE DIETARY GUIDELINES TO REDUCE CANCER RISK

1. *Maintain a desirable body weight.* Overweight has been linked with cancers of the breast, uterus, colon, prostate, and gallbladder.

2. *Eat a varied diet.* A varied diet, eaten in moderation, offers the best hope for lowering cancer risk.

3. *Include a variety of both vegetables and fruits in the daily diet.* Consumption of vegetables and fruits is associated with a decreased risk of lung, prostate, bladder, esophageal, and stomach cancers.

4. *Eat more high-fiber foods, such as whole-grain cereals, legumes, vegetables, and fruits.* Colon cancer is low in populations who live on a diet high in fiber.

5. *Decrease total fat intake.* Substantial evidence now suggests that excessive fat intake increases the risk of developing cancers of the breast, colon, and prostate. The National Cancer Institute and American Cancer Society now both recommend reducing total fat intake from the current average of approximately 40 to 30 percent or less of total caloric intake.

6. *Limit consumption of alcoholic beverages.* Alcohol has also been implicated in the development of cancers of the liver, pancreas, colon, and, most recently, breast.

7. *Limit consumption of salt-cured, smoked, and nitrite-preserved foods.* There is limited evidence that salt-cured, pickled, or nitrite-cured foods may increase the risk of stomach and esophageal cancers in countries where these foods are common in the diet.

ditions characterized by growth of cells that have lost their usual growth restraints and thus multiply and spread." Normal healthy cells grow, divide, and replace themselves in an orderly way. Sometimes, however, for reasons which are still not fully understood, cells lose their ability to control their growth and begin to multiply abnormally. In the process, they can develop their own network of blood vessels that siphon nourishment away from tissues and organs.

Because cancer cells grow and multiply out of control, they constantly seek more nourishment. In siphoning off energy from normal, healthy cells, cancerous cells deprive them of needed nutrition. This is probably why, in many cases of advanced cancer, a person suffers debilitating loss of weight and strength — a condition called cachexia — even when consuming an adequate amount of food.

Despite uncertainties regarding the exact contribution of diet and nutrition to cancer risk, Shils states that there is growing evidence that changes in dietary patterns help reduce the risk for certain types of cancer. As a result, the National Cancer Institute recently joined with eight other voluntary and government organizations to issue a report about diet and disease that all the participating agencies could support.

## THE NIXON CANCER DIET

The Nixon Cancer Diet is detailed in Dr. Daniel W. Nixon's *The Cancer Recovery Eating Plan*. Nixon is Folk professor of experimental oncology and director of cancer prevention and control at the Hollings Cancer Center at the Medical University of South Carolina. Formerly, he was an associate director of the Cancer Prevention Research Program of the National Cancer Institute. He currently serves as a consultant to the American Cancer Society, and editor in chief of *Cancer Prevention*.

### Basic Nutritional Approach

Nixon's book presents the most comprehensive discussion of up-to-date information on the role of diet and nutrition in cancer treatment and prevention. Nixon stresses that while diet plays an important role in modulating the development, growth, and spread of cancer, diet most likely does not cause cancer by itself. Cancer is the result of a combination of poor diet along with genetic, environmental, and other factors that can lead to some cancers.

Likewise, Nixon points out, diet alone is not by itself a useful treatment for any existing cancer. Nevertheless, he suggests that nutrition working together with other factors can contribute to both cancer-risk reduction and chances of remission of specific types of cancer.

An important helpful feature of this book is the fact that Nixon distinguishes between the more than one hundred types of cancer. He stresses that the diet one adopts should always depend on what type of cancer a patient has. He notes that the nature of the relationship between the cancer and nutrition tends to fall into one of three groups: 1) tumors of "overnutrition" (such as breast cancer); 2) tumors of "undernutrition"; 3) cancers where other factors tend to overwhelm any effect of nutrition. Some cancers, he observes, have no known nutritional connection.

## General Recommended Foods

*Fiber.* Nixon cites an impressive number of studies which suggest that fiber can reduce the risk of cancer. Water-insoluble fiber has been associated with decreased cellular activity and decreased polyp formation in the gut, and thereby is thought to help prevent colon cancer. Fiber also acts as a laxative and reduces the amount of time food remains in the intestinal tract. It may also bind with carcinogens in the gut and render them harmless. A final benefit is that fiber may alter gut bacteria and acidity so that fewer carcinogens are produced. The water-soluble group (gums, pectin, and others) also tend to lower cholesterol levels in the blood which may reduce the risk of some cancers. Nixon stresses that Americans should consume as much as 35 grams of fiber daily to prevent cancer.

*Carbohydrates.* A number of cross-national studies, according to Nixon, have shown that high intake of carbohydrate-rich foods, especially vegetables and fruits, has a cancer-protective effect. These foods tend to be high vitamin and chemopreventive compounds, high in fiber, and low in fat, all of which are preventive measures for cancer.

## Generally Eliminated or Restricted Foods

*Fat.* Fat, according to Nixon, has a dual role in cancer. It may act both as a promoter of cancer and as a modulator of the growth of existing cancer. He presents a substantial amount of evidence that high-fat diets can cause breast and colon cancer. Conversely, he notes that a lowfat, low-calorie diet can inhibit the development of certain types of tumors and even slow the growth of established tumors in laboratory animals.

Scientists do not yet know which types of fat (saturated, unsaturated, omega-3 fatty acids, and so on) are directly linked to different cancers. Therefore, Nixon recommends that total fat be restricted to reduce cancer risk. He notes that 30 percent of daily total calories as fat is too high, and cautions everyone to consume less than 20 percent. For persons recovering from breast, colon, and prostate cancer, he emphasizes that 15 percent fat is even better. He also notes that most Americans consume fat that comes from animal products and that "animal fat is the major problem in our diets."

*Cholesterol.* A diet high in fats also increases blood cholesterol levels, although Nixon states that it is not clear precisely what role, if any, cholesterol might play in cancer. There is evidence, however, he suggests, that farnesyl, a substance created as the liver synthesizes cholesterol, may have some role in the earliest stages of cancer development. Farnesyl may interact with oncogenes (the genes through which cancer begins) and create byproducts which trigger cancer cells to activate. If the farnesyl hypothesis is true, Nixon contends that consuming less cholesterol may reduce oncogene byproducts.

*Protein.* According to Nixon, the link between excess protein consumption and cancer has not been definitively established. Nevertheless, he cites several population studies which found a relationship between high consumption of animal protein (meat and dairy products) and breast cancer. He also notes that laboratory studies have shown that when breast tumors are induced in animals by carcinogens, feeding the animals more protein leads to increased tumors. Some epidemiological studies have also linked animal protein intake to colon cancer, prostate cancer, and endometrial cancer. Nixon hypothesizes that one reason that cancer causes cachexia might be the interference of the cancer with the body's ability to turn food into lean protein and muscle tissue.

Although Nixon does not recommend a strict vegetarian diet because it lends itself to nutritional deficits, he does state that "limiting meat consumption to six ounces weekly has as much anticancer benefit as the total exclusion of meat from the diet." He writes, "There is strong evidence that complete lowfat vegetarianism is the best diet to help prevent and perhaps even reverse heart disease." He therefore recommends that everyone consider at least two meat-free days a week, which helps reduce total fat intake and increases fiber intake.

Nixon only provides dietary guidelines for those cancers which he and other researchers have found can either be prevented, or treated with nutritional therapy: breast, colorectal, or prostate cancer, as well as cancer of the lung, head, neck, esophagus, cervix, bladder, or skin.

*Sodium (Salt).* Nixon states that although there is no known direct connection between sodium intake and cancer, excess sodium can aggravate high blood pressure, which, in turn, often increases the risk of heart attack, stroke, and kidney disease. It also poses complications for cancer patients undergoing hormonal therapy, because excess sodium intake can cause their bodies to accumulate fluids — thus raising their blood pressure. Also, certain chemotherapeutic agents can damage the heart and kidneys, and salt and fluid overload often exacerbates such damage.

## Diet for Breast Cancer

Breast cancer, according to Dr. Nixon, has the closest scientific link with excess dietary fat. Nixon does not promise that reducing fat will help patients whose disease has progressed despite other therapy. Reducing fat consumption will help in the early stages of breast cancer, however, especially if patients are being given adjutant chemotherapy and hormonal therapy.

Nixon's diet for breast cancer focuses on replacing fats with fiber-rich foods. Restricting fat intake will normally decrease calories (which provide energy for tumors to grow). It will also reduce tumor-stimulating fatty acids and circulating estrogen levels. The relationship between fiber and breast cancer is still unclear, Nixon cautions, although he suggests that high-fiber intake reduces estrogen levels by changing the way food is absorbed in the gut.

Foods that contain beta-carotene (such as fruits and vegetables) are low in fat and high in fiber and other chemopreventive compounds. Studies suggest that certain forms of vitamin A may prevent second primary tumors in breast cancer.

*Recommended Foods.* 1) Increase fiber intake to 25 grams per day or more; 2) Increase foods that contain beta-carotene.

*Restricted Foods.* Reduce fat intake to no more than 20 percent of total calories.

## Diet for Colorectal Cancer

According to Nixon, three food components have been definitely linked with colon cancer: fiber, fat, and calcium. He cites studies which have shown that countries with high-fat, low-fiber diets have higher rates of colorectal cancer than countries where people consume high levels of fiber and less fat. He suggests that consuming high levels of dietary fiber may inhibit large-bowel cancer by hurrying food through the gut and helping to increase the bulk of stool. Fiber may also bind with other substances in the gut that could become a source of cancer, modifying or neutralizing them so that they can do no harm.

*Recommended Foods.* 1) Increase fiber intake to 30 to 35 grams per day; 2) Select a variety of fruits and vegetables; 3) Emphasize calcium-rich foods; 4) Stress beta-carotene–rich foods; 5) Include allium vegetables such as garlic, onions, and leeks.

*Eliminated or Restricted Foods.* 1) Decrease fat consumption to no more than 20 percent of daily calories.

## Diet for Prostate Cancer

Despite the strong suspicion of a link between diet and prostate cancer, Nixon states "there have been very few clinical trials to test diet's role in prevention or as an adjunct to treatment of the disease." Nevertheless, he adds that it is known that "like colorectal, breast and other cancers, the more fat in the diet, the greater the chance of developing prostate cancer."

*Recommended Foods and Supplements.* 1) Because prostate cancer is associated with aging, Nixon advises patients to ask their physician about taking a multivitamin supplement which includes vitamin E, an important antioxidant that may not be present in sufficient quantity in a lowfat diet.

*Eliminated or Restricted Foods.* 1) Lower dietary fats to 20 percent or less of total calories and increase foods containing beta-carotene.

Nixon's contention was indirectly proven recently in laboratory studies with mice. Researchers at Memorial Sloan-Kettering Cancer Center in New York injected human prostate cancer cells into special laboratory mice. The mice were then divided into four groups, and each group received different levels of fat, ranging from a high of 40.5 percent to a low of 2.3 percent fat per calories. Tumor growth was two and a half times greater in mice on the high-fat diet than in mice on the lowest-fat diet. Dr. William R. Fair, director of the study, states in the October 3, 1995, issue of the *San Francisco Chronicle* that the difference in tumor growth reflected levels of a prostate-specific antigen (PSA) in the rodents' blood. High levels of PSA are often indicative of cancer growth. Fair suggested that his study raises the possibility that a lowfat diet can play a role in both the prevention and treatment of prostate cancer, although he warned that his findings remain to be verified in human clinical trials.

## Basic Diet for Squamous Cancers (Cancer of the Lung, Head, Neck, Esophagus, Cervix, Bladder, or Skin)

Squamous cell cancers arise from cells that cover organs and form the lining of tissue surfaces. Most lung cancers have been directly linked to tobacco use. Skin cancer is caused by excess sunlight, and cervical cancer has been linked with a particular group of viruses. All squamous cell cancers, according to Nixon, require similar nutritional plans and his diet is recommended for all of them.

As with other cancers, Nixon cautions that nutritional changes have the best chance of helping in the early stage of squamous cell cancers and premalignant lesions. Once these cancers metastasize, they have a much poorer chance of responding to dietary changes.

Diets high in fruits and vegetables will contain antioxidant vitamins and other chemopreventives that may act to deprive squamous cells of the energy they need to spread. Specifically, fruits and vegetables contain important beta-carotene, a known chemopreventive. Vegetables such as garlic, onions, and leeks contain allium compounds with chemopreventive properties. He also suggests that vitamin E and a multivitamin supplement may boost immunity in older patients.

*Recommended Foods.* 1) Increase fruits and vegetables to 11 or more servings per day.

*Eliminated or Restricted Foods.* 1) Lower fat intake to 25 percent of daily calories.

## Vitamin and Mineral Supplements

Although several vitamins are now known to be important in cancer, Nixon states that their exact role in specific cancers is still not known. He notes that a number of clinical trials are currently in progress to test the use of vitamins (especially antioxidants) to prevent cancer. Much of the attention is focused on vitamin A and synthetic counterparts of vitamin A, as well as

## FOOD SUBSTITUTION RECOMMENDATIONS TO REDUCE DIETARY FAT

Nixon offers the following suggestions to reduce dietary fat and lower the risk of cancer:

1. Replace whole eggs in baking recipes with two egg whites.
2. Use nonfat yogurt instead of sour cream, heavy cream, oil, or mayonnaise. For cooked dishes that require sour cream, substitute the same amount of nonfat yogurt plus a 1/2 teaspoon of flour.
3. Use nonfat yogurt cheese and use in place of cream cheese to top bagels or to make cheesecake, or use nonfat cream cheese.
4. Use evaporated skim milk in coffee or hot tea, cream-based soups, stews, and salad dressings.
5. In baking recipes, replace whole milk with skim milk or nonfat buttermilk.
6. Substitute an equivalent portion of applesauce for oil in muffins, cakes, brownies, and sweetbreads.
7. Substitute unsweetened cocoa for Baker's chocolate.
8. Reduce 1/2 cup nuts in recipes to 1 tablespoon nuts.
9. Replace ground beef with ground turkey and chicken in recipes; reduce the meat to 3 ounces per person.

vitamins C and E. Nixon also notes that vitamins can reduce the side effects of cancer therapies. One example is taking folic acid supplements while undergoing chemotherapy with methotrexate which can reduce bone marrow damage and severe mouth sores. Patients with promyelocytic leukemia, for example, have experienced some remissions after taking transretinoic acid, a form of vitamin A.

Nixon adds that vitamins A, C, and E may also help remove potentially harmful oxidative compounds from cells which are capable of damaging DNA and may, in this way, cause cancer. These vitamins are called "anti-oxidants" because they inhibit the harmful activity of free radicals and prevent oxidative damage. The extent of their ability to prevent cancer is still not fully known. Some vitamins and vitamin precursors such as beta-carotene appear to hinder the development of skin cancer and upper digestive tract cancers, as well as cervical cancer in its earliest stages.

## Calcium

Nixon cites research studies that suggest a possible link between calcium deficiencies and cancer. Epidemiological studies, for example, have shown that the more milk a person drinks, the lower their risk of colon cancer, and vice versa. Calcium has also been shown in laboratory studies to decrease the cell division activity in the colon-lining cells. Calcium may also bind and inactivate carcinogens in the stool. As detailed in Chapter 17, excellent sources of calcium besides nonfat dairy products include asparagus, broccoli, Great Northern and navy beans, okra, spinach, and soybean products (tofu).

## Physical Activity

According to Nixon, the most important benefit of physical activity for cancer, especially for women with breast cancer, is that it decreases their overall body fat. Exercise helps decrease body fat and increase lean body mass which may foster a more favorable hormone balance in early breast cancer — and perhaps other hormonally sensitive cancers as well. Several studies have also suggested that exercise helps overcome cancer cachexia, the condition in which persons suffer debilitating weight loss and strength, even when they eat an adequate amount of food. Exercise may improve the body's conversion of glucose to useful energy and make it more sensitive to insulin.

Exercise, Nixon adds, may also help prevent colon cancer for a variety of reasons. He stresses that anyone with cancer should discuss his or her exercise program with his or her health care provider, although even if a person's physical capacity is very limited, any form of exercise will improve quality of life.

## Behavioral Modification

Nixon notes that stress and anxiety affect the functioning of the body, but pinning down exactly how is very difficult. Some research has also found that people survive cancer longer when they used relaxation and imaging techniques, but random trials are lacking to prove this. Nixon cites one study in which a group of melanoma patients experienced an increase in immune function when they participated in support groups that focused on coping and relaxation skills. Importantly, their natural killer cells increased in activity while they participated in group work. Nixon cautions, however, that techniques such as "imaging" the immune system fighting against cancer cells, relaxation tapes, and other mind therapies are not yet known to have real clinical value.

## THE SIMONE CANCER DIET

The Simone Cancer Diet was developed by Charles B. Simone, M.D., and outlined in his book, *Cancer and Nutrition: A Ten-Point Plan to Reduce Your Risk of Getting Cancer*. Dr. Simone is a nationally renowned cancer specialist and currently directs the Simone Cancer Center in Lawrence-ville, New Jersey. He has conducted research at the National Cancer Institute.

### Basic Nutritional Approach

Simone asserts that nearly 60 percent of all women's cancers and 40 percent of all men's cancers are related to nutritional factors alone. Nutritional factors, he adds, "are most closely associated with the following cancers in order of their prevalence in the U.S.: gastrointestinal cancers, breast cancer, prostate cancer and endometrial cancer."

Simone's basic nutritional approach is outlined in his ten-point plan for reducing the risk of cancer and heart disease:

1. Maintain an ideal body weight. Lose weight even if it is just five to seven pounds.
2. Decrease the number of daily calories.
3. Eat a lowfat, low-cholesterol diet consisting mainly of fish rich in omega-3 fatty acids; poultry without skin; and skim-milk products (not whole, 2%, or 1% milk). Limit red meat, including luncheon meat. Limit oils and fats.
4. Eat plenty of fiber (25 to 30 grams a day). Include fruits, vegetables, cereals, and supplements of fiber to obtain a consistent amount each day (guar gum, bran, etc.). High-fiber cereals are best.
5. Supplement the diet with vitamins and minerals in the proper doses recommended by your physician.
6. Eliminate salt and food additives.
7. Limit barbecued, smoked, or pickled foods.
8. Avoid caffeine.

## Recommended Foods: Fiber

Simone's diet is high in fiber because, like many cancer specialists, he has found that it protects against colorectal cancer, breast cancer, heart disease, diverticular disease, obesity, and diabetes. A low incidence of cancer is seen in people who consume large amounts of carotene-rich foods and cruciferous vegetables such as cabbage, broccoli, cauliflower, and Brussels sprouts. Fiber's protective action, Simone explains, is due to the fact that it binds bile acids, cholesterol, lipids, poisons, and carcinogens. It also increases the weight and mass of stool, which, in effect, dilutes carcinogens. And it decreases the gastrointestinal transit time so that the carcinogens are excreted more quickly. Finally, it helps keep the intestinal flora healthy.

He especially recommends high-fiber cereals and vegetables of the Brassicaceae family, which provide fiber and induce enzymes to destroy certain carcinogens. These include Brussels sprouts, broccoli, and cabbage. Dieters are advised to eat whole or lightly milled grains such as rice, barley, and buckwheat. Whole-wheat bread and wheat pasta, cereals, crackers, and other grain products should also be eaten.

## Eliminated or Restricted Foods

*Fats.* Dietary fat found in red meat, luncheon meats, and all dairy products promotes and probably initiates carcinogenesis, according to Simone. He reviews several studies that suggest an association between consumption of dietary fat and the occurrence of cancer at several sites, most notably the breast, prostate, and colorectal area, the endometrium, and to a lesser extent, the ovaries. High-fat consumption is related not only to the high incidence of breast cancer but also to high mortality rates. Some studies show a correlation with saturated fats, but other studies show a correlation with both saturated and unsaturated fats. Low breast cancer rates, on the other hand, are observed among populations who consume lowfat diets.

Therefore, Simone's diet eliminates all oils and fats including butter, margarine, meat fat, lard, and all oils. Both saturated and polyunsaturated fats are prohibited. Either eliminating or severely restricting these oils, he notes, is especially important for breast cancer patients. The best way to eliminate fats, he adds, is to replace fatty foods with high-fiber foods because they have been shown to increase the fecal excretion of estrogen and to decrease the plasma concentration of estrogen. This replacing fats with fiber dietary approach might also be helpful, he suggests, for colorectal, prostate, and endometrial cancer patients.

Simone cautions that dieters must restrict their consumption of garnishes and sauces by using products that do not have fats, oils, or egg yolks. Dry white wine may be used in cooking, along with ketchup and vinegar. Dieters must also restrict salad dressings, pickle relishes, gravies, fatty sauces, mayonnaise, sandwich spreads, and other products containing fats or oils.

*Red Meat.* Simone's diet suggests that dieters restrict their meat consumption to six ounces once every ten days. He eliminates all fatty meats such as bacon, hamburger, spareribs, sausage, luncheon meats, sweetbreads, hot dogs, kidney, brains, liver, etc. He also suggests completely eliminating all smoke and salt-cured foods. Barbecued and charcoal-broiled foods should also be restricted.

*Dairy Products.* Simone advises dieters to consume only nonfat dairy products such as skim milk, skim-milk cheese, skim powdered milk, evaporated skim milk, nonfat yogurt, and buttermilk. Dieters are permitted only two egg whites per week or a cholesterol-free egg substitute a couple of times a week. Whole and lowfat milk and the products made from them are completely eliminated, including cream, half and half, all cheeses containing fat, whipped cream, etc. Whole eggs are also eliminated.

*Sugar.* A high dietary intake of refined sugar was one of the dietary components linked to the increased incidence of breast cancer in several studies. Simone therefore restricts or eliminates all cooked, canned, or frozen fruit with added sugar; all jams and jellies; fruit syrups with added sugar, fruit juices with added sugar, bleached white flour; and grain products made with added fats, oils, or egg yolks. He recommends that dieters gradually eliminate all butter rolls, commercial biscuits, muffins, doughnuts, sweet rolls, cakes, egg bread, cheese bread, and commercial mixes containing dried eggs and whole milk from their diet.

*Proteins.* High amounts of daily protein, Simone explains, have been found to cause a high incidence of carcinogenesis in animals. In many animal studies carcinogenesis was suppressed when animals were fed levels of protein that were at the minimum or below the minimum required for optimal growth. Simone suggests that high protein intake has been linked indirectly with breast cancer and colorectal cancer. There has also been a weaker association between high protein intake and other cancers, specifically pancreatic cancer, prostate cancer, and endometrial cancer. As a result, he severely restricts animal protein in his diet.

*Food Carcinogens.* Simone cites research by UC Berkeley researcher Bruce Ames that indicates that some plants have certain molecules to protect them against microorganisms and insects, and some of these are carcinogenic or mutagenic in humans. The following are a few Simone mentions and they are listed with their carcinogens in parentheses: black pepper (piperine and sarole), bruised celery (psoralen), herbal teas (pyrolizidine), mushrooms (hydrazines), and all foods containing mold (aflatoxin) or bacteria (nitrosamines). Many of these are occasional contaminants, whereas others are normal components of relatively common foods. Foods that pose the greatest risk of cancer in humans, according to Simone, are the mycotoxins (aflatoxin) and nitrous compounds from bacteria.

*Coffee.* Simone also notes that some foods such as caffeine also contain mutagens, which are chemical compounds that cause heritable changes in the genetic material of cells. Many vegetables contain mutagenic flavonoids, and mutagens are also produced in charred and smoked foods. Mutagens can also be produced at lower temperatures. Others, like coffee and horseradish, contain quinones and allyl isothiocyanate, although he believes the risk of developing cancer from mutagens in humans is minimal.

*Food Additives.* Simone warns that currently there are more than 3,000 intentional food additives, some of which are potentially carcinogenic. One of these, nitrite, is converted in the body to a very potent carcinogen, nitrosamine. In addition, there are more than 12,000 unintentional additives found in packaging, food processing, and other phases of the food industry. The worst of these, he warns, are vinyl chloride and diethylsilbestrol, which are used in food packaging and processing and in the foods fed to many livestock.

## Weight Loss, Obesity, and Cancer

Simone, like Nixon, notes the increasing evidence that excess weight and obesity are directly linked to cancer. According to Simone, obesity is a major risk factor for the development of endometrial cancer (cancer of the inner lining of the uterus) in postmenopausal women. The reason, he suggests, is because obese postmenopausal women produce substantially more of a female hormone called estrone. This increased production is directly related to the number and size of the woman's fat cells, since estrone is manufactured in fat cells from another hormone called andros-tenedione. Estrone apparently stimulates the uterus, and this is believed to cause endometrial cancer. Similarly, postmenopausal women who take es-trogens daily for symptoms of menopause also have a higher incidence of endometrial cancer. Simone also notes that obese persons usually consume more fats in their diet, and this, as noted, is a major risk factor for breast and colon cancer. He cites animal studies which show that if food intake was reduced (the number of calories decreased) during a "critical period" after a carcinogen is introduced to induce breast cancer, the development of the cancer is inhibited. Simone suggests that leaner animals produce less of prolactin and estrogen, two hormones which in high amounts can lead to the development of cancer.

## Meal Plans and Recipes

In Chapter 23 of his book ("Diet Plan to Modify Risks") Simone outlines several easy-to-follow diets for weight reduction. He recommends that dieters initially plan to lose two to four pounds per week to achieve their ideal body weight. Once they attain their weight goal, they can easily modify their eating habits. His diet plan is a low-cholesterol, very lowfat, high-fiber diet which, he suggests, substantially reduces the risk for cancer and cardiovascular disease. He presents six tables that list food groups: milk, vegetables, fruit, meat and fish, bread and fat, and miscellaneous. He explains how dieters can trade or exchange one food item for another in the same group. He also provides a Sample Diet with number of grams, pro-tein, fat, and carbohydrates provided for each portion. His recommended Diet #1 and #2 contain approximately 1,000 calories. Diet #3 provides 1,218 calories daily; Diet #4, 1,255.

While on his recommended diets, he advises all dieters to:

1. Take a multiple vitamin/mineral complex daily.
2. Eat foods that are high in potassium, including apricots, bananas, berries, grapefruit juice, mangoes, cantaloupes, honeydews, nectar-ines, oranges, orange juice, and peaches.
3. Eat vegetables (especially raw ones) such as carrots, celery, chicory,

Chinese cabbage, cucumbers, endive, escarole, lettuce, parsley, radishes, scallions, and watercress.

4. Choose cereals and breads with high fiber content; add fiber value to breakfast by adding fruit to cereal.

5. Drink water, bouillon without fat, and salt-free club soda instead of tea and coffee.

6. Use seasonings such as paprika, garlic, parsley, nutmeg, lemon, mustard, vinegar, mint, cinnamon, and lime as substitutes for salt. Do not use salt at the table.

## Vitamin and Mineral Supplements

Simone states that by eliminating all known risk factors of cancer and practicing good nutrition supplemented with vitamins and minerals, most people can prevent many cancers. Micronutrients, he notes, have been found by cancer specialists to prevent the initiation or development of cancer. Simone recommends that adults take the following combination of vitamins and mineral supplements — certainly one of the most comprehensive multinutrient supplementation programs currently recommended by cancer specialists. Pregnant or lactating women should not follow this program, he cautions, unless it has been approved by their physician.

## Physical Activity

According to Simone, the main benefit of exercise for cancer patients is that in most cases, it produces a higher number of white blood cells, specifically granulocytes, that are needed to fight off infections and tumors. He states that exercisers have higher B and T killer cell counts. During exercise a person's temperature rises slightly which is accompanied by the production of pyrogen, an important protein produced by white blood cells that enhances lymphocyte functions. Elevated temperatures can also kill viruses — and have also been shown to kill cancer cells.

A significant number of animal studies have shown that exercise can actually inhibit cancer growth. Human studies have shown that the risk of developing breast cancer is 1.86 times higher for nonathletes than for athletes, and the risk of developing cancers of the reproductive system is 2.5 times higher. Men who do not exercise have a 1.6 higher risk of developing colon cancer than men who exercise. Like Nixon, Simone contends that the decreased incidence is probably due to the fact that increased activity causes more motility of the gastrointestinal tract. The longer the stool

## SIMONE VITAMIN/MINERAL
## SUPPLEMENTATION PROGRAM

| Nutrient | Adult Amount | Child (Age 1–4) Amount |
|---|---|---|
| Beta-carotene | 20 mg | 1 mg |
| Vitamin A (palmitate) | 5,000 IU | 834 IU |
| Vitamin D (ergocalciferol) | 400 IU | 400 IU |
| Vitamin E (di-tocopherol) | 400 IU | 15 IU |
| Vitamin C (ascorbic acid) | 350 mg | 60 mg |
| Folic acid | 400 mcg | 200 mcg |
| Vitamin B1 (thiamine) | 10 mg | 1.1 mg |
| Vitamin B2 (riboflavin) | 10 mg | 1.2 mg |
| Niacinamide | 40 mg | 9 mg |
| Vitamin B6 (pyridoxine) | 10 mg | 1.12 mg |
| Vitamin B12 (cyanobalamin) | 18 mcg | 4.5 mcg |
| Biotin | 150 mcg | 25 mcg |
| Pantothenic acid | 20 mg | 5 mg |
| Iodine | 150 mcg | 70 mcg |
| Copper (cupric oxide) | 3 mg | 1.25 mg |
| Zinc (zinc gluconate) | 15 mg | 10 mg |
| Potassium | 30 mg | 2 mg |
| Selenium (organic) | 200 mcg | 20 mcg |
| Chromium (organic) | 125 mcg | 20 mcg |
| Manganese (gluconate) | 2.5 mg | 1 mg |
| Molybdenum | 50 mcg | 25 mcg |
| Inositol | 10 mg | 0 |
| Para aminobenzoic acid | 120 mg | 0 |
| Bioflavonoids | 10 mg | 10 mcg |
| Choline (choline bitartrate) | 10 mg | 5 mg |
| L-Cysteine | 230 mg | 0 |
| L-Arginine | 5 mg | 0 |
| Histidine | N/A | 10 mg |
| Leucine | N/A | 10 mg |
| Lysine | N/A | 10 mg |
| Threonine | N/A | 10 mg |
| Calcium (calcium carbonate) | 500 mg | N/A |
| Magnesium (magnesium oxide) | 140 mg | |
| Silicon | 2 mg | |
| Boron | 2 mg | |
| L-Threonine | 2 mg | |
| L-Lysine | 2 mg | |

remains in the colon, the longer a carcinogen in the stool called fecapentaene has to exert its effect, and consequently the higher the risk for cancer in various parts of the colon which the stool contacts.

## Behavioral Modification

Simone states that stress is one of the many risk factors for the development of cancer. By itself, stress causes immunological depression, which, coupled with other risk factors, can contribute to the development of cancer. He suggests that there is a cancer-prone personality, and that persons who cope with stress better, have lower risks of cancer. He outlines several helpful relaxation exercises, including meditation and biofeedback.

## COPING WITH CHEMOTHERAPY DIET

Many books on cancer discuss chemotherapy or radiation treatment — but they often fail to describe in real human terms the pain and agony which many patients experience. A wide variety of drugs are currently employed to treat cancer, and while these often can cause the remission of the disease, they usually produce very unpleasant side effects, including the loss of appetite, nausea and vomiting, diarrhea, constipation, dehydration, and difficulty chewing or swallowing. All of these symptoms can lead to alterations in the kinds and amounts of foods they eat, as well as their body's ability to absorb and utilize what they eat. Some drugs, in addition, destroy nutrients in the body. In turn, poor nutrition often impairs both the effectiveness of chemotherapy or radiation treatment and the body's ability to defend itself against the drugs' side effects.

Nancy Bruning was diagnosed with breast cancer at the age of 31. Fortunately, she consulted a nutritionist who helped her develop a diet which specifically enhanced her ability to cope with chemotherapy. Her Coping with Chemotherapy Diet is outlined in her book, *Coping with Chemotherapy*. Bruning has counseled cancer patients informally and was a volunteer at Memorial Sloan-Kettering Cancer Center in New York. Her other books include *Swimming for Total Fitness* (with Dr. Jane Katz), *The Real Vitamin and Mineral Book* (with Shari Lieberman), and *Breast Implants: Everything You Need to Know*. She is a board member of Breast Cancer Action, an education and advocacy group based in San Francisco. She wrote her book, she states, "to collate her research and help other people live and fight cancer."

## Basic Nutritional Approach

Nancy Bruning outlines diet recommendations in Chapter 8 of her book. She states there are four important roles nutrition plays in chemotherapy:

1. *Nutrition improves tolerance of therapy:* nutrition can decrease the severity and duration of side effects such as vomiting, nausea, weakness, lowered immunity, and susceptibility to infection.
2. *Nutrition increases the effectiveness of therapy:* a good nutritional regimen allows the patient to withstand higher doses of drugs, thus increasing the effectiveness of the therapy.
3. *Nutrition speeds recovery from treatments:* a balanced chemotherapy diet helps rebuild normal tissue destroyed by chemotherapy.
4. *Nutritional therapies help regulate body weight:* many people either lose or gain weight while undergoing chemotherapy, although some women gain weight on chemotherapy, which can lead to weakness, lethargy, depression, embarrassment, and lack of self-esteem. A balanced diet can help maintain body weight and the energy patients need to stay active and positive.

## Recommended Foods

All approaches to nutritional support for the chemotherapy patient, according to Bruning, must be grounded in the concept of a well-balanced diet which contains a variety of foods that provide vitamins, minerals, protein, carbohydrates, fats, and water. Her diet focuses on the mandatory daily consumption of five food groups:

**Fruits and vegetables:** four servings (two of each)
**Meat, fish, poultry, eggs, cheese:** three servings
**Grains:** four servings
**Milk and milk products:** two servings
**Liquids:** eight to twelve glasses

According to Bruning, patients undergoing chemotherapy usually require more protein and calories than usual to help their body replace lost healthy cells and to maintain their weight, fat stores, and lean muscle mass. Even though they may not have good appetites, they should force themselves to eat well. Some patients find they have to add liquid nutritional supplements to their diets. Bruning cautions patients who lack essential nutrients that they will have to take a multivitamin/mineral supplement.

For example, supplements are absolutely necessary for patients who have lost their appetite, lost weight, who drink or smoke, or who have difficulty absorbing minerals and vitamins through their foods. Real foods, however, should be eaten to provide all nutritional requirements if possible. In extreme cases of advanced cancer or severe weight loss, some patients may need supplemental tube feedings — either through tubes inserted into the stomach or small intestine or through intravenous feedings.

*Recommended Foods.* Like Nixon and Simone, Bruning states that foods high in vitamin C and beta-carotene protect against the development of cancer and are beneficial for chemotherapy dieters. She specifically recommends: oranges, grapefruit, apricots, cantaloupes, peaches, strawberries, dark leafy green vegetables, carrots, winter squash, tomatoes, green peppers, and sweet potatoes. Cruciferous vegetables such as broccoli, Brussels sprouts, cabbage, and cauliflower contain these vitamins plus compounds called indoles that research suggests may increase the dieter's body's capacity to convert carcinogens into harmless substances.

*Fiber.* Low fiber consumption, she notes, has been linked to bowel and breast cancer, and she emphasizes that the National Cancer Center now recommends that chemotherapy patients increase their daily fiber intake. Fruits and vegetables are also high in fiber, as are whole grains such as whole-wheat bread and bran cereal.

*Glutathione-Containing Foods.* Glutathione, a biochemical component of certain foods, also deactivates many cancer-causing substances. It is found in avocados, asparagus, watermelon, fresh citrus fruits, strawberries, fresh peaches, okra, white potatoes, squash, cauliflower, broccoli, and tomatoes. Other cancer-preventing substances include bean sprouts, beans, rice, and potatoes. Some of these, she adds, also appear to reverse carcinogenesis.

## Eliminated or Restricted Foods

Foods which have been linked with cancer, or may be carcinogenic, such as pickled, smoked, and salt-cured foods are eliminated on Bruning's diet. These, she suggests, increase the incidence of stomach and esophagus cancer. Hot dogs, bologna, salami, sausages, ham, bacon, and smoked fish, for example, are prohibited. Salt is restricted to five grams per day. Alcohol, especially when combined with cigarette smoking, has been associated with higher rates of cancer of the breast, mouth, larynx, liver, and lungs, and is restricted to no more than two drinks daily.

### The Progressive Chemotherapy Diet

Bruning notes that some chemotherapy patients may not respond to her "moderate diet" and may need to increase their vitamin and mineral supplementation. Since chemotherapy patients are at a high risk for developing secondary cancers and other illnesses, Bruning advises them to adopt a more progressive diet. She specifically recommends increasing their intake of chemopreventive vitamins and minerals, either through natural foods or supplements. She contends that many cancer experts now believe aggressive vitamin and mineral supplementation can protect organs from the toxicity of chemotherapy drugs, counteract their carcinogenic activity, and improve the functioning of the immune system, which plays a role in destroying cancers cells but is severely weakened by therapy.

### Vitamin and Mineral Supplements

Bruning cites an impressive amount of evidence suggesting that vitamin and mineral supplementation may affect the progression of chemotherapy. By taking large, but not toxic doses of vitamins A, C, and E and selenium, she argues, dieters can nourish the organs that chemotherapy bombards with toxic substances and protect them against further damage. Bruning herself took large amounts of vitamins and minerals during her treatment, which formed an integral part of her overall recovery. An important result of supplementation, she notes, was that it made her feel more confident and secure and less afraid of chemotherapy and what it did to the rest of her while it killed her cancer cells.

Specifically, Bruning cites several NCI studies, for example, which indicate that vitamin E, a potent antioxidant, may protect against some of the severe side effects of chemotherapy. Also, in reasonable doses, according to Bruning, vitamin C tends to promote restoration of normal tissue strength following chemotherapy. Vitamin A in reasonable doses has been shown to be an immunostimulant under certain circumstances. The B vitamins have been shown to be useful during cell restoration and may inhibit some tumor formations.

Bruning also suggests that vitamins and minerals not only inhibit certain cancers, but may also offer some protection against the negative effects of chemotherapy and environmental toxins — and may even make the drugs more effective. For example, vitamin E may enhance the effectiveness of adriamycin; selenium may act synergistically with chemotherapy and radiation; and vitamin E and coenzyme Q may prevent cell damage, particularly of the heart, from adriamycin.

## Physical Activity

Bruning states that exercise was an important support therapy in her recovery. Regular exercise played a critically important role in her overall health, body image, self-esteem, and sense of self-sufficiency. It strengthens tissues and muscle, keeps the body limber, reduces stress, and strengthens the immune system. Exercise also releases endorphins, the morphine-like compounds released by the brain during workouts, which produce a "high" and act as a painkiller. Exercise additionally helps cancer patients feel they are maintaining control.

## Behavioral Modification

Anyone with cancer, Bruning cautions, needs to make extremely difficult psychological adjustments in order to recover. Getting emotional support is one of the most important ways to deal with chemo-related stress. Chapter 6 of her book presents an extremely helpful discussion of major forms of stress management and reduction including emotional counseling, biofeedback, deep breathing, progressive relaxation (muscle tensing and relaxing), hypnosis and self-hypnosis, visualization, and creative imaging.

## RECENT RESEARCH

A number of alternative or "holistic" cancer diets are currently being investigated by the National Institutes of Health (NIH). These include the macrobiotic diet developed by Michio Kushi, the Max Gerson cancer diet, and the diets developed by American physicians Virginia Livingston and Keith Block. These and other diet programs are comprehensively analyzed in *The Encyclopedia of Alternative Health and Medicine.*

In addition to the above-referenced chemopreventives, Nixon, Simone, and Bruning note that the following chemicals are currently being researched by the NCI for their anticancer properties:

## CHEMOPREVENTIVES

The National Cancer Institute is currently studying more than 1,000 nutrients, botanicals, and chemicals that have been shown to have cancer-preventive (chemopreventive) activity, at least in laboratory studies. Some of these, discussed in considerably more detail in the *Alternative Health and Medicine Encyclopedia,* are summarized below.

- **Vitamin B6:** 105 endometrial cancer patients, aged 45 to 65, had a 15 percent improvement in five-year survival rates compared to 105 patients who did not receive the B6 supplements. 6,300 patients with cervical, uterine, endometrial, ovarian, and breast cancers had significantly increased rates with B6 supplementation. Vitamin B6 has also proved effective in inhibiting melanoma cancer cells.
- **Folic acid supplementation** has been successfully used to cause regression in precancerous cells in patients with cervical dysplasia.
- **Combined antioxidant treatments** may extend survival times of cancer patients treated with chemotherapy or radiation. Twenty lung cancer patients in one study received antioxidant treatments of vitamins, trace elements, and fatty acids (five patients had advanced lung disease) in combination with chemotherapy and/or irradiation at regular intervals. Patients receiving antioxidants were also able to tolerate chemotherapy and radiation treatment well.
- **Shiitake mushrooms** (*lentinus edodes*) have been successfully used by Japanese physicians to shrink several different types of tumors by as much as 80 percent. Extract of *lentinus edodes* has been shown to suppress viral oncogenesis, and prevent cancer recurrence after surgery. Shiitake mushrooms prolong the lifespan of patients with advanced and recurrent stomach, colorectal, and breast cancer with minimal side effects.
- **Shark cartilage,** administered via retention enemas, reduced tumors in seven of eight cancer patients in one trial. Symptomatic improvement was observed in all eight patients, including weight gain, improved energy, and pain control. In a Cuban clinical trial, 19 terminal cancer patients experienced shrinking of their tumors after 16 weeks of therapy, with rates varying between 15 and 58 percent. No toxic side effects were reported.

## CHEMOPREVENTIVES (continued)

In a Dutch study, cervical cancer patients pretreated with shark liver oil before receiving radiation had far better survival rates than patients who did not receive the treatment. In many cases, tumors shrank significantly before radiation began, thereby rendering the radiation more effective. Several Boston hospitals associated with the Harvard Medical School use shark fin soup (available in shark cartilage capsules) to inhibit angiogenesis, the development of tiny blood vessels or capillaries through which tumors spread.

• An extract of **mistletoe** (*Iscador*) has been used for 30 years in Europe as a potential anticancer agent. Swiss scientists gave *Iscador* to 14 patients with advanced breast cancer. Twelve out of the 14 patients showed an improvement of DNA repair 2.7 times higher than before *Iscador* was administered.

• **Carnivora,** an extract of the meat-eating Venus flytrap plant (*Dionaea muscipula*), has been used on more than 2,000 patients in Europe to treat cancer, AIDS, and other immune-suppressed diseases. In an initial clinical study conducted by German physician Dr. Helmut Keller of 210 patients with a variety of cancers, all of whom had undergone unsuccessful chemotherapy or radiation, 40 percent were stabilized by *carnivora* treatment and 16 percent went into remission.

• **Traditional Chinese Medicine (TCM) botanicals:** Chinese herbs and plants from more than 120 species (belonging to 60 different families) have been used to successfully treat cancer. Juzentaihoto (or JT-48, or JTT) appears to be one of the most promising Chinese herbs for treating cancer. Patients given this herbal remedy had 3- to 10-year survival rates "significantly higher than commonly anticipated." Herbal therapy using JTT in combination with chemotherapy and hormonal therapy has been shown to extend the life (and improve the quality of life) for metastatic breast cancer patients.

• **Fu Zheng,** a Chinese herbal therapy, doubles the life expectancy of patients with rapidly advancing cancers when combined with Western treatment. The therapy, which consists of ginseng and astragalus, doubled the survival rate of patients with nasopharyngeal (nasal passage and pharynx) cancer from 24 percent to 53 percent.

Source: J. Marti, *Alternative Health and Medicine Encyclopedia.* Detroit, MI: Gale Research Inc., 1994.

## ANTICANCER CHEMICALS IN FOODS

| Chemical | Sources | Possible Protective Action |
|----------|---------|----------------------------|
| Carotene | Carrots, sweet potatoes, yams, pumpkins, squash, kale, broccoli, cantaloupe | Neutralizes free radicals and singlet oxygen radicals; enhances immune system; reverses precancer conditions; high-intake associated with low cancer rate |
| Capsicum | Cayenne pepper | Antioxidant |
| Isoflavones | Legumes: beans, peas, peanuts | Inhibits estrogen receptor; destroys cancer gene enzymes; inhibits estrogen |
| Terpene | Citrus fruit | Increases enzymes that break down carcinogens; decreases cholesterol |
| Lignans | Flaxseed, walnuts, fatty fish | Inhibits estrogen action; inhibits prostaglandins, hormones that cause cancer spread |
| Polyacetylene | Parsley | Inhibits prostaglandins; destroys benzopyrene, a potent carcinogen |
| Triterpenoids | Licorice | Inhibits estrogens, prostaglandins; slows down rapidly dividing cells, such as cancer cells |
| Quinones | Rosemary | Inhibits carcinogens or co-carcinogens |
| Various indoles | Cruciferous vegetables | Induces metabolism of estrogen to less carcinogenic forms |
| Sulfides | Garlic, onions | Stimulates removal of carcinogens by liver |
| Isothiocyanates | Mustard; radishes | Stimulates removal of carcinogens by liver |

## ANTICANCER CHEMICALS IN FOODS
### (continued)

| Chemical | Sources | Possible Protective Action |
| --- | --- | --- |
| Genistein | Soybeans, cruciferous vegetables | Antiangiogenesis |
| Ellagic acids | Grapes, raspberries | May remove or block carcinogens |
| Lycopene | Tomatoes | Antioxidant |
| Monoterpenes | Carrots, cruciferous vegetables, squash, tomatoes | Antioxidant; removes carcinogens by liver |

Over the last two decades, increasing attention has been given to the potential risk that some diets may play in causing cancer. These risks are clearly outlined in the three cancer diets reviewed in this chapter. The three authors clearly suggest that a variety of lowfat diets can play a critical role in preventing cancer and may be beneficial in treating or reversing breast and colorectal cancer. More research, however, is needed on the role of nutrition in cancer treatment. At present, no simple objective tests exist that predict who will and who will not improve with a specific dietary therapy. The best advice is that persons with cancer work closely with their physician to maximize the effect of nutrition in retarding tumor growth and to minimize the debilitating effects of cancer therapy on their nutritional status.

# References and Resources

## CHAPTER 1: HEALTHFUL NUTRITION

REFERENCES

Allen, Linsay, H., and Richard J. Wood. "Calcium and Phosphorus." In *Modern Nutrition in Health and Disease*. Philadelphia: Lea & Febiger, 1994.

American Dietetic Association. *Handbook of Clinical Dietetics*. New Haven, CT: Yale University Press, 1981.

American Medical Association. *Drug Evaluations*. Chicago: American Medical Association, 1986.

Ausman, Lynne M., and Robert M. Russell. "Nutrition in the Elderly." In *Modern Nutrition in Health and Disease*. Philadelphia: Lea & Febiger, 1994.

Balch, James F., and Phyllis Balch. *Prescription for Nutritional Healing*. Garden City Park, N.Y.: Avery Publishing Group, 1990.

Marti, James, and Andrea Hine. *Alternative Health and Medicine Encyclopedia*. Detroit: Gale Publishing Co., 1994.

Murray, Michael, and Joseph Pizzorno. *Encyclopedia of Natural Medicine*. Rocklin, CA: Prima Publishing, 1991.

U.S. Department of Agriculture. *Dietary Guidelines for Americans*. Third Edition. Washington, D.C.: U.S. Department of Agriculture.

"Vitamins and Minerals." *Nutrition Research Newsletter* (June 1992): 77.

ORGANIZATIONS

International Food Information Council Foundation. 1100 Connecticut Avenue N.W., Suite 430, Washington, D.C. 20036.

National Center for Nutrition and Dietetics. 216 West Jackson Boulevard, Chicago, IL 60606-6995.

FURTHER READING

Block, Gladys. "Vitamin C and Cancer Prevention: The Epidemiological Evidence." *American Journal of Clinical Nutrition* (January 1991).

Bricklin, Mark. "New Respect for Nutritional Healing." *Prevention* (February 1992): 31.

Butler, Kurt. *The Best Medicine: The Complete Health and Preventative Medicine Handbook.* New York, NY: Harper & Row, 1985.

Davidson, Michael. "Vitamin E and Cardiovascular Disease." Vitamin E Symposium, June 1990.

Gannon, Kathi. "The Role of Free Radicals in the Aging Process." *Drug Topics* (February 18, 1991).

Garland, Frank, and Edward D. Gorham. "Can Colon Cancer Incidence and Death Rates Be Reduced with Calcium and Vitamin D?" *American Journal of Clinical Nutrition* (July 1991): 193S.

Griffith, H. Winter. *Vitamins.* Tucson, AZ: Fisher Books, 1988.

Marshall, Charles W. *Vitamins and Minerals: Help or Harm?* Philadelphia: George F. Stickley Company, 1983.

Mills, Collins. "Zinc in Human Biology." *Journal of the American Dietetic Association* (May 1990): 756.

Newbold, H. *Meganutrients for Your Nerves.* New York: Peter H. Wyden, 1975.

Pauling, Linus. *How to Live Longer and Feel Better.* New York: W. H. Freeman and Co., 1986.

Roman, J. *Handbook of Vitamins, Minerals and Hormones.* New York: Van Nostrand Reinhold Co., 1973.

Shils, Maurice, James A. Olson, and Moshe Shike. *Modern Nutrition in Health and Disease.* Philadelphia: Lea & Febiger, 1994.

## CHAPTER 2: ANALYZING YOUR CURRENT NUTRITIONAL STATUS

REFERENCES

Goldman, B. A., and D. F. Mitchel. *Directory of Unpublished Experimental Mental Measures,* vol. 5. Dubuque, IA: William C. Brown Publishers, 1990.

Marti, James, and Andrea Hine. *Alternative Health and Medicine Encyclopedia.* Detroit: Gale Research, 1995.

Murray, Michael, and Joseph Pizzorno. *Encyclopedia of Natural Medicine.* Rocklin, CA: Prima Publishing, 1992.

Nieman, David. *Fitness and Your Health.* Palo Alto, CA: Bull Publishing Company, 1993.

Shils, Maurice, James A. Olson, and Moshe Shike. *Modern Nutrition in Health and Disease.* Philadelphia: Lea & Febiger, 1994.

Stunkard, A. J. "Eating Patterns and Obesity." *Psychiatry Quarterly* (January 1959): 284–95.

Swinburn, B., and E. Ravussin. "Energy Balance or Fat Balance?" *American Journal of Clinical Nutrition* 57 (1992): 66S–770S.

U.S. Department of Health and Human Services. *The Surgeon General's Report on Nutrition and Health.* New York: Warner Books, 1989.

PAMPHLETS

American Council on Science and Health. *Food and Life: A Nutrition Primer,* July 1990.

California Department of Health Services. *The California Daily Food Guide: Dietary Guidelines for Californians,* April 1990.

National Research Council, National Academy of Sciences. *Diet and Health: Implications for Reducing Chronic Disease Risk,* 1989.

U.S. Department of Agriculture and U.S. Department of Health and Human Services. *Nutrition and Your Health: Dietary Guidelines for Americans.* In *Home and Garden Bulletin* 232. November 1990.

U.S. Senate Subcommittee on the Tenth Edition of the RDA's Food and Nutrition Board, Commission on Life Sciences, National Research Council. *Recommended Dietary Allowances, Tenth Edition.* Washington, D.C.: National Academy Press, 1989.

ORGANIZATIONS

American Dietetic Association. 208 South LaSalle Street, Suite 1100, Chicago, IL 60604.

American Nutritionist Association. P.O. Box 34030, Bethesda, MD 20817.

American Society for Clinical Nutrition. 9650 Rockville Pike, Bethesda, MD 20814.

Food and Nutrition Information Center. National Agricultural Library, Beltsville, MD 20705.

FURTHER READING

Brody, Jane. *The Good Food Book.* New York: Bantam, 1990.

Gershoff, Stanley, and others. *The Tufts University Guide to Total Nutrition.* New York: Harper & Row, 1990.

Hamilton, Michael, and others. *The Duke University Medical Center Book of Diet and Fitness.* New York: Ballantine Books, 1990.

Herbert, Victor. *Mount Sinai School of Medicine Complete Book of Nutrition.* New York: St. Martin's Press, 1990.

Thomas, Paul R., ed. *Weighing the Options: Criteria for Evaluating Weight-Management Programs.* Washington, D.C.: National Academy of Sciences, 1995.

Willett, W. C., and others. *Nutritional Epidemiology.* New York: Oxford University Press, 1990.

## CHAPTER 3: ASSESSING YOUR CURRENT PHYSICAL STATUS

REFERENCES

Blackburn, G. L. "Comparison of Medically Supervised and Unsupervised Approaches to Weight Loss and Control." *Annals of Internal Medicine* (September 1993): 714–18.

Nieman, David C. *Fitness and Your Health.* Palo Alto, CA: Bull Publishing, 1993.

U.S. Department of Agriculture and U.S. Department of Health and Human Services. *Nutrition and Your Health: Dietary Guidelines for Americans.* In *Home and Garden Bulletin* 232 (Washington, D.C.: U.S. Department of Agriculture, November 1990).

ORGANIZATIONS

American Dietetic Association. 208 South LaSalle Street, Suite 1100, Chicago, IL 60604.

American Nutritionist Association. P.O. Box 34030, Bethesda, MD 20817.

American Society for Clinical Nutrition. 9650 Rockville Pike, Bethesda, MD 20814.

Food and Nutrition Center, National Agricultural Library, Beltsville, MD 20705.

President's Council on Physical Fitness and Health. 450 Fifth Street NW, Washington, D.C. 20001.

FURTHER READING

Butler, Kurt, and Lynn Rayner. *The Best Medicine: The Complete Health and Preventive Medicine Handbook.* New York: Harper & Row, 1985.

Guiton, Arthur. *Textbook of Medical Physiology.* New York: Harcourt Brace Jovanovich, 1991.

## CHAPTER 4: DEFINING YOUR DIET GOALS

REFERENCES

Blackburn, G. L. "Comparison of Medically Supervised and Unsupervised Approaches to Weight Loss and Control." *Annals of Internal Medicine* (September 1993): 714–18.

The Burton Goldberg Group. *Alternative Medicine: The Definitive Guide.* Puyallup, WA: Future Medicine Publishing, 1993.

Lucas, A. R., and D. M. Huse. "Behavioral Disorders Affecting Food Intake: Anorexia Nervosa and Bulimia Nervosa." In *Modern Nutrition in Health and Disease.* Philadelphia: Lea & Febiger, 1994.

Shils, Maurice, James A. Olson, and Moshe Shike. *Modern Nutrition in Health and Disease*. Philadelphia, PA: Lea & Febiger, 1994.

Thomas, Paul R., ed. *Weighing the Options: Criteria for Evaluating Weight-Management Programs*. Washington, D.C.: National Academy of Sciences, 1995.

PAMPHLETS

National Research Council, National Academy of Sciences. *Diet and Health: Implications for Reducing Chronic Disease Risk*, 1989.

National Research Council, National Academy of Sciences. *The Surgeon General's Report on Nutrition and Health*, 1988.

Public Health Service. *Recommended Dietary Allowances, Tenth Edition*, 1989.

ORGANIZATIONS

American Dietetic Association. 208 South LaSalle Street, Suite 1100, Chicago, IL 60604.

American Nutritionists Association. P.O. Box 34030, Bethesda, MD 20817.

American Society for Clinical Nutrition. 9650 Rockville Pike, Bethesda, MD 20814.

American Society of Bariatric Physicians. 5600 South Quebec, Suite 310B, Englewood, CO 80111.

Food and Nutrition Information Center. National Agricultural Library, Beltsville, MD 20705.

National Institute of Mental Health, Eating Disorders Program. Building 10, Room 3S231, Bethesda, MD 20892.

## CHAPTER 5: MEDICALLY SUPERVISED DIET PROGRAMS: VERY-LOW-CALORIE DIET (VLCD) PROGRAMS

REFERENCES

Blackburn, G. L. "Comparison of Medically Supervised and Unsupervised Approaches to Weight Loss and Control." *Annals of Internal Medicine* (September 1993): 714–18.

Blackburn, G. L., and G. A. Gray, eds. *Management of Obesity by Severe Caloric Restriction*. Littleton, MA: PSG/Biomedical, 1985.

Blundell, J. E. "Dietary Fat and the Control of Energy Intake: Evaluating the Effects of Fat on Meal Size and Postmeal Satiety." *American Journal of Clinical Nutrition* (May 1993): 55–57.

Ornish, Dean. *Eat More, Weigh Less*. San Francisco, CA: HarperCollins, 1993.

Sandoz Nutrition (Optitrim). *Medical Update on Obesity*, July/August 1992.

Scanlon, Deralee. *Diets That Work for Weight Control of Medical Needs*. Los Angeles: Lowell House, 1993.

Wadden, Thomas. "A Multidisciplinary Evaluation of Proprietary Weight Reduction Program for the Treatment of Marked Obesity." *Archives of Internal Medicine* (May 1992).

## PAMPHLETS

HMR Program for Weight Management. *Fact Sheet*, 1994.

HMR Program for Weight Management. *Research Shows*, 1994.

HMR Program for Weight Management. *The Total Health Approach to Sustained Weight Loss for High-Risk Patients*, 1994.

Medifast Program. *Medifast News*, winter 1994.

Medifast Program. *Special Report*, winter 1994.

Medifast Program. *Research Reports*, winter 1994.

National Research Council, National Academy of Sciences. *Diet and Health: Implications for Reducing Chronic Disease Risk*, 1989.

Public Health Service: *The Surgeon General's Report on Nutrition and Health*, 1992.

## ORGANIZATIONS

American Dietetic Association. 208 South LaSalle Street, Suite 1100, Chicago, IL 60604.

American Nutritionists Association. P.O. Box 34030, Bethesda, MD 20817.

American Society for Clinical Nutrition. 9650 Rockville Pike, Bethesda, MD 20814.

Food and Nutrition Information Center. National Agricultural Library, Beltsville, MD 20705.

National Institute of Mental Health, Eating Disorders Program. Building 10, Room 3S231, Bethesda, MD 20892.

## FURTHER READING

Blackburn, G. L., and G. A. Gray, eds. *Management of Obesity by Severe Caloric Restriction*. Littleton, MA: PSG/Biomedical, 1985.

Hamilton, M. *The Duke University Medical Center Book of Diet and Fitness*. New York: Ballantine, 1990.

Hirschman, Jane. *Overcoming Overeating*. Reading, MA: Addison-Wesley, 1988.

Pope, H. *New Hope for Binge Eaters*. New York: Harper/Coliphon, 1985.

Rees, Alan M., and Charlene Wiley, eds. *Personal Health Reporter*. Detroit, MI: Gale Research Inc., 1993.

Siegel, M. *Surviving an Eating Disorder*. New York: Harper & Row, 1988.

Thomas, Paul R., ed. *Weighing the Options: Criteria for Evaluating Weight Management Programs*. Washington, D.C.: National Academy of Sciences, 1995.

## CHAPTER 6: COMMERCIAL WEIGHT-LOSS DIET PROGRAMS

REFERENCES

Agras, W. S. *Eating Disorders: Management of Obesity, Bulimia, and Anorexia Nervosa.* New York: Pergamon Press, 1992.

Bennion, Lynn J., Edwin L. Bierman, and others. *Straight Talk About Weight Control: Taking the Pounds Off and Keeping Them Off.* Fairfield, OH: Consumer Reports Books, 1991.

Blackburn, G. L. "Comparison of Medically Supervised and Unsupervised Approaches to Weight Loss and Control." *Annals of Internal Medicine* (September 1993): 714–18.

Spielman, Amy B., George Blackburn, and others. "The Cost of Losing: An Analysis of Commercial Weight-Loss Programs in a Metropolitan Area." *Journal of the American College of Nutrition* (November 1992): 36–41.

Thomas, Paul R., ed. *Weighing the Options: Criteria for Evaluating Weight Management Programs.* Washington, D.C.: National Academy of Sciences, 1995.


PAMPHLETS

Jenny Craig. *Fact Sheet,* 1995.

Jenny Craig. *Personal Menu Plans and Nutritional Composition,* 1995.

Nutri/System. *Menu Plan Brochure,* 1995.

Nutri/System. *Nutri/System Information Brochure,* 1995.

Nutri/System. *Nutrient Information Brochure,* 1995.

Jenny Craig. *Overview of the Jenny Craig Personal Weight Management Program,* 1994.

Nutri/System. *Physician Brochure,* 1995.

Nutri/System. *Real Solutions: Your Twelve-Week Guide to the LIVE FOR LIFE Program,* 1995.

Nutri/System. *Standard 1200/1500 Calorie Menu Plan,* 1995.

"The Word 'Diet' Takes on New Meaning." *PR Newswire* (September 21, 1993).

Weight Watchers International. *Welcome to Weight Watchers.* Jericho, NY: Weight Watchers International, 1995.


ORGANIZATIONS

Diet Center. 921 Penn Avenue, Suite 500, Pittsburgh, PA 15222. (800) 333-2581.

Jenny Craig. 445 Marine View Avenue, Suite 300, Del Mar, CA 92014-3950. (619) 259-7000.

Nutri/System. 410 Horsham Road, Horsham, PA 19044. (215) 442-5411.

Weight Watchers. 500 North Broadway, Jericho, NY 11753. (516) 939-0400.

FURTHER READING

"A Comparison of Weight-Loss Programs." *Environmental Nutrition* (December 1990): 4–5.

ACSH. *Food and Life Primer.* Washington, D.C.: American Council on Science and Health, July 1990: 34–35.

Donahue, Peggy Jo. "Inside America's Hottest Diet Programs: Part Two — Nutri/System." *Prevention* (February 1990): 55–59, 124–133.

Edlin, Gordon, and Eric Golanty. *Health and Wellness.* Boston, MA: Jones and Barlett Publishers, 1992.

Fletcher, Anne M. "Inside America's Hottest Diet Programs: Part Five." *Prevention* (May 1990): 49, 102–04, 106–08, 110, 112.

Fletcher, Anne M. "Inside America's Hottest Diet Programs: Part Three — Weight Watchers." *Prevention* (March 1990): 554–64.

Hughes, Rebecca. "Inside America's Hottest Diet Programs: Part Four — Diet Center." *Prevention* (April 1990): 64–72.

Rees, Alan, and Charlene Willey. *Personal Health Reporter.* Detroit, MI: Gale Research Inc., 1993.

U.S. Department of Agriculture and U.S. Department of Health and Human Services. "Nutrition and Your Health: Dietary Guidelines for Americans." In *Home and Garden Bulletin* (November 1990): 3–4.

Weight Watchers International. *Corporate Backgrounder.* Jericho, NY: Weight Watchers International, Inc.

## CHAPTER 7: WEIGHT-LOSS SUPPORT GROUPS

REFERENCES

*Academia, Non-Profit Organization and Industry Team Up in All-Out Attack on Obesity.* Office of Public Affairs, Medical College of Wisconsin, April 6, 1995.

Overeaters Anonymous. *History and Structure of Overeaters Anonymous.* Rio Rancho, NM: Overeaters Anonymous, 1995.

PAMPHLETS

Overeaters Anonymous. *About OA.* Rio Rancho, NM: Overeaters Anonymous, 1995.

Overeaters Anonymous. *Overeaters Anonymous: Fifteen Questions.* Rio Rancho, NM: Overeaters Anonymous, 1995.

Overeaters Anonymous. *To the Newcomer.* Rio Rancho, NM: Overeaters Anonymous, 1995.

Take Off Pounds Sensibly. *TOPS News.* Milwaukee, WI: TOPS Club Inc., 1995.

Take Off Pounds Sensibly. *TOPS Quick Facts.* Milwaukee, WI: TOPS Club Inc., 1995.

Thomas, Paul R., ed., *Weighing the Options: Criteria for Evaluating Weight-Management Programs*. Washington, D.C.: National Academy of Sciences, 1995.

ORGANIZATIONS

Overeaters Anonymous. World Service Office, 6075 Zenith Court, Rio Rancho, NM 87124.

Take Off Pounds Sensibly. TOPS International Headquarters, 4575 South Fifth Street, P.O. Box 07360, Milwaukee, WI 53207-0360.

## CHAPTER 8: OVER-THE-COUNTER BOTANICAL DIET PROGRAMS

REFERENCES

Astrup, A. "The Effect of Ephedrine Plus Caffeine on Plasma Lipids and Lipoproteins During a 4.2 MJ/Day Diet." *International Journal of Obesity and Related Metabolic Disorders* (May 1994): 329–32.

Berkhout, Theo. "The Effect of (-)Hydroxycitrate on the Activity of the Low-Density Lipoprotein Receptor and 3-Hydroxy-3-Methylglutaryl-CoA Reductase Levels in the Human Hepatoma Cell Line." *Biochemistry Journal* (January 1992): 181–86.

Breum, L. "Comparison of an Ephedrine/Caffeine Combination and Dexfenfluramine in the Treatment of Obesity." *International Journal of Obesity and Related Metabolic Disorders* (February 1994): 99–103.

The Burton Goldberg Group. *Alternative Medicine: The Definitive Guide.* Puyallup, WA: Future Medicine Publishing, Inc., 1993.

CitriMax. "CitriMax Product Description and Guide for Health Professionals." *CitriMax Brochure*, 1994: 1–5.

CitriMax. "CitriMax: Nature's Perfect Diet Ingredient." *CitriMax Brochure*, 1995.

CitriMax. "The CitriMax All-Natural Diet Plan." *CitriMax Brochure*, 1995.

Conte, Anthony A. "A Non-Prescription Alternative in Weight Reduction Therapy." *The Bariatrician* (summer 1993): 17–19.

Daly, P., and others. "Ephedrine, Caffeine and Aspirin: Safety and Efficacy for Treatment of Human Obesity." *American Journal of Clinical Nutrition* (February 1993): S73–78.

"Ephedrine, Xanthines, Aspirin and Other Thermogenic Drugs to Assist the Dietary Management of Obesity." Proceedings of an international symposium. *International Journal of Obesity and Related Metabolic Disorders* (February 1993): Suppl. S1–83.

"Health Tips." *The Johns Hopkins Medical Letter* (June 1995): 7.

Kolata, Gina. "Metabolism Found to Adjust for a Body's Natural Weight." *New York Times*, March 9, 1995: A1.

Lamb, Steven. "A Fresh Approach to Weight Loss." *American Health* (May 1995): 36.

Lewis, Y. "Isolation and Properties of Hydroxycitric Acid." In *Methods in Enzymology, Citric Acid Cycle.* John M. Lowenstein, ed., Volume 13. New York, NY: Academic Press, 1969.

Mowrey, Daniel B. *Fat Management: The Thermogenic Factor.* Lehi, UT: Victory Publications, 1994.

Mowrey, Daniel B. "The Major Scientific Breakthrough of the 90's: Reducing Body Fat Through Thermogenesis." In *Health Store News* (October/November 1994): 1–5.

Toubro, S., A. Astrup, and others. "The Effect and Safety of an Ephedrine/Caffeine Compound Compared to Ephedrine, Caffeine and Placebo in Obese Subjects on an Energy-Restricted Diet. A Double-Blind Trial." In *International Journal of Obesity and Related Metabolic Disorders* (April 1992): 269–77.

RESOURCES

Dullo, Abdul G. "Ephedrine in the Treatment of Obesity." *American Journal of Clinical Nutrition* (November 1993): S1–2.

Dullo, Abdul G., and Lucien Girardier. "Adaptive Role of Energy Expenditure in Modulating Body Fat and Protein Deposition During Catch-Up Growth After Early Undernutrition." *American Journal of Clinical Nutrition* (November 1993): 614.

Dullo, Abdul G., and D. Miller. "Ephedrine, Caffeine and Aspirin: Over-the-Counter Drugs That Interact to Stimulate Thermogenesis in the Obese." *Nutrition* (May 1989): 7–9.

"Fat-Burning Substances Can Assist Weight Loss." *Better Nutrition for Today's Living* (June 1994): 13.

Laville, Martine, et al. "Decreased Glucose-Induced Thermogenesis at the Onset of Obesity." *American Journal of Clinical Nutrition* (June 1993): 851.

Maffeis, Claudio. "Meal-Induced Thermogenesis in Lean and Obese Prepubertal Children." *American Journal of Clinical Nutrition* (April 1993): 481.

"Nutrients Are Useful for Weight Reduction." *Better Nutrition for Today's Living* (November 1992): 22.

Pasquali, R. "Clinical Aspects of Ephedrine in the Treatment of Obesity." *American Journal of Clinical Nutrition* (February 1993): S65–68.

Rabin, Anne, and others. "Decreased Postprandial Thermogenesis and Fat Oxidation But Increased Fullness After a High-Fiber Meal Compared with a Low-Fat Fiber Meal." *American Journal of Clinical Nutrition* (June 1994): 1386–89.

Westrate, Jan. "Resting Metabolic Rate in Diet-Induced Thermogenesis: A Methodological Reappraisal." *American Journal of Clinical Nutrition* (November 1993): 592.

FURTHER READING

Cloutre, Dallas. *Getting Lean with Anti-Fat Nutrients*. San Francisco: Pax Publishing, 1993.

Simon, Harvey B. *Staying Well*. Boston: Houghton Mifflin, 1992.

Thomas, Paul R., ed. *Weighing the Options: Criteria for Evaluating Weight Management Programs*. Washington, D.C.: National Academy of Sciences, 1995.

## CHAPTER 9: POPULAR BOOK DIET PROGRAMS

RESOURCES: RECOMMENDED RECIPES AND COOKBOOKS

Bienenfeld, Florence. *Mother Nature's Garden: Healthy Vegan Cooking*. Freedom, CA: Crossing Press, 1994.

Carper, Jean. *Food — Your Miracle Medicine: How Food Can Prevent and Cure Over 100 Symptoms and Problems*. New York: HarperCollins, 1994.

Hurley, Judith, and Patricia Hausman. *The Healing Foods*. New York: Dell, 1994.

Lemlin, Jeanne. *Quick Vegetarian Pleasures*. New York: HarperCollins, 1992.

Pasquale, Bruno, Jr. *Italian Light and Easy: More Than 100 Delicious and Healthy Low-Fat, Low-Calorie Recipes*. Chicago: Contemporary Books, 1993.

Pepin, Jacques. *Jacques Pepin's Simple and Healthy Cooking*. Emmaus, PA: Rodale Press, 1994.

Reader, Diane. *Healthy Meal Planning for People on Sodium-Restricted Diets*. Minnetonka, MN: Diabetes Center, 1992.

## CHAPTER 10: DIETS FOR WOMEN

REFERENCES

Gittleman, Ann Louise. *Super Nutrition for Women*. New York: Bantam Books, 1991.

Mallek, Henry. *The Woman's Advantage Diet*. New York: Simon & Schuster, 1989.

Marti, James E., and Andrea Hine. *The Alternative Health and Medicine Encyclopedia*. Detroit, MI: Gale Research Inc. and Invisible Press, 1994.

"Research Finds Fat Can Be Fatal." *Chicago Tribune*, September 14, 1995: A24.

Shils, Maurice, James A. Olson, and Moshe Shike. *Modern Nutrition in Health and Disease*. Philadelphia: Lea & Febiger, 1994.

Somer, Elizabeth. *Nutrition for Women*. New York: Henry Holt and Company, 1993.

"Super Nutrition for Women (Interview with Ann Louise Gittleman)." *American Fitness* (September/October 1992): 18.

PAMPHLETS

American College of Obstetricians and Gynecologists. *Estrogen Use,* 1988.

American College of Obstetricians and Gynecologists. *Gynecological Problems: Dysmenorrhea,* 1985.

American College of Obstetricians and Gynecologists. *Premenstrual Syndrome,* 1985.

ORGANIZATIONS

National Women's Health Network. 1325 G Street NW, Washington, D.C. 20005.

## CHAPTER 11: DIETS FOR CHILDREN

REFERENCES

Children's Nutrition Research Center, Baylor College of Medicine. *Nutrition and Your Child.* 1993.

Epstein, L. H., and others. "Ten-Year Follow-Up of Behavioral, Family-Based Treatment for Obese Children." *JAMA* 264 (1990): 2519–23.

Epstein, L. H. "Exercise and Obesity in Children." *Journal of Applied Sports Psychology* 4 (1992): 120–33.

"Family Treatment Can Reduce Obesity in Children." *The Meninger Letter* (February 1995): 3.

Gong, Elizabeth J., and Felix P. Heald. "Diet, Nutrition, and Adolescence." In *Modern Nutrition in Health and Disease.* Philadelphia: Lea & Febiger, 1994.

Gortmaker, S. L., and others. "Inactivity, Diet, and the Fattening of America." *Journal of the American Dietetic Association* 90 (1990): 1247–52.

Heird, William C. "Nutritional Requirements During Infancy and Childhood." In *Modern Nutrition in Health and Disease.* Philadelphia: Lea & Febiger, 1994.

"High Schoolers Sit More Than They Sweat, Study Finds." *Marin Independent Journal* (December 5, 1994): A6.

Klesges, R. C., and others. "Effects of Television on Metabolic Rate: Potential Implications for Childhood Obesity." *Pediatrics* 91 (1993): 281–86.

Mellin, L. M., and others. "Children and Adolescent Obesity: The Nurse Practitioner's Use of the SHAPEDOWN Method." *Journal of Pediatric Health Care* (July-August 1992): 187–93.

Mellin, L. M. "To: President Clinton. Re: Combating Childhood Obesity." *Journal of American Dietetics Association* 93 (1993): 265–66.

Mellin, L. M., and others. "Adolescent Obesity Intervention: Validation of the Shapedown Program." *Journal of the American Dietetic Association* (March 1987): 333–38.

National Center for Health Statistics. *Healthy People 2000 Review* (Hyattsville, MD: Public Health Service), 1995.

Prince, Harold, and Francine Prince. *Feed Your Kids Bright.* New York: Simon & Schuster, 1987.

Shils, Maurice, James A. Olson, and Moshe Shike. *Modern Nutrition in Health and Disease.* Philadelphia: Lea & Febiger, 1994.

Squires, Sally. "Too Many Youngsters Too Fat, Report Says." *San Francisco Chronicle* (October 6, 1995): A5.

Stunkard, A. J. "An Adoption Study of Human Obesity." *New England Journal of Medicine* 314 (1986): 193–98.

Taras, H., and others. "Television's Influence on Children's Diet and Physical Activity." *Development Behavioral Pediatrics* 10 (1993): 176–80.

Thomas, Paul R., ed. *Weighing the Options.* Washington, D.C.: National Academy Press, 1995.

"TV Advertising Aimed at Kids Is Filled with Fat." *Wall Street Journal* (November 9, 1993): 7.

"U.S. Teenagers Growing Fatter — Need Exercise." *San Francisco Chronicle* (November 11, 1994): A11.

Waxman, M., and A. J. Stunkard. "Caloric Intake and Expenditure of Obese Boys." In *Journal of Pediatrics* 96 (1980): 187–93.

ORGANIZATIONS

Alan Guttmacher Institute. 11 Fifth Avenue, New York, N.Y. 10003.

Health Research Group, 2000 P Street NW, Washington, D.C. 20036.

The Children's Nutrition Research Center (CNRC). 1100 Bates Street, 2nd Floor, Houston, TX 77030-2600.

Shapedown Weight Management Program for Children and Adolescents. 117 Library Place, San Anselmo, CA 94960.

## CHAPTER 12: DIETS FOR THE ELDERLY

REFERENCES

Allen, Linsay H., and Richard J. Wood. "Calcium and Phosphorus." In *Modern Nutrition in Health and Disease.* Philadelphia: Lea & Febiger, 1994.

Ausman, Lynne M., and Robert M. Russell. "Nutrition in the Elderly." In *Modern Nutrition in Health and Disease.* Philadelphia: Lea & Febiger, 1994.

The Burton Goldberg Group. *Alternative Medicine: The Definitive Guide.* Puyallup, WA: Future Medicine Publishing, Inc., 1993.

Feltin, Hendler. *The Complete Guide to Anti-Aging Nutrients.* New York: Simon and Schuster, 1990.

Marti, James E., and Andrea Hine. *The Alternative Health and Medicine Encyclopedia.* Detroit: Gale Research Inc. and Invisible Press, 1994.

Somer, Elizabeth. *Nutrition for Women*. New York: Henry Holt Publishers, 1993.

Walford, Roy. *Maximum Life Span*. New York: W. W. Norton & Company, 1983.

RESOURCES

National Research Council, National Academy of Sciences. *Diet and Health: Implications for Reducing Chronic Disease Risk*, 1989.

ORGANIZATIONS

Alzheimer's Disease Education and Referral Center. P.O. Box 8250, Silver Spring, MD 20807-8250.

National Osteoporosis Association. 1625 Eye Street NW, Washington, D.C. 20006.

National Council on Aging. Family Caregivers Program, 600 Maryland Avenue SW, Washington, D.C. 20024.

National Institute on Aging Information Center. 2209 Distribution Circle, Silver Springs, MD 20910.

## CHAPTER 13: VEGETARIAN DIET PROGRAMS

REFERENCES

"Cholesterol-Lowering Effects of an Uncooked Vegan Diet." In *Nutritional Research Newsletter* 12 (April 1993): 39.

Gong, Elizabeth J., and Felix P. Heald. "Diet, Nutrition and Adolescence." In *Modern Nutrition in Health and Disease*. Philadelphia: Lea & Febiger, 1994.

Koop, C. Everett. *U.S. Surgeon General's Report on Nutrition and Health*. Washington, D.C.: U.S. Public Health Service, 1988.

Kushi, Michio, and Alex Jack. *The Book of Macrobiotics: The Universal Way of Health, Happiness and Peace*. New York: Japan Publications, 1987.

Marti, James, and Andrea Hine. *Alternative Health and Medicine Encyclopedia*. Detroit: Gale Research, 1994.

Nelson, Jennifer, and others. *The Mayo Clinic Diet Manual*. St. Louis, MO: Mosby-Year Book Inc., 1994.

Null, Gary. *Vegetarian Handbook: Eating Right for Total Health*. New York: St. Martin's Press, 1987.

Shils, Maurice, James A. Olson, and Moshe Shike. *Modern Nutrition in Health and Disease*. Philadelphia: Lea & Febiger, 1994.

RESOURCES

The American Dietetic Association. *Eating Well — The Vegetarian Way*. Chicago: American Dietetic Association.

*Vegetarian Journal*. Published by the Vegetarian Resource Group, P.O. Box 1463, Baltimore, MD 21203.

## CHAPTER 14: HIGH-PERFORMANCE-SPORTS DIETS

REFERENCES

Burke, Louise. *The Complete Guide to Food for Sports Performance.* Sydney, Australia: Allen & Unwin, 1992.

Hultman, Eric, Roger C. Harris, and Lawrence L. Spriet. "Work and Exercise." In *Modern Nutrition in Health and Disease.* Philadelphia: Lea & Febiger, 1994.

Nieman, David. "More Strength, More Endurance." *Vibrant Life* (May/June 1992): 34.

Nieman, David. *Fitness and Your Health.* Palo Alto, CA: Bull Publishing Company, 1993.

Somer, Elizabeth. *Nutrition for Women.* New York: Henry Holt & Company, 1993.

RESOURCES

President's Council on Physical Fitness and Sports. "Healthy People 2000: National Health Promotion and Disease Prevention Objectives." Washington, D.C.: President's Council on Physical Fitness and Sports.

President's Council on Physical Fitness and Sports. "Physical Activity and Fitness." Washington, D.C.: President's Council on Physical Fitness and Sports.

Shape Up America! "On Your Way to Fitness: A Practical Guide to Achieving and Maintaining Healthy Weight and Physical Fitness." Hanover, N.H.: The Koop Foundation, 1994.

ORGANIZATIONS

National Center for Nutrition and Dietetics/The American Dietetic Association. 216 West Jackson Blvd., Chicago, IL 60606-6995.

President's Council on Physical Fitness and Sports. 701 Pennsylvania Ave. NW, Suite 250, Washington, D.C. 20004.

## CHAPTER 15: DIETS FOR OSTEOPOROSIS

REFERENCES

Allen, Linsay H., and Richard J. Wood. "Calcium and Phosphorus." In *Modern Nutrition in Health and Disease.* Philadelphia: Lea & Febiger, 1994.

Ausman, Lynne M., and Robert M. Russell. "Nutrition in the Elderly." In *Modern Nutrition in Health and Disease.* Philadelphia: Lea & Febiger, 1994.

"The Bare-Bones Facts for Avoiding Osteoporosis." *Tufts University Diet and Nutrition Letter* (June 1994): 3–6.

Blackburn, George. "Shake Down Your Cholesterol and Blood Pressure (Skim Milk)." *Prevention* (August 1992): 101.

Brody, Jane. "New Clues in Balancing the Risk of Hormones After Menopause." *New York Times,* June 15, 1995.

Brody, Jane. "Personal Health." *New York Times,* July 14, 1993.

Butler, Kurt, and Lynn Rayner. *The Best Medicine: The Complete Health and Preventive Medicine Handbook.* New York: Harper & Row, 1985.

"Calcium." *Mayo Clinic Health Letter.* May 1995: 4.

Dover, Clare (in association with the British National Osteoporosis Society). *Osteoporosis.* London, England: Ward Lock, 1994.

Gaby, Alan. *Preventing and Reversing Osteoporosis.* Rocklin, CA: Prima Publishing, 1994.

Murray, Michael, and Joseph Pizzorno. *An Encyclopedia of Natural Medicine.* Rocklin, CA: Prima Publishing, 1991.

Omi, N. "Evaluation of the Effect of Soybean Milk and Soybean Milk Peptide on Bone Metabolism." *Journal of Nutritional Science and Vitaminology* (April 1994): 201–11.

Ornish, Dean. *Dr. Dean Ornish's Program for Reversing Heart Disease.* New York: Random House, 1990.

Rozek, Jan. *Keys to Understanding Osteoporosis.* Barron's Educational Series, 1992.

ORGANIZATIONS

National Osteoporosis Association. 1625 Eye Street NW, Washington, D.C. 20006.

## CHAPTER 16: DIETS FOR ARTHRITIS

REFERENCES

The Burton Goldberg Group. *Alternative Medicine: The Definitive Guide.* Puyallup, WA: Future Medicine Publishing, Inc., 1993.

"Herbs That Help Beat Arthritis Aches." *Your Health* (February 22, 1994): 45–46.

Prosch, Gus J. "Dr. Gus J. Prosch's Dietary Recommendations for the Rheumatoid Arthritic." *Supplement to the Art of Getting Well: Proper Nutrition for Rheumatoid Arthritis.* Franklin, TN: The Rheumatoid Disease Foundation, 1994.

Scala, James. *The Arthritis Relief Diet.* New York: New American Library, 1991.

Sobel, Dava, and Arthur C. Klein. *Arthritis: What Works.* New York: St. Martin's Press, 1989.

PAMPHLETS

Arthritis Foundation. *Basic Facts: Answers to Your Questions.* Atlanta, GA: Arthritis Foundation.

Arthritis Foundation. *Exercise and Your Arthritis.* Atlanta, GA: Arthritis Foundation, 1991.

ORGANIZATIONS

Arthritis Foundation. P.O. Box 19000, Atlanta, GA 30326.

National Institute on Aging Information Center. 2209 Distribution Circle, Silver Spring, MD 20910.

The Rheumatoid Disease Foundation. 5106 Old Harding Road, Franklin, TN 37064.

## CHAPTER 17: DIETS FOR CORONARY ARTERY DISEASE

REFERENCES

American Heart Association. *Fact Sheet on Heart Attacks: Stroke and Risk Factors.* 1987.

American Heart Association. *Heart and Stroke Facts.* Dallas, TX: American Heart Association, 1992.

DeBakey, Michael E., Antonia M. Gotto, Lynne W. Scott, and John P. Foreyt. *The Living Heart Diet.* New York: Simon & Schuster, 1986.

Grundy, Scott. *American Heart Association Low-Fat, Low-Cholesterol Cookbook.* New York: Random House, 1992.

Kieswetter, H. "Effects of Garlic-Coated Tablets in Peripheral Arterial Occlusive Disease." *Clinical Investigator* 71 (1991): 383–86.

Kolata, Gina. "Study Finds Fish-Heavy Diet Offers No Heart Protection." *New York Times,* April 13, 1995.

Marti, James, and Andrea Hine. *Alternative Health and Medicine Encyclopedia.* Detroit, MI: Gale Publishing, 1994.

Ornish, Dean. *Dr. Dean Ornish's Program for Reversing Heart Disease.* New York: Ballantine Books, 1990.

Stipp, David. "Vitamin E Link Is Seen in Lowering Heart Disease Risk." *Wall Street Journal,* May 20, 1993.

ORGANIZATIONS

American Heart Association. 7320 Greenville Avenue, Dallas, TX 75231.

FURTHER READING

The Burton Goldberg Group. *Alternative Medicine: The Definitive Guide.* Puyallup, WA: Future Medicine Publishing, Inc., 1993.

National Heart, Lung, and Blood Institute. *Eating to Lower Your High Blood Cholesterol.* NIH pub. no. 89-2920 (June 1989): 5–6.

## CHAPTER 18: DIETS FOR TYPE I AND TYPE II DIABETES

REFERENCES

Algert, Susan, and others. *The UCSD Healthy Diet for Diabetics.* Boston: Houghton Mifflin, 1988.

Anderson, J. W. *Plant Fiber in Foods.* Lexington, KY: HCF Nutrition Research Foundation, 1990.

Anderson, James W., and Geil, Patti Bazel. "Nutritional Management of Diabetes Mellitus." In *Modern Nutrition in Health and Disease.* Philadelphia: Lea & Febiger, 1994.

Beaser, Richard S. "Diabetes Research Update." *Diabetes in the News.* January/February 1991: 9–10.

Beaser, Richard. *Joslin Diabetes Manual,* 12th Edition. Philadelphia: Lea & Febiger, 1989.

Brody, Jane. "The Diabetic Fat of Choice May Be Monounsaturated." *New York Times* (May 25, 1994): B9.

Corica, F., and others. "The Role of Magnesium in Glucose Homeostasis: Therapeutic Implications." *Clinica Terapeutica* (July 1993): 45–55.

Mirsky, Stanley. *Controlling Diabetes the Easy Way.* New York: Random House, 1981.

Passwater, Richard. *GTF Chromium.* New Canaan, CT: Keats Publishing Inc., 1982. First clinical discussion of the possible benefits of chromium in the treatment of diabetes.

Somer, Elizabeth. *Nutrition for Women.* New York: Henry Holt & Co., 1993.

"Wellness Facts." *University of California at Berkeley Wellness Letter,* May 1995: 1.


PAMPHLETS

American Diabetes Association. *Adults: Diabetes and You,* 1989.
American Diabetes Association. *Children: Diabetes and You,* 1987.
American Diabetes Association. *Seniors: Diabetes and You,* 1987.
American Diabetes Association. *What You Need to Know About Diabetes,* 1989.
HCF Diabetes Foundation. *The HCF Exchanges: The High Carbohydrate (HCF) Nutrition Plan,* 1987.


ORGANIZATIONS

American Diabetes Association. National Service Center, P.O. Box 25757, 1600 Duke Street, Alexandria, VA 22314.

Diabetes and Nutrition News, HCF Diabetes Foundation. P.O. Box 22124, Lexington, KY 40522.

International Diabetes Center. 5000 West 39th Street, Minneapolis, MN 55416.

Joslin Diabetes Center. One Joslin Place, Boston, MA 02215.

Juvenile Diabetes Foundation. 60 Madison Avenue, New York, N.Y. 10010-1550.

National Diabetes Information Clearinghouse. P.O. Box NDIC. Bethesda, MD 20892.

University of Michigan Diabetes Research and Training Center. S2310 Old Main Hospital, 1500 East Medical Center Drive, Ann Arbor, MI 48109.

FURTHER READING

American Diabetes Association. *Diabetes in the Family, Revised Edition.* Englewood Cliffs, NJ: Prentice-Hall, 1987.

American Diabetes Association, and American Dietetic Association. *Family Cookbook.* Volume III. Englewood Cliffs, NJ: Prentice-Hall, 1987.

## CHAPTER 19: FOOD ALLERGY ELIMINATION DIETS

REFERENCES

Braly, James. *Dr. Braly's Diet and Nutrition Revolution.* New Canaan, CT: Keats Publishing, 1992.

The Institute of Food Technologists' Expert Panel on Food Safety and Nutrition. "Food Allergies and Other Food Sensitivities." *Contemporary Nutrition* 10 (1985): 1–2.

Mandel, Marshall. *Dr. Marshall Mandell's Five-Day Allergy Relief System.* New York: Simon & Schuster, 1979.

Nelson, Jennifer, and others. *The Mayo Clinic Diet Manual.* St. Louis, MO: Mosby-Year Book Inc., 1994.

Sampson, Hugh A. "Food Allergy." In *Modern Nutrition in Health and Disease.* Philadelphia: Lea & Febiger, 1994.

Shils, Maurice, James A. Olson, and Moshe Shike. *Modern Nutrition in Health and Disease.* Philadelphia: Lea & Febiger, 1994.

PAMPHLETS

American Academy of Allergy and Immunology. *Adverse Reactions to Foods: A Parent's Guide to Problem Foods,* 1990.

American Academy of Allergy and Immunology. *Food Additives: Diagnosis and Treatment,* 1988.

American Academy of Allergy and Immunology. *Helpful Hints for the Allergic Patient,* 1990.

American Academy of Allergy and Immunology. *What Is an Allergic Reaction?* 1990.

American Council on Science and Health. *Food Allergies,* 1989.

Asthma and Allergy Foundation of America. *Allergy in Children.*

Asthma and Allergy Foundation of America. *Food Allergy.*

The Food Allergy Network. *Food Allergy News.* A bimonthly newsletter with recipes published by The Food Allergy Network, 4744 Holly Ave., Fairfax, VA 22030.

## CHAPTER 20: DIETS FOR HYPERTENSION (HIGH BLOOD PRESSURE)

REFERENCES

Appel, L. "Does Supplementation of Diet with 'Fish Oil' Reduce Blood Pressure?" *Archives of Internal Medicine* (June 28, 1993): 1429–38.

Atkins, Robert. "Lowering Cholesterol: Seventeen Natural Ways to Bring Cholesterol Under Control." *Well-Being Journal* (May/June 1994): 1,5.

Balch, James, and Phyllis Balch. *Prescription for Nutritional Healing.* Garden City Park, NY: Avery Publishing Group Inc., 1990.

Burr, M. "Dietary Fiber, Blood Pressure, and Plasma Cholesterol." *Nutrition Research* (May 1985): 465–72.

Cutler, J. "Combinations of Lifestyle Modifications and Drug Treatment in Management of Mild-Moderate Hypertension." *Clinical and Experimental Hypertension* (November 1993): 1193–1204.

Eliasson, K. "A Dietary Fiber Supplement in the Treatment of Mild Hypertension." *Journal of Hypertension* (February 1992): 195–99.

Geleijnse, J. "Reduction in Blood Pressure with a Low-Sodium, High-Potassium, High-Magnesium Salt in Older Subjects with Mild to Moderate Hypertension." *British Medical Journal* (August 13, 1994): 233–37.

Haga, H. "Effects of Dietary Magnesium Supplementation on Diurnal Variations of Blood Pressure." *Japanese Heart Journal* (November 1992): 785–800.

"Hypertension." *Johns Hopkins Medical Letter.* September 1989.

"Hypertension: Lower Your Blood Pressure Without Drugs." *Mayo Clinic Nutrition Letter* (May 1990): 2–3.

Iso, H. "Effectiveness of a Community-Based Education Program on Blood Pressure Reduction." *Japanese Journal of Public Health* (March 1993): 147–58.

Keeswater, H. "Hypertension." *Clinical Investigator* (July 1991).

Krotkiewski, M. "Effects of a Sodium-Potassium Ion-Exchanging Seaweed Preparation in Mild Hypertension." *The American Journal of Hypertension* (June 1991): 483–88.

Margolis, Simeon, and Hamilton Moses III, eds. *The Johns Hopkins Medical Handbook.* New York: Rebus Inc., 1993.

Marti, James, and Andrea Hine. *The Alternative Health and Medicine Encyclopedia.* Detroit, MI: Gale Research Inc., 1994.

Moser, Marvin. *Lower Your Blood Pressure and Live Longer.* New York: Random House, 1989.

Murray, Michael, and Joseph Pizzorno. *Encyclopedia of Natural Medicine*. Rocklin, CA: Prima Publishing, 1991.

Ornish, Dean. *Dr. Dean Ornish's Program for Reversing Heart Disease*. New York: Ballantine Books, 1990.

Passfall, J. "Different Effects of Eicosapentaenoic Acid and Olive Oil on Blood Pressure, Intracellular Free Platelet Calcium, and Plasma Lipids in Patients with Essential Hypertension." *Clinical Investigator* (August 1993): 620–33.

Rowan, Robert L. *How to Control High Blood Pressure Without Drugs*. New York: Ballantine Books, 1986.

Schwartz, Harry. "Initial Therapy for Hypertension — Individualizing Care." *Mayo Clinic Proceedings* (January 1990): 73–87.

Sha, M. "Hypertension Prevention Trial (HPT): Food Pattern Changes Resulting from Intervention of Sodium, Potassium, and Energy Intake." *Journal of the American Dietetic Association* (January 1990): 69–76.

Shils, Maurice, James A. Olson, and Moshe Shike. *Modern Nutrition in Health and Disease*. Philadelphia: Lea & Febiger, 1994.

Shulman, Neil B., Elijah Saunders, and W. Dallas Hall. *High Blood Pressure: The Clear, Complete, Up-to-Date Guide to Tests, Treatments, Dangers and Cures*. New York: Dell Publishing, 1993.

Singh, R. "Can Guava Fruit Intake Decrease Blood Pressure and Blood Lipids?" *Journal of Human Hypertension* (February 1993): 33–38.

Singh, R. "Dietary Modulators of Blood Pressure in Hypertension." *European Journal of Clinical Nutrition* (1990): 319–27.

Stevens, V. "Weight-Loss Intervention in Phase 1 of the Trials of Hypertension Prevention." *Archives of Internal Medicine* (April 12, 1993): 849–58.

PAMPHLETS

American Heart Association. *About High Blood Pressure*, 1986.

American Heart Association. *Feeling Fine: Living with High Blood Pressure as We Grow Older*, 1989.

National High Blood Pressure Information Center. *High Blood Pressure and What You Can Do About It*, 1987.

National High Blood Pressure Information Center. *High Blood Pressure: Your Doctor's Advice Could Save Your Life*, 1987.

ORGANIZATIONS

American Heart Association. 7320 Greenville Avenue, Dallas, TX 75231.

National High Blood Pressure Education Program. 4733 Bethesda Ave., Bethesda, MD 20814.

FURTHER READING

Cooper, Kenneth H. *Overcoming Hypertension*. New York: Bantam Books, 1990.

Grundy, Scott, and Mary Winston, eds. *Low-Fat, Low-Cholesterol Cookbook*. Dallas: American Heart Association, 1989.

Harper, Jean. *The Food Pharmacy Guide to Good Eating*. New York: Bantam Books, 1991.

Rees, Alan, and Charlene Willey. *Personal Health Reporter*. Detroit: Gale Research Inc., 1993.

Saltman, Paul, Joel Gurin, and Ira Mothner. *The University of California San Diego Nutrition Book*. Boston: Little, Brown & Company, 1993.

## CHAPTER 21: DIETS FOR HYPOGLYCEMIA

REFERENCES

Airola, Paavo. *Hypoglycemia: A Better Approach*. Sherwood, OR: Health Plus Publishers, 1994.

Auer, R. "Hypoglycemia: Brain Neurochemistry and Neuropathy." *Bailleires Clinical Endocrinology and Metabolism* (July 1993): 611–25.

Balch, James, and Phyllis Balch. *Prescription for Nutritional Healing*. Garden City Park, N.Y: Avery Publishing Group, 1990.

The Burton Goldberg Group. *Alternative Medicine: The Definitive Guide*. Puyallup, WA: Future Medicine Publishing, Inc., 1993.

Krimmel, Edward, and Patricia Krimmel. *The Low Blood Sugar Cookbook Diet*. Memphis, TN: Franklin Publishers, 1992.

Martin, Clement G. *Low Blood Sugar: The Hidden Menace of Hypoglycemia*. New York: Simon & Schuster, 1969.

Mirsky, Stanley. *Controlling Diabetes the Easy Way*. New York: Random House, 1981.

Shils, Maurice, James A. Olson, and Moshe Shike. *Nutrition in Health and Disease*. Philadelphia: Lea & Febiger, 1994.

ORGANIZATIONS

National Diabetes Information Clearinghouse. Box NDIC, 9000 Rockville Pike, Bethesda, MD 20892.

Dr. John W. Tinera Memorial Hypoglycemia Lay Group. 149 Spindle Road, Hicksville, N.Y. 11801.

FURTHER READING

Barnett, Carol. *Life with Diabetes: Diabetes Defined*. Ann Arbor, MI: Michigan Diabetes Research Center, University of Michigan, 1987.

Somer, Elizabeth. *Nutrition for Women*. New York: Henry Holt & Co., 1993.

## CHAPTER 22: DIETS FOR IRRITABLE BOWEL SYNDROME

REFERENCES

The Burton Goldberg Group. *Alternative Medicine: The Definitive Guide.* Puyallup, WA: Future Medicine Publishing, Inc., 1993.

Murray, Michael, and Joseph Pizzorno. *Encyclopedia of Natural Medicine.* Rocklin, CA: Prima Publishing, 1991.

Nelson, Jennifer. *Mayo Clinic Diet Manual: A Handbook of Nutrition Practices.* Seventh Edition. New York, NY: Mosby, 1994.

Peikin, Steven. *Gastro Intestinal Health.* New York, NY: HarperCollins, 1991.

Scanlon, Deralee, and Barbara Cottman Becnel. *The Wellness Book of I.B.S.* New York: St. Martin's Press, 1989.

Shils, Maurice, James A. Olson, and Moshe Shike. *Nutrition in Health and Disease.* Philadelphia, PA: Lea & Febiger, 1994.

Shimberg, Elaine Fantle. *Relief from IBS.* New York, NY: Ballantine Books, 1988.

PAMPHLETS

National Digestive Disease Information Clearinghouse. *Irritable Bowel Syndrome,* 1992.

ORGANIZATIONS

Intestinal Disease Foundation, Inc. 1323 Forbes Avenue, Suite 200, Pittsburgh, PA 15219

National Digestive Disease Information Clearinghouse. Box NDDIC, 9000 Rockville Pike, Bethesda, MD 20892.

National Foundation for Ileitis and Colitis. 444 Park Avenue South, New York, N.Y. 10016.

FURTHER READING

"Irritable Bowel Syndrome — Can Medication Help?" *Harvard Medical School Health Letter* (January 1989): 2–4.

Malagelada, Juan. "About Stomach Ulcers." *National Digestive Disease Information Clearinghouse Fact Sheet.* NIH Pub. No. 87-676. January 1987: 1–3.

Margolis, Simeon, and Hamilton Moses III, eds. *The Johns Hopkins Medical Handbook.* New York: Rebus Inc., 1993.

Newberry, Benjamin H., Janet Madden, and Thomas Gertsenberger. *A Holistic Conceptualization of Stress and Disease.* New York: AMS Press, Inc., 1991.

Rees, Alan, and Charlene Wiley. *Personal Health Reporter.* Detroit, MI: Gale Research Inc., 1993.

Scala, James. *Eating Right for a Bad Gut Diet: The Complete Nutritional Guide to Ileitis, Colitis, Crohn's Disease, and Inflammatory Bowel Disease.* New York: Penguin Books, 1990.

## CHAPTER 23: MULTIPLE SCLEROSIS DIETS

REFERENCES

Balch, James, and Phyllis Balch. *Prescription for Nutritional Healing.* Garden City Park, NY: Avery Publishing Group, 1990.

The Burton Goldberg Group. *Alternative Medicine: The Definitive Guide.* Puyallup, WA: Future Medicine Publishing, Inc., 1993.

Donsbach, Kurt, and H. Rudolph Alsleben. *Multiple Sclerosis, Muscular Dystrophy and ALS.* New York: The Rockland Corporation, 1993.

Graham, Judy. *Multiple Sclerosis: A Self-Help Guide to Its Management.* Rochester, VT: Healing Arts Press, 1989.

Sibley, William A. *Therapeutic Claims in Multiple Sclerosis.* New York: Demos Publications, 1992.

Swank, Roy. "Multiple Sclerosis: Fat-Oil Relations." *Nutrition* (September/October 1991): 368–76.

Swank, Roy, and Barbara Brewer Dugan. *The Multiple Sclerosis Diet Book: A Low-Fat Diet for the Treatment of MS.* New York: Doubleday, 1987.

ORGANIZATIONS

Helping Multiple Sclerosis, Inc. P.O. Box 1, Darien, CT 06820.

Kalsow Medical Self-Care Centers. 795 Alamo Pintado Road, Solvang, CA 93464.

The Medical Rehabilitation Research and Training Center for Multiple Sclerosis. Albert Einstein College of Medicine, 1300 Morris Park Avenue, Bronx, N.Y. 10461.

Multiple Sclerosis Self-Help Project. P.O. Box 7573, Berkeley, CA 94707.

National Multiple Sclerosis Society. 205 East 42nd Street, New York, N.Y. 10017.

The Mary Ingraham Bunting Institute of Radcliffe College, 34 Concord Avenue, Cambridge, MA 02138.

## CHAPTER 24: CANCER AND CHEMOTHERAPY DIETS

REFERENCES

Bruning, Nancy. *Coping with Chemotherapy.* New York: Ballantine Books, 1993.

The Burton Goldberg Group. *Alternative Medicine: The Definitive Guide.* Puyallup, WA: Future Medicine Publishing, Inc., 1993.

Marti, James E., and Andrea Hine. *The Alternative Health and Medicine Encyclopedia.* Detroit: Gale Research, Inc., and Invisible Press, 1994.

Nixon, Daniel W. *The Cancer Recovery Eating Plan.* New York: Random House, 1994.

Simone, Charles B. *Cancer and Nutrition.* Garden City Park, NY: Avery Publishing Group, 1992.

U.S. Congress Office of Technology Assessment. *Unconventional Cancer Treatments.* Washington, D.C.: Government Printing Office, September 1990.

ORGANIZATIONS

American Cancer Society. 1599 Clifton Road NE, Atlanta, GA 30329.

National Cancer Institute. Office of Cancer Communications, Building 31, 9000 Rockville Pike, Bethesda, MD 20892.

Syracuse Cancer Research Institute. Presidential Plaza, 600 East Genesee Street, Syracuse, N.Y. 13202.

# Index

Abrams, Steven, 168, 169
acidophilus. *See* dairy products
Addison's disease (hypoglycemia and), 67
adolescents
  girls, and calcium levels, 29, 62, 165,
    168–69
  iron requirements, 29
  obesity in, 36, 179, 183
  weight-loss programs for, 90, 108, 181,
    183
  *See also* children
Aging, White House Conference on
  (1994), 186. *See also* elderly, the
AIDS, 431
Airola, Paavo, 366–72
alcohol consumption
  for arthritics, 270, 273
  for athletes, 223, 238
  and cancer, 409, 427–28
  in commercial weight-loss and OTC
    programs, 102, 121
  for diabetics, 303, 312
  for the elderly, 188, 201
  and food allergies, 323, 331
  in heart diets, 285, 291, 296
  and hypertension, 337, 341, 345
  and hypoglycemia, 361, 363
  and IBS, 388
  for men ("moderate"), 218
  monitoring of, 34
  and MS, 394
  and osteoporosis, 101, 250, 260
  at "Reward Meal," 133
  surgeon general's recommendations,
    29
  in vegetarian diet, 218
  for women, 102, 157, 160, 162, 218
    and osteoporosis, 101, 250
    during pregnancy, 29, 160
Alcoholics Anonymous, 113, 117
algae, 213, 219
Algert, Susan, 300
alkaline salts (in allergy elimination diet),
  325, 327, 335
allergies. *See* food allergies; food allergy
  elimination diets
All-Family Menu Plan, 178–79
Alliance for Aging Research, 202–3
aloe vera juice, 390
Alsleben, H. Rudolph, 392, 404–6
*Alternative Health and Medicine Encyclope-
  dia*, 213, 297, 336, 430
*Alternative Medicine: The Definitive Guide*
  (Goldberg Group), 121, 278, 372,
  389, 407
American Academy of Allergy and Immu-
  nology, 316
American Academy of Nutrition, 153
American Academy of Pediatrics, 169
American Association of Retired Persons
  (AARP), 186, 196
American Cancer Society, 341, 409, 410
American College of Sports Medicine,
  106, 237, 242
American Council on Science and Health,
  30
American Diabetes Association (ADA),
  123, 300
  food exchange system of, 301, 305, 357
  nutritional guidelines of, 310–11

American Dietetic Association (ADA), 123, 237, 240, 241
  *Journal of,* 95, 179
  and vegetarian diets, 205, 211, 217, 220
*American Health* magazine, 167, 314
American Heart Association (AHA), 149, 238, 280, 347
  diets, 64, 281, 343
  Step One and Step Two, 287–92
*American Heart Association Low-Fat, Low-Cholesterol Cookbook* (Grundy and Winston), 287–92
American Holistic Medical Association, 257
*American Journal of Public Health,* 184
American Medical Association *Journal,* 182
American Medical Writers Association, 374
Ames, Bruce, 421
amino acids, "essential," 11, 212, 213, 216. *See also* proteins
amphetamines and blood pressure, 346
Anderson, James W., 299
anemia, 210
  iron-deficiency, 157, 201, 236, 317–18
*Annals of Internal Medicine,* 42, 93
anorexia nervosa (AN), 50–51, 53
antacids and mineral loss, 22, 23
Anti-Aging Plan, 185, 186–91. *See also* elderly, the, diets for
*Anti-Aging Plan, The* (Walford), 186
antioxidants, 18, 23, 60, 297, 414, 415
  and chemotherapy, 428, 430
  free radicals combated by, 203, 235, 416
  pepper (capsicum), 432
  *See also* vitamin(s)
appetite (vs. hunger), 35
appetite suppressants, 121–22, 125
ARMS (Action for Research into Multiple Sclerosis, UK), 392, 399, 403
arteriosclerosis risk, alcohol and, 201
arthritis
  calcium deficiency and, 273–74, 275
  dairy products and (pros and cons), 270, 272
  incidence and effects of, 264–65
  osteoarthritis, 63, 264–65

rheumatoid arthritis (RA), 264, 265, 271–72, 274, 277
  yucca and, 278–79
arthritis diets, 63–64, 264–78
  basic nutritional approaches, 266, 271–72, 274–75
  behavior modification with, 271, 278
  exercise with, 270–71, 278
  fluid intake in, 268, 269, 275
  meal habits, 277
  recent research, 278
  recommended foods, 267–69, 272, 275–76
  restricted or eliminated foods, 269–70, 273, 276
  vitamin/mineral supplements to, 270, 271, 273–74, 276–78
*Arthritis Relief Diet, The* (Scala), 265–66
Arthritis Survey Diet, 274–78
*Arthritis: What Works* (Klein and Sobel), 274
ascorbic acid. *See* vitamin C
aspirin
  in ECA weight-loss formula, 121, 124, 125–26
  and vitamin C, 277
atherosclerosis, 285, 336, 340
  cholesterol and, 13, 64, 208, 280
  prevention or reversal of, 141, 194
  *See also* coronary artery disease (CAD) diets
athletes
  caloric intake, 244
  diets and fluid requirements for, *see* sports diets
  and fasting, avoidance of, 335
  mineral needs and deficiencies, 61, 228–29, 235–36, 243
  Olympic contestants, 136, 222
  protein needs, 216, 224, 232, 241, 245
  and steroids, 245
  vegetarian, 216, 228
  women, 229–36
Australian Institute of Sport, 222

Bailey, Covert, 129, 143–46, 147, 148
bakery goods. *See* bread/bakery goods
Balch, James and Phyllis, 372, 389–90
Barnard, R. James, 315
Baylor College of Medicine, 165, 281

beans. *See* legumes; soybean products

Beaser, Richard, 308–13

Becnel, Barbara Cottman, 378

behavior modification, 52, 120, 341. *See also individual diet plans*

*Best Medicine, The: The Complete Health and Preventive Medicine Handbook* (Butler and Rayner), 249

beta-carotene. *See* vitamin A as beta-carotene

beverages
   alcohol, *see* alcohol consumption
   for arthritics, 269, 275–76
   for athletes, *see* sports drinks
   for children ("worst"), 177
   coffee and tea, *see* caffeine
   herbal teas, 371, 394, 406
   macrobiotic, 208
   milk, *see* milk
   sugar-rich sodas, 170. *See also* soft drinks
   water, 10–11, 160, 170, 184. *See also* fluid intake

"binge" eating, 51, 52, 57, 115, 156

Bingham, Robert, 273, 278

Biosphere 2 diet, 186–91

Bjornstrop, Per, 145

Blackburn, George L., 43, 49, 84, 93, 97, 262–63

blood sugar. *See* glucose (dextrose)

blood sugar, low. *See* hypoglycemia

bodybuilding. *See* muscle mass

body composition
   how to measure, 40
   vs. pounds, as measure of health, 100

body fat, calories equivalent to one pound of, 54. *See also* body weight; weight control

body height and frame size, how to measure, 39–40

body mass index (BMI), 42
   nomogram for, 43

body shape (waist-to-hip ratio, WHR), 138–39
   how to measure, 40–42

body weight
   how to measure, 38
   ideal (IBW), 53
   metabolism and, 45
   muscle tissue vs. fat, 126, 145
   *See also* weight control; weight loss

book diet programs. *See* popular book diet programs

*Book of Macrobiotics, The: The Universal Way of Health, Happiness and Peace* (Kushi and Jack), 205

botanical diet programs. *See* over-the-counter (OTC) botanical diets

botanical supplements, 371, 372, 389–90
   garlic, 175, 297, 390, 414, 415
   peppermint oil, 377, 389
   traditional Chinese medicine (TCM), 431
   *See also* herbs and spices

brain dysfunction (hypoglycemia and), 67

Braly, James, 317, 328–35

bran. *See* fiber

bread/bakery goods
   diet recommendations or restrictions
      cancer, 419–20
      children, 174, 177
      the elderly, 188
      heart disease, 284, 290
      MS, 393, 396, 401
   as "worst" food, 177

breakfast, importance of, 34–35, 230, 277

breakfast foods, 177, 213, 268. *See also* grains and cereals

Breast Cancer Action (advocacy group), 425

*Breast Implants: Everything You Need to Know* (Bruning), 425

Breum, L. 127

brewer's yeast, 368–69

Brigham and Women's Hospital (Boston), 163, 297

*British Medical Journal,* 352

British National Osteoporosis Diet, 255–57

Brody, Jane, 313

Bruning, Nancy, 425–29

bulimia nervosa (BN), 50, 51–53

Burke, Louise, 62, 222–29

Butler, Kurt, 249

cachexia. *See* weight loss

cadmium, exposure to, 250

caffeine
   and cholesterol, 242, 291
   decaffeinated coffee or coffee substitute, 394, 406

caffeine (*cont.*)
in EC and ECA weight-loss formulas, 121, 125–27
intake restrictions, 124
for arthritics, 269, 273
for athletes, 242
in food allergies, 331
in heart diet, 291
in hypertension, 337
in hypoglycemia, 363
in IBS, 388
in MS, 394, 406
and mutagens, 421
in osteoporosis, 260
so ft drinks, 363
tea, 291, 363, 388
for women, 101, 157
tea permitted, 269
withdrawal symptoms, 363
calcium/calcium deficiency, 21, 210, 253, 255
arthritis, 273–74, 275
athletes, 61, 229, 236
calcium absorption, 21–22, 254
fat or steroid interference with, 194, 277
food inhibition of, 157
calcium-phosphorus ratio in soft drinks, 22, 258
calcium supplements, 254, 273–74 (*see also* osteoporosis)
and cancer, 413, 414, 417
children, 58, 164, 165, 168–69, 175, 176, 179
dietary tips, 256
elderly persons, 185, 202
gluten foods and, 157
and heart disease, 21
and hypertension, 337, 344–45, 349
and iron absorption, 23, 254
RDA, 27, 168, 185
sources of calcium, 256
dairy products, 21, 30, 210, 255–56, 262–63, 272
15 best, 257
grains, 251
soybean products, 219–20, 255
vegetable, 21, 167, 187, 213, 215, 219, 251, 256
vegetarian diet, 175

ways of adding calcium to diet, 253, 254, 256
women's needs, 29, 62, 158, 168, 201, 250, 262
and deficiencies, 157, 202, 236, 249
*Calcium Plus Workbook, The* (Whitlock), 158
calories, 10
in American Heart Association diet, 288
athletes' requirements, 244
"counting," 32–33, 137, 338
elderly requirements, 59–60, 185
equivalent to one pound of body fat, 54
in fats and sugars, 12
how to eliminate, 339
low- and very-low-calorie diets (LCDs and VLCDs), 55, 73–96, 284–86
measuring need for, 44–48
meat as source of, 213
and "nutrient-dense" foods, 10
surgeon general's recommendation, 29
Campbell, Colin, 184
Canada's Food Guide to Healthy Eating, 99
cancer
breast, colorectal, prostate, and squamous, 413–15
endometrial, 421–22
fat consumption and, 12, 13
fiber and, 69, 409, 411, 413–14, 419, 427
hypoglycemia and, 67
incidence of, 408
meat-cooking techniques and, 212, 420
obesity and, 73, 163, 182, 421–22
pesticides and, 184
vegetarians and, 221
vitamins and, 17, 221
*See also* carcinogens
cancer and chemotherapy diets, 408–33
anticancer chemicals in foods, 427, 432–33
basic nutritional approaches, 410–11, 418, 426
behavior modification with, 417–18, 425, 429
for breast cancer, 413
calcium and, 413, 414, 417
chemopreventives, 408, 415, 428–29, 430
for colorectal cancer, 413–14

cancer and chemotherapy diets (*cont.*)
coping with chemotherapy diet, 425–29
exercise with, 417, 423, 425, 429
fluid intake in, 426
meal plans, 422–23
nutritional connection with, 410–11
obesity and, 73, 163, 182, 421–22
progressive chemotherapy diet, 428
for prostate cancer, 414–15
recent research, 429–33
recommended foods, 411, 413, 414, 415, 419, 426–27
to reduce risk, 69–70, 101, 140, 141, 409–10
among elderly, 185, 190
NCI guidelines, 409
vegetarians and, 187, 204, 211
restricted or eliminated foods, 411–13, 414–15, 419–21, 427–28
for squamous cancers, 415
vitamin/mineral supplements to, 414, 415–16, 423, 424, 427, 428–29
*Cancer and Nutrition: A Ten-Point Plan to Reduce Your Risk of Getting Cancer* (Simone), 418
*Cancer Prevention* magazine, 410
*Cancer Recovery Eating Plan, The* (Nixon), 410
canned foods. *See* processed foods
*Carbohydrate Addict's Diet, The* (Heller and Heller), 129, 132–35
carbohydrates, 11–12
and cancer, 411
carbohydrate loading, 225–28, 230–31, 233, 239
complex, 11–12, 29, 34, 244, 267
15-gram starches, 306
guidelines for consumption, 29, 30, 34
for arthritics, 267
for diabetics, 310
for the elderly, 193
for replenishing, 231
simple, *see* sugars
sources of, 11–12, 34
high-carbohydrate foods, 239, 339, 358
in sports diet, 224, 225–28
stored (glycogen), 12, 21, 122, 227, 231, 233, 244

*See also* high-carbohydrate, lowfat diets; low-carbohydrate diets
carbonated drinks. *See* soft drinks
carcinogens
cooking techniques and, 155, 212, 420
food, 409, 421, 427
food combating, 427, 432–33
cardiovascular, definition of, 280. *See also* heart disease, risk of
carpal tunnel syndrome, 278
CATS (coffee, alcohol, tobacco, sugar) and allergies, 331. *See also* food allergies
cellulose, 14, 34. *See also* fiber (soluble and insoluble)
Center for Disease Control and Prevention, 106
Center for Weight and Eating Control, 132
cereals. *See* breakfast foods; grains and cereals
chemopreventives, 408, 415, 428–29, 430
chemotherapy diets, 425–29
children
cancer in, 184
cholesterol levels of, 165, 169, 173
fat consumption by, 169–70
fiber needs of, 167–68
restricted, 176
food allergies of, 318, 328
fruit and vegetable consumption by, 165–68
limitation of sugar intake of, 29, 167, 170
obesity in, 36, 58, 164, 165, 179, 181–82, 183
and osteoporosis, 168
protein needs of, 175, 176–77, 217
RDAs for, 26–27, 164, 171–72
school lunches for, 170–71, 184
vegetarian, 175, 176, 217, 220
vitamin/mineral needs and deficiencies, 20, 58, 168–79 *passim*, 220 (*see also* calcium/calcium deficiency; iron/iron deficiency)
"worst foods for," 177–78
*See also* adolescents
children's diet programs, 58–59, 103, 164–84
basic nutritional approaches, 172–73, 180

children's diet programs (*cont.*)
  behavior modification with, 182
  eligibility and cost, 179–80
  exercise with, 182–83
  family counseling in, 182
  food diary in, 182
  monitoring weight loss in, 181–82
  and new foods, 171
  parent programs as part of, 179–80, 182, 183–84
  recent research, 183–84
  recipes, 178–79
  recommended or required foods, 165–69, 173–75, 180
  restricted or eliminated foods, 169–70, 176–78, 181
  vitamin/mineral supplements to, 164, 170, 171–72, 179, 219, 220
Children's Nutrition Research Center (CNRC), 164
  Diet Plan of, 59, 165–72
Chinese medicine, traditional (TCM), 431
chips, 393, 396
chlorella, 213
chloride, 21, 52, 240
chocolate eliminated from MS diet, 396
cholecalciferol. *See* vita min D
cholesterol, 13
  adult level, 293
  and atherosclerosis/heart disease, 13, 33, 64, 208, 280
  caffeine and, 242, 291
  and cancer, 412
  carbohydrates and, 135
  children's level, 165, 169, 173
  exercise and, 190
  fats and, 12, 33, 194, 208, 340
  fiber and, 187
  fish and, 289, 394
  and gallstones, 94
  guava fruit and, 354
  HDL ("good"), 13, 94, 126–27, 190, 201, 285, 354
  and hypertension, 345
  high serum levels, 41, 54–55
  LDL ("bad"), 12, 13, 56, 96, 122, 190
  measurement of, 280
  organ meats and, 290
  OTC programs and, 122, 126–27
  reduction of, in diet, 293–94, 380

soybean substitutes and, 169
  surgeon general's recommendation, 29, 33
  vegetarian diet and, 218
  VLCDs and, 96
choline, 179
Chopra, Deepak, 391
chromium as diet supplement, 179, 369
cirrhosis of the liver, 194
CitriMax All-Natural Diet Plan, 121–23
*Clinical Investigator* (periodical), 297
*Clinica Terapeutica* (Italian periodical), 314
Clinton Administration, 164
Clymer Health Clinic, 380
cobalamin. *See* vitamin B12
*Co-Dependent Parent, The* (Becnel), 378
coenzyme Q, 429
coffee (decaffeinated and regular). *See* caffeine
"comfort" foods, 384
commercial mixes. *See* processed foods
commercial weight-loss programs, 97–112
  for adolescents, 108, 183
  alcohol restrictions, 102
  basic nutritional approaches, 99–100, 104, 108, 111–12
  behavior modification as part of, 102, 106, 109
  cost and eligibility, 98, 99, 103, 104, 107, 110, 111
  counseling in, 100, 101, 102, 107–8
  exercise included in, 101, 102, 105–6, 109
  fluid intake in, 101, 108, 112
  food diary in, 109
  group support as part of, 106, 109
  kosher, 80, 91, 108
  medically supervised, 111
  physician referral required, 98, 103, 107, 110
  special programs in, 100–101, 108, 112
  transition phase in, 100
  vegetarian, 80, 91, 100–101, 108
  vitamin/mineral supplements to, 101, 109, 111
*Complete Guide to Food for Sports Performance, The* (Burke), 222
condiments, flavorings, sauces, salad dressings, 175, 189
  "worst" for children, 177

Connor, William and Sonja, 129, 141–43
*Controlling Diabetes the Easy Way* (Mirsky), 304–8, 356
*Controlling Your Food Allergies* (Mandell), 324
cookbooks, 129, 149–50
    American Heart Association, 287–92
    *See also* recipes
cooking techniques
    in arthritis diets, 268, 272
    carcinogenic results, 155, 212, 420
    in diabetic diet, 300
    in elderly persons' diet, 195
    for IBS, 380
    with oil, 402
    to reduce fat or cholesterol consumption, 169–70, 240, 251, 267, 268, 277, 293–94, 380
*Coping with Chemotherapy* (Bruning), 425
copper/copper deficiency, 20, 158, 176, 179, 210
corn allergy, 323
corn syrup, 11, 323. *See also* sugars
coronary artery disease (CAD), vegetarians and, 221
coronary artery disease (CAD) diets, 64–65, 141, 185, 190, 204, 280–97
    basic nutritional approaches, 281–82, 287–88, 292–93
    behavior modification with, 286, 291–92, 296–97
    exercise with, 286, 291, 296
    prevention diet, 293–94
    recent research, 297
    recipes, 285, 291, 295
    recommended foods, 282–83, 288–90, 294–95
    restricted or eliminated foods, 283–84, 290–91, 295
    reversal diet, 292–93
    total calories in, 288
    vitamin/mineral supplements to, 295, 297
counseling in commercial diet programs, 100, 101, 102, 107–8
    in VLCDs, 82, 85, 86, 88, 91, 92
crackers, 174, 393, 396, 419. *See also* bread/bakery goods
Craig, Jenny and Sid, 97, 98, 107–10, 183
Crawford, Michael, 399

dairy products
    acidophilus, 368, 390
    as calcium source, *see* calcium/calcium deficiency
    diet recommendations or restrictions
        arthritis, 270, 272
        cancer, 420, 426
        children, 174, 177
        elderly, 192–93, 200
        heart disease, 284, 290
        hypoglycemia, 368
        MS, 393, 395, 400
        osteoporosis, 250–51, 262–63
    disorders caused by, 209, 214
    guidelines for consumption of, 30, 174
    as protein source, 331, 368
    substitutes for, 284
    yogurt, 255, 256, 272, 400
    *See also* lactose intolerance; milk
Daley, Rosie, 129, 149–50
Daly, P. A., 125
Dalman, Annette, 83, 84
DBPCFC (double-blind, placebo-controlled oral food challenges), 317
Debakey, Michael, 281–86, 287, 288
delicatessen food, "worst" for children, 177
dental cavities, sugar and, 29, 218
Department of Agriculture, U.S. (USDA), 30, 40, 153, 184, 204, 218, 238
    Food Guide Pyramid, 99, 164, 165, 172–73
    National Food Consumption Surveys, 184
Department of Health and Human Services, U.S., 30, 204
Desert Arthritis and Medical Clinic (California), 278
desserts, 193, 208
    for diabetics, 305–6
    for hypoglycemics, 362
    "worst" for children, 177
dextrose. *See* glucose
DF (dexfenfluramine), 127
diabetes
    and eligibility for diet programs, 73, 80, 98, 107, 110, 124
    and heart disease, 280
    hypoglycemia and, 355
    incidence of (Types I and II), 298–99

diabetes (*cont.*)
  obesity and, 41, 73, 93, 95, 182, 299
  and Syndrome X, 94
  U.S. Dietary Goals, 309
  vegetarians and, 221
  in women, 298
  *See also* hypoglycemia; insulin
Diabetes Control and Complications Trial,
  308
diabetes diets, 65, 108, 141, 298–315
  basic nutritional approaches, 300, 304–
    5, 309–10
  behavior modification with, 313
  exercise with, 299, 303–4, 305, 308,
    312–13, 314–15
  fluid intake in, 308
  food exchange system for meal plan-
    ning, 301, 305
  "intensive" therapy in, 309, 310, 311
  nutritional guidelines, 309–10
    ADA, 310–11
  recent research, 313–14
  recipes, 300, 302–3
  recommended foods, 301, 305–7
  restaurant meals, 302
  restricted or eliminated foods, 301–2,
    307
  timing of meals and snacks, 307, 312
  vegetarian, 311
  vitamin/mineral supplements to, 303,
    307–8, 314
  weight gain in, 311–12
DiBartolomeo, Joseph J., 111
diet(s)
  allergy, *see* food allergy elimination, *be-
    low*
  all-family menu plan, 178–79
  arthritis, 63–64, 264–78
  athletic performance, *see* sports, *below*
  basis of comparison, 2–3
  cancer risk reduction, *see* cancer; cancer
    and chemotherapy diets
  and causes of death, 28, 163
  children's, 58–59, 103, 164–84
  choosing and maintaining, suggestions
    for, 69, 70
  commercial programs, 97–112
  coronary artery disease prevention, 64–
    65, 141, 185, 190, 204, 280–97
  "crash," 95

diabetes, 65, 108, 141, 298–315
diet goals, 49–70
elderly persons', 59–60, 185–203
exercise included with, *see* exercise
failure of, 137, 146
food allergy elimination, 66, 91, 215,
  258–60, 316–35
frequent meals or snacks, 34–35, 122,
  124, 140, 160, 230. *See also* snacks
"good," 30
"heart reversal," 83
high-carbohydrate, *see* high-carbohydrate, lowfat diets
hypertension, 66–67, 141, 190, 336–54
hypoglycemia, 67, 108, 355–72
irritable bowel syndrome (IBS), 68, 373–
  90
kosher, 80, 91, 108
lactose-intolerance, 77, 80, 100, 101–2
low- and very-low-calorie (LCD and
  VLCD), 55, 73–96
low-carbohydrate, 132–38
lowfat, high-carbohydrate, *see* highcar-
  bohydrate, lowfat diets
macrobiotic, 61, 204, 205–15
medically supervised programs, 73–96,
  111, 121
monitoring, *see* food diary
for multiple sclerosis (MS), 68, 391–407
nutrition guidelines and assessment, 30–
  39
osteoporosis prevention, 60, 62–63, 101,
  190 , 249–63
over-the-counter (OTC) botanical, 121–
  28
salt-restricted, 21. *See also* salt
side effects (ketogenic), 75, 78
sports, 61–62, 135–38, 222–45
stress and, 36–37
time, place, and mood and, 35–37
vegetarian, *see* vegetarian diets
vitamins/minerals in or added to, *see*
  minerals and trace elements; vita-
  min/mineral supplements; vitamin(s)
weight control, 50–57. *See also* weight
  loss
for women, 57–58, 62–63, 100, 101,
  153–63, 178
"yo-yo," 47, 115
"zone-favorable," 135–38

*Diet, Nutrition, and Cancer Prevention: The Good News* (NCI booklet), 221

*Dietary Guidelines for Americans* (USDA), 218

diet books, 129–50

Diet Center (commercial diet program), 97, 98–102

Diet for Women Over 50, 196–202

diet pills and high blood pressure, 346

diet supplements
bars and crackers, 89, 92, 93
brand foods, 99–100, 104, 106
brewer's yeast, 368–69
EPA capsules, 266
liver tablets, 400
powdered/liquid
in chemotherapy, 426
for hypoglycemia, 372
in sports diets, 224, 226, 231
in VLCDs, 75, 76, 81, 89, 90, 92
wheat germ oil, 405
*See also* botanical supplements; vitamin/mineral supplements

diuretics (and potassium loss), 201

diverticulitis, risk of, 190, 221

DNA, 16, 17, 24, 416

Donsbach, Kurt, 392, 404–5

Dover, Clare, 255–57

Dr. Barry Sears's Zone Sport Diet, 62, 129, 135–38

*Dr. Braly's Diet and Nutrition Revolution* (Braly), 328

*Dr. Dean Ornish's Program for Reversing Heart Disease* (Ornish), 263, 292–97

*Dr. Mandell's Five-Day Allergy Relief System* (Mandell), 317, 324

drugs
diet pills, 346
over-the-counter, 121, 124, 125–26, 277
prescription
for arthritis, 277
blood pressure medication, 341, 345–46, 347
and osteoporosis, 250
for weight loss, 127–28
recreational, 346

Dugan, Barbara Brewer, 392

du Pré, Jacqueline, 391

Durning, Annie, 300

East West Foundation, 205

*Eating Right for a Bad Gut* (Scala), 266

Eating Well—The Vegetarian Way (American Dietetic Association), 205

EC, ECA. *See* ephedra-based formulas

egg allergy elimination diet, 318–19

eggs
allergy to, 214
diet recommendations or restrictions, 173, 290, 394, 420, 426
"substitutes" for, 270, 319

eicosanoids, 135–36, 137. *See also* fatty acids

elderly, the
alcohol for, 188, 201
diet and disease risk of, 185, 190
fiber needs of, 187–88, 193
fluid intake of, 193–94
and gallstones, 94
lactose intolerance in, 200
metabolism of, 45, 145
noneligible for diet program, 73
protein needs of, 193, 195, 198
tips for, 195
vitamin/mineral needs and deficiencies, 20, 185, 191, 195–96, 200, 202–3

elderly, the, diets for, 59–60, 185–203
basic nutritional approaches, 186–87, 191–92, 197
behavior modification with, 202
exercise with, 190, 196, 201–2
meal plans, 198–200
recent research, 202–3
recommended or required foods, 187–88, 189, 192–94, 197–98
restricted or eliminated foods, 188, 194, 195
vitamin/mineral supplements to, 188, 190, 192, 194–96, 200–201, 202–3

electrolytes. *See* sports drinks

Eliasson, K., 352

emotional state. *See* stress

*Encyclopedia of Natural Medicine* (Murray and Pizzorno), 36, 337, 352, 389

energy expenditure. *See* exercise

energy intake. *See* calories

*Enter the Zone* (Sears), 129, 135

EPA (eicosapentaenoic acid), 266, 267

EPA (Environmental Protection Agency) survey, 184
ephedra (mahuang), 57, 121, 124, 125
ephedra-based formulas (EC and ECA), 121, 125–27
Epstein, Leonard, 182
*Essential Guide to Vitamins and Minerals, The* (Somer), 159, 229
estrogen and progesterone replacement therapy, 63, 94, 138, 262, 422
estrogen deficiency, 158, 249, 419
exercise, 54, 69
  for arthritics, 270–71, 278
  with cancer diet, 417, 423, 425, 429
  for children, 180, 182–83
  and cholesterol, 190
  in commercial weight-loss programs, 101, 102, 105–6, 109
  for diabetics, 299, 303–4, 308, 312–13, 314–15
  for the elderly, 190, 196, 201–2
  energy expenditure, resting and physical (REE, PEE) and metabolism, 45, 46–47, 48
  and fasting (pro and con), 327, 335
  garlic and, 297
  and heart disease, 286, 291, 296
  with hypertension diet, 341–42, 346, 351
  with hypoglycemia diet, 365–66, 371–72
  with IBS diet, 377, 383, 388
  importance of, 96, 140
  and metabolism, 145, 228
  and MS, 396–97, 398, 403–4, 406
  and obesity, 145
  and osteoporosis, 254–55, 257, 261
  with OTC programs, 123, 125
  in popular book diet programs, 131–32, 136–37, 140, 145–50 *passim*
  in preparing for sports competition, 225–26, 245
  and protein requirements, 224
  support groups and, 120
  surgeon general's recommendation, 29
  and vitamin/mineral needs, 228–29, 235–36
  with VLCDs, 77, 81, 86, 89, 95–96
  for women, 57, 140, 158–59, 160, 163
  *See also* sports diets

Fair, William R., 414–15
family counseling (children's diet), 182
Family Heart Study, 141
farnesyl hypothesis (cancer), 412
fast food. *See* junk food; restaurant meals
fasting
  in allergy elimination diets, 327, 330, 335
  avoidance of, by athletes and exercisers, 335
  in hypoglycemia, 372
fat, body. *See* body fat
fat cells, 56, 57, 138–40
fats, dietary, 12–13
  and atherosclerosis, 340
  and calcium absorption, 194
  consumption of (U.S.), 28
    by children, 169–70, 178
    and disease, 12, 13, 419
    guidelines for, 30, 33, 194, 218
    not as factor in weight gain, 137
    as "number one enemy," 145
    surgeon general's recommendation, 29, 30
  diet recommendations or restrictions
    athletes, 223
    cancer, 409, 411–12, 413, 419–20
    children, 174
    food allergies, 330–31
    IBS, 385
    MS, 393, 395, 402
  as essential for body function, 12
  high-fat diet, 136
  how to decrease in diet
    at home, *see* cooking techniques
    in restaurant meals, 302
  hydrogenated (hardened), avoidance of, 273, 290–91, 395
  and insulin levels, 131
  lowfat diet, *see* high-carbohydrate, low-fat diets
  metabolism of, 33, 138
  as protein source, 331
  saturated, 12–13, 331, 419
    and cholesterol, 12, 33, 208, 340
    and MS, 404
  small children's need of, 173
  unsaturated, 12
    monounsaturated, 12, 341

fats *(cont.)*
  polyunsaturated, 12, 173, 194, 340–41, 402, 419
  *See also* oils
fatty acids, essential (EFA)
  in arthritis diet, 271
  and eicosanoids, 135–36, 137
  in MS diet, 397, 399
  polyunsaturated (PUFAs), 194, 406
  and prostaglandins, 12, 266
  saturated, 208
  sources of, 275, 367, 385, 390
  *See also* fats, dietary
*Feed Your Kids Bright* (Prince and Prince), 172–79
Feltin, Marie, 60, 186, 196–202
Ferguson, Sybil, 97, 98
fiber (soluble and insoluble), 13–14, 60
  for arthritics, 268, 275
  athletes' needs, 224
  bran, 330, 375, 401
  and cancer, 69, 409, 411, 413–14, 419, 427
  for children, 166, 167–68, 176
  for diabetics, 301, 306–7, 311
  for the elderly, 187–88, 193
  and food allergies, 330
  in heart diet, 294–95
  and hypertension, 352
  and hypoglycemia, 358
  and IBS, 374, 375–76, 385
  recommended consumption, 14, 29, 34, 122, 143
    in VLCDs, 78, 83, 92
  for women, 156
fish
  and acidity, 272
  allergy to, 319–20
  in chemotherapy diet, 426
  cholesterol in, 289, 394
  fatty, as anticancer agent, 432
  fish oils, 173, 274–75
  in MS diet, 394–95, 400–401
  as protein source, 30, 33, 147, 267, 331
  shellfish, 272, 289, 394, 400
  as source of polyunsaturated fats/ fatty acids, 173, 275, 385
  "worst" kind for children, 178
fish or shellfish allergy diet, 319–20

*Fitness and Sports Medicine: An Introduction* (Nieman), 238
*Fitness and Your Health* (Nieman), 36, 38, 237
*Fit or Fat Target Diet, The* (Bailey), 129, 143–46
flavorings. *See* condiments, flavorings, sauces, salad dressings; herbs and spices
fluid intake and calcium absorption, 254. *See also individual diet plans*
fluoride, 29
folic acid or folate. *See* vitamin B9
food additives. *See* processed foods
food allergies, 210, 214, 316–23
  calcium and, 21
  in children, 318, 328
  commonest allergic foods, 318, 329
  diseases related to, 317, 328
  fixed or cyclic, 324, 326
  "hidden" ingredients, 318, 319, 321, 331
  symptoms of, 316, 317, 328
  testing for, 317, 329
  *See also* gluten intolerance; lactose intolerance
food allergy elimination diets, 66, 91, 215, 258–60, 316–35
  alkaline salts used in, 325, 327, 335
  basic nutritional approach, 324
  corn allergy, 323
  egg allergy, 318–19
  exercise during (pros and cons), 327, 335
  fasting in, 327, 330, 335
  fish or shellfish allergy, 319–20
  fluid intake in, 325, 327
  and food diary, 335
  milk allergy, 320. *See also* lactose intolerance
  recommended or required foods, 320, 330
  restricted or eliminated foods, 325–26, 330–31
  rotation diet, 332, 335
  sample diets, 326, 333–34
  soy and peanut allergy, 321
  vitamin/mineral supplements to, 317–25 *passim*, 328, 331–32, 335
  wheat allergy, 322–23
Food Allergy Network (FAN), 333

Food and Drug Administration (FDA), 17, 73, 125, 127, 273
  packaging requirements, 32
  removes minerals from market, 274
Food and Nutrition Board, 45, 179, 385
food carcinogens. *See* carcinogens
food diary, how to keep, 31–37. *See also* individual diet plans
food exchange system, 301, 305
  in commercial diet programs, 100, 105, 108
Food Guide Pyramid (USDA), 99, 164, 165
  inadequacy of vitamins/minerals in, 164, 173
food labels and food label terms, 32, 319, 321, 322
food pyramid, 147–48. *See also* Food Guide Pyramid (USDA)
Food Specific Immune Complex test (FICA), 329–30
footstrike hemolysis, 236
Foreyt, John, 281
Fortune 500 companies, 105
frame size, how to determine, 39–40
free radicals. *See* antioxidants
fructose, 11. *See also* sugars
fruit
  as anticancer agent, 431, 432
  children's consumption of, 167
  diet recommendations or restrictions
    arthritis, 268, 269, 272
    cancer, 409, 414, 415, 426, 427, 432–33
    diabetes, 305
    heart disease, 289
    hypoglycemia, 368
    in macrobiotic diet, 207–8
    MS, 394, 401
    osteoporosis, 251
  dried, 130, 189, 215
  frozen, 189
  glutathione-containing, 427
  guava, 353–54
  pesticides on, 184
  raw, 380
Fu Zheng (Chinese herbal therapy), 431

Gaby, Alan, 257–62
gallbladder disease/gallstones, 73, 317

  obesity and, 93–94
  vegetarians and, 221
Gallup Organization survey, 117
*Garcinia cambogia* (tropical fruit), 121
Garg, Abhimanyu, 314
garlic, onions, leeks. *See* vegetables (allium)
gastrocolic reflex, 374
*Gastrointestinal Health* (Peikin), 383
Gastrointestinal Health Diet, 383–89
Geleijnse, J. M., 352
genetic factors (in obesity), 55, 56, 120
ginger (for digestive relief), 389. *See also* botanical supplements
Gittleman, Ann Louise, 57, 153–59, 163
glucose (dextrose), 11, 12
  in diabetes, 298–99, 303, 313
  foods stabilizing levels of, 187
  and glucose intolerance, 56
  insulin and (G/I ratios), 94–95
  *See also* sugars
glutathione, 427
gluten intolerance, 157, 298, 317, 322
  diet accommodating, 80
glycogen. *See* carbohydrates (stored)
Goldman, B. A., 36
Gong, Elizabeth, 164
Gotto, Antonio, 281
Graham, Judy, 392, 397–404
grains and cereals
  as calcium source, 251
  diet recommendations or restrictions
    arthritis, 268
    cancer, 419, 426
    children, 174
    heart disease, 282, 284, 289
    hypoglycemia, 3679
    MS, 393, 396, 401
  *See also* breakfast foods; fiber
Grasse, Barbara, 300
group support. *See* support groups Grundy, Scott M., 287–92
guava fruit, 353–54

Hall, W. Dallas, 343
H.A.L.T., 117
Harris, Roger C., 243, 244
Harris, S., 363–64
Harvard Medical School, 42, 125
Harvard School of Public Health, 297
Havala, Suzanne, 217

HCA (hydroxycitric acid), 121, 122, 125, 127
HDL cholesterol. *See* cholesterol
Heald, Felix, 164
*Health Media of America's Nutrition Report* (monthly), 159
Health Restoration Institute (Mexico), 404
*Healthy Way* (periodical), 264
Healthy Woman's Diet (HWD), 159–63
  adapted for the elderly, 191–96
  for athletes, 229–36
heart disease, risk of
  bulimia and, 51–52
  calcium and, 21
  and cholesterol intake, 33
  coronary (CHD), 221, 280. *See also* coronary artery disease (CAD) diets
  hypertension and, 336
  hypoglycemia and, 67
  obesity and, 41, 55, 73, 163, 280, 288
  salt and, 194
  smoking and, 280, 285–86, 296
  for women, 140, 163
  *See also* atherosclerosis
Heilman, Joan, 356
Heller, Richard and Rachel, 129, 132–35, 136
herbal therapy, Chinese, 431
herbal weight-loss formulas, 57, 121–28 *passim*
herbs and spices, 57
  as appetite suppressant, 121
  in children's sweets, 175
  ginger, for digestive complaints, 389
  and herbal teas, 371, 394, 306
  pepper as antioxidant, 432
  rosemary as anticancer agent, 432
  as salt substitute, 276, 351
  as seasoning, for elderly, 189, 195
  in treating IBS, 389–90
  as vitamin/mineral source (children's diet), 175
  *See also* botanical supplements
herpes, 317
high blood pressure. *See* hypertension; hypertension diets
*High Blood Pressure* (Shulman et al.), 343
*High Blood Pressure Relief Diet, The* (Scala), 266

high-carbohydrate foods. *See* carbohydrates
high-carbohydrate, lowfat diets, 130–31, 141–48, 159–62
  for arthritics, 266–70, 274–76
  and cancer, 411
  for children, 58, 165–71, 176, 180–84
  cookbooks for, 149–50, 287–92
  for diabetics, 301–15
  for the elderly, 186–89, 191–95, 197–200
  exercise recommendations, 136–37, 140, 145–46, 148–49
  food pyramid, 147–48, 165
  for heart disease, 280–97
  for hypertension, 338–41
  for hypoglycemia, 357–60
  for IBS, 379–80, 384–85
  for MS, 392–97
  for osteoporosis, 250–53
  recommended foods, 130, 142, 147, 180–81
  restricted or eliminated foods, 130–31
  theory challenged, 132–38, 155–56, 173, 176–77, 313–14
  *See also* sports diets; vegetarian diets
high-fat diet, 136
Hippocrates, 317
H. J. Heinz Company, 103, 106
HMR (Health Management Resources) VLCD program, 74–79, 96
Hoffer, Abram, 317
Holistic Medicine Research Foundations, comparison of diets by, 2
honey, 11, 368. *See also* sugars
*How to Control High Blood Pressure without Drugs* (Rowan), 337
Hultman, Eric, 243, 244
hunger level, 35, 56, 134
hydrochloric acid, 21
hypertension
  and disease risk, 280, 336
  "essential," 336
  factors contributing to, 51–52, 66, 336–37, 341, 345, 346. *See also* stress
  incidence of, 66, 336
  obesity and, 41, 54, 93, 182, 336, 338
  and overeating, 182
  and potassium supplements, 201
  secondary, 336
  symptoms of, 338

hypertension (*cont.*)
  therapies for, 353
  vegetarians and, 221
hypertension diets, 66–67, 141, 190, 336–54
  basic nutritional approaches, 337–38, 343–44, 347–48
  behavior modification with, 342, 346–47, 351–2
  exercise with, 341–42, 346, 351
  medications used in, 341, 345–46, 347
  menu plan, 338–39
  recent research, 352–54
  recommended foods, 339–40, 344–45, 348–49
  restricted or eliminated foods, 339, 340–41, 349–50
*Hypoglycemia: A Better Approach* (Airola), 366
hypoglycemia, 56, 317, 355–56
hypoglycemia diets, 67, 108, 355–72
  basic nutritional approaches, 357, 362–63, 366–67
  behavior modification with, 366
  botanical supplements used with, 371, 372
  eating habits, 369
  exercise with, 365–66, 371–72
  fluid intake in, 369
  meal planning and menus, 359–60, 363–65, 370
  recent research, 372
  recommended foods, 357–58, 362, 367–69
  restricted or eliminated foods, 358–59, 363, 369–70
  vitamin/mineral supplements to, 360–61, 365, 370–71, 372
hypothyroidism, 55–56

immune function tests, 31
Independent Living Primary Care Program, 196
infants, iron deficiency in, 20, 170. *See also* children
insulin
  imbalance, 56–57, 131, 134, 157
  resistance, 94–95, 299
  response, 131, 132, 133, 135, 136
insulin-dependent and non-insulin de-
  pendent (Types I and II) diabetes. *See* diabetes; diabetes diets
insurance, medical, 74, 75, 87
Inter-Health Company, 121–22
*International Journal of Obesity and Related Metabolic Disorders*, 125, 126–27
International Olympic Committee, 242
*In the Kitchen with Rosie* (Winfrey and Daly), 129, 149–50
iodine, 24, 27, 158, 179
iron/iron deficiency, 23, 27
  and anemia, 157, 201, 236, 317–18
  anti-iron foods, 1796–77
  athletes, 16, 228–29, 236, 243
  children and adolescents, 29, 179
  excess iron, 210
  food sources of iron, 29, 167, 210, 237, 369, 400
    and iron absorption, 23, 156, 215, 220
    "nutrient-dense," 10
  iron absorption, vitamin C, or calcium and, 23, 215, 229, 254 (*see also* food sources, *above*)
  women, 20, 29, 156, 157, 201, 202, 236
irritable bowel syndrome (IBS), 318, 378
  incidence of, 373–74
irritable bowel syndrome (IBS) diets, 68, 373–90
  basic nutritional approaches, 374–75, 379, 384
  behavior modification with, 377–78, 388–89
  eating habits, 376, 383
  exercise with, 377, 383, 388
  fluid intake in, 385
  and food diary, 375
  food sensitivities or intolerances, 380–81
  meal plans and menu, 381–82, 386, 387, 389
  medications and, 376–77, 383
  professional therapy for, 376–77, 378
  recent research, 389–90
  recipes, 386
  recommendations, dietary, 389
  recommended foods, 375–76, 379
  restricted or eliminated foods, 374, 376, 380, 385–86
  two-week master program, 384–85, 386–87

irritable bowel syndrome (IBS) diets (*cont.*)
  vitamin/mineral supplements to, 382–83, 387

Jack, Alex, 205
Japan Women's University (Tokyo), 263
Jenny Craig diet program, 97, 98, 107–10
  for adolescents, 108, 183
*Johns Hopkins Medical Letter,* 336
Johnson & Johnson "Real Solutions" plan, 111, 112
Joslin Diabetes Center, Inc. (Boston), 304, 308, 356
*Journal of Human Hypertension,* 353
*Journal of Hypertension,* 352
Journal of Nutritional Science and Vitaminology, 263
*Journal of the American Dietetic Association,* 95, 179
Journal of the American Medical Association, 182
Judy Graham Self-Help MS Diet, 397–404
junk food, 167, 181, 258
"junk food recipes," 178–79

Kapler, Michael, 219
Kardong, Don, 222
Katz, Harold, 97, 110
Katz, Jane, 425
Keller, Helmut, 431
*Keys to Understanding Osteoporosis* (Rozek), 250
Kenny, Skip, 136
kidney disease, hypertension and, 336
kidney stones, 318
  calcium and, 221, 254, 263, 349
  vegetarians and, 221
Kieswetter, H., 297
Kirili, Linda, 104
Klein, Arthur C., 274
Koop, C. Everett, 204
KOPS (Keep Off Pounds Sensibly), 120
kosher diets, 80, 91, 108
Kushi, Michio, 61, 204, 205–10, 211, 213, 216
Kushi Institute, Kushi Foundation, 205

laboratory tests (of nutritional status), 31
lactose, 11. *See also* sugars

lactose intolerance, 200, 381
  diets accommodating, 77, 80, 100, 101
  and IBS, 374
LCDs (low-calorie diets), 55. *See also* VLCDs (very-low-calorie diets)
LDL cholesterol. *See* cholesterol
lecithin, sources of, 367
Lee, John, 262
legumes
  as anticancer agent, 432
  diet recommendations or restrictions, 174, 282, 289, 386, 402
licorice, 337, 346, 372, 432
Lieberman, Shari, 425
*Lifeline* (OA journal), 114, 116
linoleic acid, 12, 405, 406
lipoproteins, low- and high-density (LDL and HDL). *See* cholesterol
*Living Heart Diet, The* (Debakey et al.), 281–86
low blood sugar. *See* hypoglycemia
*Low Blood Sugar: The Hidden Menace of Hypoglycemia* (Martin), 361
low-calorie diets, 55, 284–86. *See also* VLCDs (very-low-calorie diets)
Low-Calorie Living Heart Diet, 284–86
low-carbohydrate diets, 132–38, 362–64
  criticized, 366
Lowenstein, John M., 121
*Lower Your Blood Pressure and Live Longer* (Moser), 347
lowfat, high carbohydrate diets. *See* high-carbohydrate, lowfat diets
*Low-Fat, Low-Cholesterol Cookbook* (Grundy and Winston), 287–92

Mac, Phillip, 373–74
McDougall, John, 129–32
*McDougall Program for Maximum Weight Loss, The,* 129
macrobiotic diets, 61, 204, 205–15
Macrobiotics International, 205
magnesium, 21–22, 27, 254
  athletes' needs, 61, 235–36
  children's needs, 176, 179
  diabetics, supplements for, 314
  FDA and supplements, 274
  women, supplements for, 158, 250
mahuang. *See* ephedra
maltose, 11. *See also* sugars

Mandell, Marshall, 317, 323–28, 335
manganese, 124, 158, 176, 179
Manson, JoAnn, 163
Manz, Esther S., 118
maple syrup, 11. *See also* sugars
Martin, Clement C., 361–66
May, C., 317
Mayo Clinic Allergy Diet, 318–23
*Mayo Clinic Diet Manual, The*
  and allergy elimination diets, 318–20,
    322, 331, 335
  elderly population surveyed by, 185
  IBS discussed in, 373
  vegetarian diet endorsed by, 205, 215,
    216, 217
*Mayo Clinic Health Letter,* 257
Mayo Clinic Vegetarian Diet, 61, 215–21
meals, frequent. *See* diet(s)
mealtimes, 35, 376
meat
  as calorie source, 213
  diet recommendations or restrictions
    arthritis, 267, 269, 272
    cancer, 412, 420, 426
    children, 173–74, 178
    heart disease, 289, 290
    hypertension, 340
    IBS, 380
    macrobiotic/vegetarian, 208, 213–14
    MS, 395, 396, 400
    popular book diet program, 148
  as iron source, 156, 170, 177, 400
  organ meats (pro and con), 290, 400
  overconsumption of, and obesity, 213
  as protein source, 148, 213–14. *See also*
    proteins
Medical College of Wisconsin (Milwaukee), 120
medical insurance, 74, 75, 87
medically supervised programs, 111, 121
MEDIFAST (VLCD program), 88–93
Mellin, Laura M., 164, 179–82
Memorial Sloan-Kettering Cancer Center,
  414, 425
men
  basic menu for, 178
  calorie needs of, 45, 46, 47
  fat cells of, 138–39
  "moderate" alcohol consumption, 218

  RDAs for, 26–27
  WHR and disease risk, 42
menstruation. *See* women
metabolism
  basal and resting (BMR, RMR), 45–46,
    47, 48, 57, 145
  and body weight, 45
  digestive, 47–48
  exercise and, 145, 228
  of fat, 33, 138
  low, insulin and, 56
  meal times and, 35
  total needs, 48
  women's, 57
methionine (amino acid), 212
Metropolitan Life Insurance Company
  standards, 40
"micronutrients," vitamins as, 14
milk, 174
  allergy to, 320, 331. *See also* lactose intol-
    erance
  for arthritics, 275
  raw whole, 272, 368
  skim, 262–63, 290, 294
  *See also* dairy products
milk allergy elimination diet, 320
minerals and trace elements, 20–24
  and chemotherapy, 428–29
  children's needs, 179
  deficiencies, 22, 34, 61, 176, 210
  children, women, and elderly, 20, 156–
    58, 175, 186 (*see also* vitamin/min-
    eral supplements)
  elderly persons' needs, 196, 202
  FDA removes from market, 274
  female athletes' needs, 235–36
  food processing and, 173
  food sources, 20–24, 175, 210, 369
    meat, 156, 170, 177
    vegetables, legumes, and grains, 167,
      207, 213, 215, 219–21, 251, 367
  RDAs for, 24–25, 27, 168, 173, 185
    children, 171
  toxicity, 210
  *See also entries for individual minerals and
    trace elements*
Mirsky, Stanley, 304–8, 356–61
mistletoe extract (chemopreventive), 431
Mitchel, D. F., 36

mixes. *See* processed foods
*Modern Nutrition in Health and Disease* (Shils et al.), 52, 164, 243, 298, 299, 316, 408
molasses, 11, 215. *See also* sugars
molybdenum as diet supplement, 179
monitoring
  alcohol consumption, 34
  diet, *see* food diary
  weight loss, 181–82
monosaccharides, 358. *See also* sugars
monosodium glutamate (MSG), 351
Moser, Marvin, 347–52
Motil, Kathleen, 170
multiple sclerosis (MS), 318
  constipation as problem, 401, 402
  conventional view challenged, 398
  incidence of, 391
  symptoms of, 391–92
  weight as issue, 398
multiple sclerosis (MS) diets, 68, 391–407
  additional therapies, 406–7
  basic nutritional approaches, 392, 399, 404–5
  behavior modification with, 397, 404
  exercise with, 396–97, 398, 403–4, 406
  fatty acids (PUFAs) in, 406
  recent research, 406–7
  recipes, 396
  recommended foods, 393–95, 399–402, 405
  restricted or eliminated foods, 395–96, 402–3, 405–6
  vitamin/mineral supplements to, 396, 403, 407
*Multiple Sclerosis: A Self-Help Guide to Its Management* (Graham), 397
*Multiple Sclerosis Diet Book, The: A Low-fat Diet for the Treatment of MS* (Swank and Dugan), 392
*Multiple Sclerosis, Muscular Dystrophy and ALS* (Donsbach and Alsleben), 404
Murray, Michael, 36, 337, 352, 389
muscle mass
  age, and loss of, 45
  diet, and loss of, 145, 146
  EC (ephedrine-caffeine) formula and, 126
  and female bodybuilding, 232, 234–35
  and muscle-building, 145, 148. *See also* exercise
  protein and, 245
mutagens, 421

National Academy of Sciences, 30, 197, 385
National Cancer Institute (NCI), 221, 410
  dietary guidelines, 238, 385, 409, 427
  studies, 408, 428
National Center for Health Statistics, 164
National Center for Nutrition and Dietetics, 231
National Cholesterol Education Program (NCEP), 221
National High Blood Pressure Education Program Award, 347
National Institutes of Health (NIH), 168, 250, 257, 298, 308, 429
National Multiple Sclerosis Society, 391, 398, 402
National Osteoporosis Foundation, 249, 250
National Osteoporosis Society (Britain), 255
National Research Council, 238, 243
Nelson, Jennifer, 215–21, 318, 323
*New American Diet, The* (Connor and Connor), 129, 141–43
*New England Journal of Medicine,* 163
*New Fit or Fat, The* (Bailey), 147
*New York Times,* 297, 313
niacin. *See* vitamin B3
Nidetch, Jean, 97, 103
Nieman, David, 36, 38, 39, 41, 42, 45
  and sports medicine diet, 62, 226, 237–43
nightshade plants. *See* vegetables
nitrites. *See* processed foods
Nixon, Daniel W., 410–18
Null, Gary, 61, 205, 210–15, 216
"nutrient-dense" foods, 10, 59
nutrients, 10–24
  tests measuring, 30
Nutri/System diet program, 97, 98, 110–12
nutrition, assessment of and guidelines for, 30–39. *See also* diet(s)
*Nutritional Monograph, A, for Taking Pounds Off Sensibly,* 119

*Nutritional Therapy for the 1990s* (Gaby et al.), 258
*Nutrition and Your Child* (quarterly), 165, 167
*Nutrition Desk Reference* (Somer), 159, 229
*Nutrition for Women: The Complete Guide* (Somer), 159, 229
Nutrition Screening Initiative (1991), 185
nuts, nut butters, and seeds
  as anticancer agent, 432
  diet recommendations or restrictions, 174, 289, 367, 401
  peanut allergy, 321, 322
  peanut oil, 321, 331

obesity
  adolescent, 36, 179, 183
  botanical formulas and, 125–26
  and calorie intake, 32–33
  in children, 36, 58, 164, 165, 179, 181–82, 183
  diet goals for, 54–55
  exercise and, 145
  genetic factors in, 55, 56, 120
  health problems arising from, 41, 54, 73, 93–94, 163, 299, 336, 421–22
  high-fat foods and, 12
  insulin and, 56–57, 94–95, 131, 134
  meat consumption and, 213
  and metabolism, 45
  morbid, 55
  TV and, 36, 183–84
  waist-to-hip ratio (WHR) and, 41
  *See also* overeating; weight loss
oils
  cooking technique, 402
  corn, 323
  diet recommendations or restrictions, 174, 189, 208, 341, 393, 402, 419–20
  fish, 173, 274–75
  hydrogenated (hardened), avoidance of, 273, 290–91, 395
  peanut (cold-pressed), 321, 331
  peppermint, 377, 389
  primrose, 397
  vegetable (cold-pressed), 368
  wheat germ, 405
  *See also* fats, dietary
Olson, James A., 298
Olympic contestants. *See* athletes

Omi, N., 263
OPTIFAST (VLCD) program, 73, 74, 86–88, 95, 96
OPTITRIM (VLCD) program, 74, 84–86
Ornish, Dean, 83, 263, 281, 292–97
Oshawa, George, 205
osteoporosis, 157, 158–59, 168, 194, 249–50, 318
  allergies and, 258
  and calcium supplements, 201, 213, 250, 253–54
  estrogen and progesterone therapy, 63, 262
  fat intake and, 194
  incidence of, 258
  smoking and, 158, 250, 388
  vegetarians and (pros and cons), 221, 263
osteoporosis diets, 62–63, 101, 190, 249–63
  basic nutritional approaches, 250, 255, 258
  behavior modification with, 255
  exercise with, 254–55, 257, 261
  meal planning and menus, 252–53
  recommended foods, 250–51, 255–56, 258–60, 262–63
  restricted or eliminated foods, 251–52, 260
  vegetarian, 263
  vitamin/mineral supplements to, 250, 253–54, 261
*Osteoporosis* (Dover), 255
*Outsmarting Diabetes: A Dynamic Approach for Reducing the Effects of Insulin-Dependent Diabetes* (Beaser), 308–13
*Outsmarting the Female Fat Cell* (Waterhouse), 129, 138–40
Overeaters Anonymous (OA), 113–18, 132
overeating
  compulsive, 113–17 *passim*
  emotional state and, 36–37, 115, 182
  *See also* obesity
over-the-counter drugs. *See* drugs
over-the-counter (OTC) botanical diets, 121–28
  basic nutritional approaches, 122, 124
  eligibility for, 122, 124
  exercise recommended with, 123, 125

over-the-counter (OTC) botanical
    diets (*cont.*)
  fluid intake in, 121, 124
  physician referral recommended, 122
  recent research, 125–27
  recommended foods, 125
  restricted foods, 125
  sample menu plan, 123
  two major types (lipogenic and thermo-
    genic), 125
  vitamin/mineral supplements to, 123

pantothenic acid. *See* vitamin B5
*Parents Who Help Their Children Overcome
    Drugs* (Becnel), 378
Parker, David, 42
pasta, 267, 393, 396, 419
pastry. *See* bread/bakery goods
Pauling, Linus, 317
peanuts. *See* nuts, nut butters, and seeds
Peikin, Steven R., 383–89
Pelletier, Jean-Paul, 264
peppermint oil. *See* oils
pesticides, 184, 214
phosphorus, 27, 158, 176, 250, 254
  calcium ratio (soft drinks), 22, 258
phylloquinone. *See* vitamin K
physical status, assessment of, 38–48
  worksheet for, 39
Pizzorno, Joseph, 36, 337, 352, 389
plastic packaging, 325, 421
popular book diet programs, 129–50
  basic nutritional approaches, 129–30,
    132–39, 141–44
  cookbooks, 129, 149–50
  exercise recommendations, 131–32, 136–
    37, 138, 140, 145–50 *passim*
  guidelines, 133
  recommended foods, 130, 147–48
  restricted or eliminated foods, 130–31
  vegetarian, 143
  vitamin/mineral supplements to, 131,
    144
potassium
  beverages containing, 232–33, 240. *See
    also* sports drinks
  deficiency of, 52, 201
  sources of, 22, 339–40, 344, 349
potassium chloride, 21, 331
Pouliot, Michelle, 56–57

poultry, 394, 426
  as protein source, 267, 331
  as substitute for red meat, 289
  "worst" kind for children, 178
Powter, Susan, 129, 140, 146–49
Pratt, Kathleen, 274
*Pregnancy, Children and the Vegan Diet*
    (Kapler), 219
pregnancy and lactation, 160
  and alcohol, 29, 160
  iron deficiency in, 20, 156
  milk recommended, 174
  protein needs, 175
  RDAs, 26–27
  smoking and, 162
  vegetarians and, 219, 220
  vitamin needs in, 16, 17, 158, 162, 220,
    423
  and weight-loss diet restrictions, 73, 79,
    98, 103, 107, 110, 124
    special diets, 108, 178
  *See also* women
prescription drugs. *See* drugs
*Prescription for Nutritional Healing* (Balch
    and Balch), 372, 389
*Preventing and Reversing Osteoporosis*
    (Gaby), 257
*Prevention* magazine, 262
Prince, Harold and Francine, 59, 164, 172–
    79
Prior, Jerilynn C., 262
Pritikin diet, 155
processed foods
  and allergies, 318–25 *passim,* 331
  canned, 177, 189, 393, 396
  cholesterol in, 13
  dried fruit, 130, 189, 215
  eliminated from diet for:
    arthritis, 273
    cancer, 420, 421
    children, 177
    the elderly, 188, 194
    heart disease, 284, 289, 290
    MS, 395–96
    osteoporosis, 258
  food additives, 162, 260
    nitrites, 409, 421
  frozen fruit and vegetables, 189, 268,
    277
  mixes, 177, 393, 395, 420

processed foods (*cont.*)
    packaging of, 325, 421
    permitted in MS diet, 393
    salt in, 344, 351
    saturated fats in, 12–13
    soy products in, 321
    sugar in, 12, 34
    vitamin/mineral loss from, 173
progesterone therapy, 262
Prosch, Gus J., 271–74
prostaglandins, 12, 266
proteins
    algae as source of, 213
    adult needs, 11
    animal, 30, 33, 148, 175, 267, 272, 331
        (*see also* dairy products; fish; meat;
        poultry)
    athletes' needs, 216, 224, 232, 241, 245
    best source in allergy diet, 331
    and cancer, 412, 420–21
    children's needs, 175, 176–77, 217
    complementary, 175, 211, 214, 216
    "complete," 175, 186–87, 211, 216–17
    complex carbohydrates (starches) con-
        taining, 12
    elderly persons' needs, 193, 195, 198
    guidelines for consumption, 30, 33
    "incomplete," 216
    meaning of word, 11
    milk, and allergies, 320
    and muscle mass, 245
    in osteoporosis diet, 251
    pasta as source of, 267
    RDAs for, 26
    vegetables, 211–19 *passim*, 263, 331
        in Biosphere diet, 186
        "hydrolyzed," 321
        value questioned, 175, 204
    women's needs, 175, 198, 232
PSA (prostate-specific antigen), 414–15.
    *See also* cancer
pyridoxine. *See* vitamin B6

*Quantum Healing* (Chopra), 391
Quick, Richard, 136

Ravussin, E., 33
Rayner, Lynn, 249
RDAs (recommended dietary allowances),
    26–27

for children, 26–27, 171–72
    exceeded, 164
vitamin/mineral, 19, 24–27, 168, 171–
    72, 185, 203
VLCD formulas compared to, 77–79,
    82–83, 91–92
Real Solutions Program (Johnson &
    Johnson), 111, 112
*Real Vitamin and Mineral Books, The*
    (Bruning and Lieberman), 425
recipes
    all-family menu plan, 178–79
    for diabetics, 300, 302–3
    heart diet, 285, 291, 295
    IBS diet, 386
    "junk food," 178–79
    macrobiotic, 209
    MS diet, 396
    *See also* cookbooks
refined foods, 131. *See also* processed foods
*Relief from IBS* (Shimberg), 374
Report on Nutrition and Health (1988),
    204
restaurant meals
    and allergies, 319, 321
    for children, 181
    fast food, 171, 321
    how to reduce fat in, 302
    take-out, "worst" for children, 177
retinols (vitamin A derivative), 14
Reversing Heart Disease Diet, 292–97
Reward Meal (in carbohydrate addict's
    diet), 133
rheumatoid arthritis (RA). *See* arthritis
Rheumatoid Disease Foundation, 271
riboflavin. *See* vitamin B2
RNA, 16, 17, 24
rosemary, as anti-cancer agent, 432
Royal Veterinary and Agricultural Univer-
    sity (Copenhagen), 126, 127
Rowan, Robert L., 337–42, 344
Rozek, Jan, 250–55

St. Helena Hospital and Health Center
    (California), 130
salt, 21, 23
    diet recommendations or restrictions
        allergies, 331
        arthritis, 276
        cancer, 409, 412–13, 427

salt (*cont.*)
    children, 170
    diabetes, 301
    the elderly, 194
    hypertension, 337, 343–44, 350–51
    processed foods, 344, 351
    surgeon general's, 29
    vegetarian, 218
    women, 155
  iodized, 24
  salt substitutes, 276, 349, 351, 352
  salt tablets, 223
  *See also* sodium
Saltman, Paul, 156
*San Francisco Chronicle,* 414
Saunders, Elijah, 343
Scala, James, 265–71, 272
Scanlon, Deralee, 374, 378–83
Schilling test (of vitamin B12), 31
Scott, Lynne, 281
seafood. *See* fish
Sears, Barry, 62, 129, 135–38
seaweeds, sea vegetables (kombu; nori;
    arame), 189, 207, 209, 219
seeds. *See* nuts, nut butters, and seeds
selenium, 24, 27, 210, 369
  diet supplements, 124, 158, 179
  and chemotherapy, 428–29
self-esteem, 52, 90, 119. *See also* behavior
    modification
Shapedown Weight-Loss Program for
    Children, 164, 179–83
shark cartilage, 430–31
shiitake mushrooms (as chemopreventive),
    430
Shike, Moshe, 298
Shils, Maurice, 164, 298, 408, 410
Shimberg, Elaine Fantle, 374–78
Shulman, Neil B., 343
Sibley, William A., 406
Silver Sage (manufacturers), 123
Simone, Charles B., 418–25
Singh, R., 353–54
sleep disorders (insulin and), 56
smoking
  and allergies, 331
  and arthritis, 273
  and cancer, 428
  and gallstones, 94
  and heart disease, 280, 285–86, 296

  and hypertension, 336, 341, 345
  and hypoglycemia, 363
  and IBS, 388
  and osteoporosis, 158, 250, 388
  prohibited during fast, 327
  sensitivity to nightshade and, 276
  women and, 157, 158, 162, 163
snacks, 133, 207, 217
  as aid in diet, 34, 95, 122, 160, 161, 192
  for athletes, 230
  for diabetics, 307, 312
  and obesity, 36, 183
  "worst" for children, 178
Sobel, Dava, 274
Socrates, 28
sodas. *See* soft drinks
sodium, 23, 254
  as electrolyte, 240
  monitoring of, in VLCDs, 79, 83
  reduced intake recommended, 29, 78,
    310–11, 412–13
    for hypertensives, 337, 340, 350–51
  sodium chloride, 21, 23
  *See also* salt
soft drinks, 269, 362
  caffeine-containing, 363
  calcium-phosphorus ratio in, 22, 258
  sugar-rich, 170
  *See also* beverages
Somer, Elizabeth, 153, 159–63, 185, 191–
    96, 229–36, 314
sorbitol, 11. *See also* sugars
soup, in macrobiotic/vegetarian diet, 207,
    213
soybean products
  allergy to, 321
  as anticancer agent, 432
  and cholesterol, 169
  and osteoporosis, 263
  as protein source, 214
  in vegetarian diets, 206–79, 209, 212–
    13, 214, 219–20
  as vitamin/mineral source, 209, 214,
    219–20, 255
spices. *See* herbs and spices
Spielman, Amy B., 97
spiritual component of program, 115, 117,
    347
spirulina, 209, 213, 372
sports diets, 61–62, 135–38, 222–45

sports diets (*cont.*)
  and alcohol, 223, 238
  basic nutritional approaches, 223, 238
  and caffeine, 242
  fluid requirements, 225, 226, 227, 231, 232–33, 239–41, 244
  food hints, 240
  menu plans, 227–28, 233–35, 242–43
  preparing for competition, 225–28, 233, 245
  recent research, 243–45
  recommended foods, 223–24, 230–33, 239–41
  restricted foods, 225
  vitamin/mineral supplements to, 222, 228–29, 235–36, 242, 245
  for women, 229–36
  *See also* athletes
sports drinks, 231, 233
  electrolyte-replacement, 232–33, 240–41, 244
  *See also* water
Spriet, Lawrence L., 243, 244
sprouts, 367
Stanford men's swim team, 136
staples, dry and canned, in elderly persons' diet, 189
starches. *See* carbohydrates (complex)
steroid use, 245, 277
*Stop the Insanity* (Powter), 129, 146–49
stress
  and disease, 280, 342, 377–78, 388–89, 425
  and overeating, 36–37, 115, 182
stroke, risk of, 54, 64, 336, 346
Struff, Janice, 166, 167–68
substance abusers and VLCDs, 79
sugars (simple carbohydrates), 11–12
  corn sugar, syrup, or starch, 11, 323
  diet recommendations or restrictions
    allergies, 331
    arthritis, 273
    athletes, 225, 239
    cancer, 420
    the elderly, 188
    hypertension, 340
    MS, 394, 396
    osteoporosis, 260
    women, 157
  excessive consumption of, 56, 157, 194

  guidelines for consumption, 29, 30, 34
  honey, 11, 368
  and hypertension, 337
  molasses, 11, 215
  in processed foods, 12, 34
  substitutes for, 178, 276, 301, 349, 362, 368
  sugar-rich beverages, 170
  "worst" for children, 178
  *See also* desserts
sulfur, 23
*Super Nutrition for Women* (Gittleman), 153–54
*Supplement to the Art of Getting Well: Proper Nutrition for Rheumatoid Arthritis* (Rheumatoid Disease Foundation), 271
support groups, 113–20
  basic nutritional approaches, 114, 119
  behavior modification in, 120
  cancer patient, 417
  in commercial weight-loss programs, 106, 109
  cost and eligibility, 114, 118
  exercise recommended by, 120
  group support within, 114–15, 116, 117, 119–20
  and medical research, 120
  in VLCDs, 76, 77, 81–89 passim
*Surgeon General's Report on Nutrition and Health*, 28–30, 33, 296
Swank, Roy, 392–97
*Swank Low-Fat Diet* (Swank), 392
sweeteners (sugar substitutes), 178, 276, 301, 349
sweets (for children), 175. *See also* desserts
*Swimming for Total Fitness* (Bruning and Katz), 425
Swinburn, B., 33
Syndrome X, 93, 94
synthetic foods. *See* processed foods

take-out food. *See* restaurant meals
TCM (traditional Chinese medicine), 431
tea. *See* caffeine; herbs and spices
television, 180, 183
  and obesity, 36, 183–84
Texas Children's Hospital (Houston), 165
*Therapeutic Claims in Multiple Sclerosis* (Sibley), 406

Thermogenics Plus weight-loss program, 121, 123–25
thiamin. *See* vitamin B1
thyroid, inactive (hypothyroidism), 55–56
Tobian, Louis, 349
tocopherol. *See* vitamin E
*Top News* (TOPS magazine), 118
TOPS (Take Off Pounds Sensibly), 113, 118–20
Toubro, S., 126
*Townsend Letter for Doctors,* 257
trace elements. *See* minerals and trace elements
triglycerides, 96, 126–27, 135
Tufts University Diet and Nutrition Letter, 202, 249

University of California, San Diego, School of Medicine, 300
*University of California at Berkeley Wellness Letter,* 315
University of Kansas Medical School, 329
University of Messina (Italy), 314
University of Montreal, 264
University of Pittsburgh School of Medicine, 182
University of Texas Medical Center (Dallas), 313
*USCD Healthy Diet for Diabetes, The: A Comprehensive Guide and Cookbook* (Algert et al.), 300–304

Van Pelt, Stephen, 226
vegetable oils, 368. *See also* oils
vegetables
    allium (garlic, onions, leeks), 175, 297, 390, 414, 415
    as anticancer agent, 427, 432, 433
    children's consumption of, 165–68
    diet recommendations or restrictions
        arthritis, 268–69, 272, 275
        cancer, 409, 414, 415, 419, 426, 427, 432–33
        children, 174
        diabetes, 306
        the elderly, 187
        heart disease, 284, 289
        hypoglycemia, 358, 367
        MS, 394, 401
    as fiber source, 166, 385

frozen, 189, 268, 277
glutathione-containing, 427
nightshade family, 209, 267–73 *passim,* 276, 277
processed, 284, 393
as protein source, *see* proteins
raw, 380
sea, 189, 207, 209, 219
as vitamin/mineral source, 14–18 *passim,* 167, 209, 215, 219–21, 367. *See also* calcium/calcium deficiency
"worst" kind for children, 178
*See also* legumes
vegetarian diets, 60–61, 130–31, 187, 204–21
    athletes on, 216, 228
    basic nutritional approaches, 206, 211, 216
    behavior modification with, 210
    commercial or popular book diet plans modified for, 80, 91, 100–101, 108, 131, 143
    for diabetics, 311
    for heart disease, 294
    macrobiotic, 61, 204, 205–15
    Mayo Clinic endorses, 205, 215, 216, 217
    menu plans, 215, 217–18
    and osteoporosis, 263
    recent research, 221
    recommended or required foods, 206–8, 211–13, 216–18, 220
    restricted or eliminated foods, 208–9, 213–14, 218
    rotational, 215
    vitamin/mineral supplements to, 17, 101, 131, 175, 209–10, 213, 214–15, 218–20, 228
*Vegetarian Handbook: Eating Right for Total Health* (Null), 211
vegetarians
    amino acid requirements of, 11
    children, 175, 176, 217, 220
    disease risk for, 187, 204, 221, 263
    with MS, 401
    types of, 205
    vitamin deficiency in, 16. *See also* vegetarian diets
Venus flytrap plant (*Dionaea muscipula*), 431

viral infections, 318
vitamin(s)
    antioxidant, *see* antioxidants
    and cancer risk, 17, 221
    as chemopreventives, 430
    children's needs, *see* children
    deficiency of, *see individual vitamin list-
        ings below*
    elderly needs, *see* elderly, the
    food processing and, 173
    in herbs, 175
    natural vs. synthetic, 361
    RDAs for, 19, 24–25, 26–27
        children, 172, 173
        the elderly, 185, 203
    supplemental, *see* vitamin/mineral sup-
        plements, *below*
    toxicity of, 19, 20, 243
    vegetable sources of, 14–18 *passim*, 209
    women's needs
        athletes, 235–36
        during pregnancy or lactation, 16, 17,
            158, 162, 220, 423
vitamin A, 14, 26, 185, 251
    and cancer, 221, 413, 415–16, 428
    deficiency, 19, 162, 176, 202, 271
    interaction with other vitamins/miner-
        als, 15, 18, 24
    sources, 14, 167, 400
    synthetic, 273, 415
    toxicity, 19, 243
vitamin A as beta-carotene, 14, 158
    as antioxidant, 203
    and cancer, 60, 221, 413, 414, 419
    deficiency, 162
    sources, 14, 60, 215
vitamin B1 (thiamin), 15, 27, 400
    deficiency, 19, 61, 185, 202
vitamin B2 (riboflavin), 15–16, 27, 219
    deficiency, 19, 185
    sources, 15, 320, 321, 400
vitamin B3 (niacin), 15–16, 27, 320
    deficiency, 19, 185
vitamin B5 (pantothenic acid), 16, 124,
        320, 321
    deficiency, 19
    discoverer of, 325
vitamin B6 (pyridoxine), 16, 27, 167, 277,
        320, 400, 430
    deficiency, 19, 61, 162, 185

*Vitamin B6: The Natural Healer* (Gaby),
        257–58
vitamin B9 (folic acid, folate), 16–17, 27,
        167, 400
    and chemotherapy, 416, 430
    deficiency, 17, 20, 58, 157, 176, 185
vitamin B12 (cobalamin), 16, 17, 27, 31,
        185, 295, 407
    deficiency, 20, 58
    sources, 17, 131, 209, 213–15 *passim*,
        219, 320, 321, 400
vitamin C (ascorbic acid), 17, 27, 124, 203,
        251
    aspirin and, 277
    and cancer, 17, 221, 416, 428
    deficiency, 20, 58, 61, 162, 185
    and iron absorption, 23, 215, 229
    sources, 17–18, 60, 167, 209, 215, 402
    toxicity, 20
vitamin D (cholecalciferol), 18, 26, 220,
        250, 254, 262
    deficiency, 20, 157, 185, 236, 271
    sources, 18, 320, 321
    synthetic, 273
    toxicity, 20, 243
vitamin E (tocopherol), 18, 26, 167, 215,
        277
    as antioxidant, 20, 203, 235
    and cancer, 414, 416, 428, 429
    deficiency or toxicity, 20, 243
    and heart disease, 297
vitamin K (phylloquinone), 18, 26, 390
    deficiency or toxicity, 20, 157, 243
vitamin/mineral supplements
    for anorexics, 51
    for arthritics, 270–74 *passim*, 276–78
    for athletes, 222, 228–29, 235–36, 243,
        245
    with cancer diets, 414, 415–16, 423,
        424, 427, 428–29
    for children, 164, 170, 171–72, 179,
        219, 220
    with commercial weight-loss diets, 101,
        109, 111
    with coronary artery disease diet, 295,
        297
    for diabetics, 303, 307–8, 314
    and digestive disorders, 317–18
    for the elderly, 188, 190, 192, 194–96,
        200–201, 202–3

vitamin/mineral supplements (*cont.*)
and food allergies, 317–25 *passim,* 328, 331–32, 335
and heart disease, 295, 297
for hypoglycemia, 360–61, 365, 370–71, 372
for IBS, 382–83
for MS, 396, 403, 407
and osteoporosis, 250, 253–54, 261, 318
with popular book diets, 131, 144
and toxicity, 19, 20
for vegetarians, *see* vegetarian diets
Vitamin and Mineral Insurance Formula, 325
with VLCDs, 92
for women, 58, 158, 160, 162
*See also* diet supplements
VLCDs (very-low-calorie diets), 55, 73–96
advantages/disadvantages, 79, 83–84, 86, 88, 92–93
behavior modification with, 75, 81, 84, 86–91 *passim,* 93
and blood sugar (glucose) levels, 95
compared to RDAs, 77–79, 82–83, 91–92
cost of, 74, 75, 80, 85, 87, 89
and counseling, 82, 85, 86, 88, 91, 92
effectiveness of, 93
eligibility for, 73, 75, 79, 80–81, 85, 87, 89
exercise programs with, 77, 81, 86, 89, 95–96
fluid intake with, 76
group support meetings as part of, 76, 77, 81–89 *passim*
insurance coverage of, 74, 75, 87
medical benefits of, 96
medical supervision of, 73, 93
nutritional analysis, 77–79, 82–83, 85, 87–88, 91–92
physician referral required, 74, 80, 87
transition phase in, 76, 82, 84, 86, 89, 90–91, 95
vitamin/mineral supplements to, 92
vomiting (by bulimics), 51–52

waist-to-hip ratio (WHR), 40–42
Walford, Ray, 60, 185, 186–91
*Wall Street Journal,* 297

water
contamination of (by pesticides), 184
as nutrient, 10–11, 160, 170
*See also* fluid intake
Waterhouse, Debra, 129, 138–40, 145, 148
*Weighing the Options: Criteria for Evaluating Weight-Management Programs* (Blackburn), 49, 55, 94, 179, 183
weight control
determining ideal weight, 42–44
fat intake and, 33
meal patterns and, 34–35
measuring body weight, 38–42
surgeon general's recommendations, 29
weight gain
in diabetics, 311–12
as diet goal, 50–53
fat not factor in, 137
men vs. women, 138–39
weight maintenance as diet goal, 53–54
*See also* obesity; weight loss
weight loss
for adolescents, 90, 108, 181–83
cachexia (in advanced cancer cases), 410, 412
children's diet programs, 58–59, 103, 164–84
commercial diet programs, 97–112
as diet goal, 54–57
for the elderly, 59–60, 185–203
herbal formulas, 57, 121–28 *passim*
medically supervised programs (VLCDs), 55, 73–96
for men, comparative ease of, 139
monitoring (in children's program), 181–82
over-the-counter (OTC) botanical diet programs, 121–28
popular book diet programs, 129–50
prescription drugs for, 127–28
rapid, discouragement of, 97
support groups, 113–20
for vegetarians, *see* vegetarian diets
will power and, 117
for women, difficulty of, 57, 145–46. *See also* women's diets
Weight Watchers International (WW), 97, 98, 103–6, 132

*Wellness Book of I.B.S., The* (Scanlon), 374, 378–79
wheat allergy elimination diet, 322–23. *See also* gluten intolerance
wheat germ oil, 405
White House Conference on Aging (1994), 186
Whitlock, Evelyn, 158
Williams, Roger, 317, 325
Winfrey, Oprah, 73, 95, 129, 149–50
Wing, Rena, 95
Winston, Mary, 287
*Woman's Guide to Good Health After 50* (Feltin), 196
women
    anorexic and bulimic, 50–51
    athletes, 229–36
    bodybuilders, 232, 234–35
    calorie needs, 45, 46, 47
    diabetes in, 298
    diet restrictions, 157–58, 162
        alcohol, *see* alcohol consumption
        caffeine, 101, 157
    and estrogen replacement therapy, 63, 94, 138, 262, 422
    exercise for, 57, 140, 158–59, 160, 163
    fat cells of, 57, 138–40
    heart disease among, 140, 163
    insulin imbalance in, 56–57
    and menstruation
        irregularity or cessation, 50, 51, 157, 236
        nutrient depletion by, 101
    metabolism of, 57
    and osteoporosis, 62–63, 101, 157, 158–59, 168, 201, 213, 249. *See also* osteoporosis diets
    postmenopausal, and cancer, 422
    protein needs, 175, 198, 232
    RDAs for, 26–27
    smoking by, 157, 158, 162, 163
    "super foods" for, 156
    vitamin/mineral needs or deficiencies, 16, 17, 158, 162, 220, 235–36, 432.
        *See also* calcium/calcium deficiency; iron/iron deficiency
    vitamin/mineral supplements for, 58, 158, 160, 162
    waist-to-hip ratio (WHR) of, 42
    and weight-loss difficulty, 57, 145–46
    weight-loss plan for, 138–40
    *See also* pregnancy and lactation
women's diets, 57–58, 100, 101, 153–63, 178
    for athletic performance, 229–36
    basic nutritional approaches, 154–55, 159–60
    essential fatty acids in, 155–56
    exercise with, 140, 158–59, 160, 163
    fluid intake in, 101
    to prevent or reduce osteoporosis, 62–63
    recent research, 163
    recommended foods, 156, 160–62
    restricted or eliminated foods, 157–58, 162
    vitamin/mineral supplements in, 158, 160, 162
    Women Over 50, 196–202
WTB (Weigh to Be) VLCD program, 80–81, 82, 83
WTL (Weigh to Live) VLCD program, 79–84

xylitol (sugar alcohol), 11

yogurt. *See* dairy products
yohimbe (herb), 57
yucca and arthritis, 278–79

zinc/zinc deficiency, 24, 124, 210
    athletes, 61
    and bone calcification, 250, 254
    children, 20, 58, 175, 176, 179
    the elderly, 185
    toxicity, 210
    women, 158, 162
    zinc food sources, 24, 220–21, 400
Zone Sports Diet, 62, 135–38